Companion for
OBSTETRICS and GYNECOLOGY
Practical Examination

Companion for
OBSTETRICS and GYNECOLOGY
Practical Examination

Sixteenth Edition

Haresh U Doshi
MD (Gynec) PhD FICOG Diploma (USG)
PGDMLS PGCML PGDCR PGDHHM

Professor and Head
Department of Obstetrics and Gynecology
Gujarat Cancer Society Medical College
Ahmedabad, Gujarat, India

Foreword
NT Vani

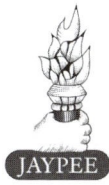

JAYPEE BROTHERS MEDICAL PUBLISHERS
The Health Sciences Publisher
New Delhi | London

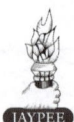 **Jaypee Brothers Medical Publishers (P) Ltd**

Headquarters
EMCA House
23/23-B, Ansari Road, Daryaganj
New Delhi 110 002, India
Landline: +91-11-23272143, +91-11-23272703
+91-11-23282021, +91-11-23245672
E-mail: jaypee@jaypeebrothers.com

Corporate Office
4838/24, Ansari Road, Daryaganj
New Delhi 110 002, India
Phone: +91-11-43574357
Fax: +91-11-43574314
E-mail: jaypee@jaypeebrothers.com

Overseas Office
J.P. Medical Ltd
83 Victoria Street, London
SW1H 0HW (UK)
Phone: +44 20 3170 8910
E-mail: info@jpmedpub.com

EU GPSR Authorised Representative
Logos Europe, 9 rue Nicolas Poussin
17000, La Rochelle, France
Phone: +33 (0) 6 67 93 73 78
E-mail: contact@logoseurope.eu

Website: www.jaypeebrothers.com
Website: www.jaypeedigital.com

© 2020, Jaypee Brothers Medical Publishers

The views and opinions expressed in this book are solely those of the original contributor(s)/author(s) and do not necessarily represent those of editor(s) of the book.

All rights reserved. No part of this publication may be reproduced, stored or transmitted in any form or by any means, electronic, mechanical, photocopying, recording or otherwise, without the prior permission in writing of the publishers.

All brand names and product names used in this book are trade names, service marks, trademarks or registered trademarks of their respective owners. The publisher is not associated with any product or vendor mentioned in this book.

Medical knowledge and practice change constantly. This book is designed to provide accurate, authoritative information about the subject matter in question. However, readers are advised to check the most current information available on procedures included and check information from the manufacturer of each product to be administered, to verify the recommended dose, formula, method and duration of administration, adverse effects and contraindications. It is the responsibility of the practitioner to take all appropriate safety precautions. Neither the publisher nor the author(s)/editor(s) assume any liability for any injury and/or damage to persons or property arising from or related to use of material in this book.

This book is sold on the understanding that the publisher is not engaged in providing professional medical services. If such advice or services are required, the services of a competent medical professional should be sought.

Every effort has been made where necessary to contact holders of copyright to obtain permission to reproduce copyright material. If any have been inadvertently overlooked, the publisher will be pleased to make the necessary arrangements at the first opportunity. The **CD/DVD-ROM** (if any) provided in the sealed envelope with this book is complimentary and free of cost. **Not meant for sale**.

Inquiries for bulk sales may be solicited at: jaypee@jaypeebrothers.com

Companion for Obstetrics and Gynecology: Practical Examination

First Edition: 1985
Sixteenth Edition: **2020**
Reprint: 2025
ISBN 978-93-89776-74-4
Printed at SDR Printers

Dedicated

*To the Students of
Obstetrics and Gynecology*

Foreword

Since Dr Haresh joined as a first year resident with us many years back, his sincerity getting deeply involved in the concerns of patients and students, and his ability to teach became quite obvious. Students would flock around him and persistently goad him to teach. Whenever he got an opportunity to talk to students, going to or coming back from undergraduate and postgraduate exams, he made a deep study of their talk, studiously cataloguing the facts and fallacies and *Companion for Obstetrics and Gynecology: Practical Examination* is the natural outcome.

It is very gratifying that the book is in its Sixteenth edition. Obviously the book has been found very useful. Dr Haresh through his continued involvement with the student and teacher population, has kept up updating the text and deleting the redundant or erroneous information and adding what is new and of current interest.

Whereas I have not been able to spell an A in print, Haresh, my one-time resident and now a colleague makes me proud through this publication.

I wish him all the best.

NT Vani
MD (Bom) FRCS (Edin)
Ex Honorary Professor of Obstetrics and Gynecology
BJ Medical College and Civil Hospital
Ahmedabad, Gujarat, India

Preface to the Sixteenth Edition

Since the first edition in 1985, 35 years have passed by now. I did not think at that time that this book will become so popular and widely accepted by students. The book is now in its Sixteenth edition. Obviously the book is found useful by not only UG and PG students but also by practicing doctors and teachers.

I have continued the original style of listing and tabulating the points in a simplified manner and yet it is intended to provide a compact aid for revision of complete course for practical exam. The whole book is revised and updated. Additions are done in the chapters on Contraception, Drugs, Obstetric Cases, Specimens and Miscellaneous. New chapter *Induction of Labor* is added.

I am very much indebted to my esteemed teacher, Professor Dr Narendra Vani, for his invaluable guidance which helped me in coming out with this book. I am also grateful to my other teachers with whom I have worked Professor Dr (Miss) LB Trivedi, Dr RS Patel and Dr (Mrs) LG Dutta.

I am also grateful to Dr Kirti M Patel, Director, Gujarat Cancer Society Medical College, for his full academic support.

I express my sincere thanks to all my students of present and past for their tremendous love and faith in me.

Finally I remain indebted to my wife Manisha and my children Binal and Fenil, who served as my quality controllers.

Haresh U Doshi

Contents

1. Instruments — 1
2. Catheters — 32
3. Suture Materials and Needles — 38
4. Obstetric Forceps and Vacuum Extractor — 45
5. Contraception — 56
6. Medical Termination of Pregnancy — 77
7. Drugs — 87
8. Obstetric Operations — 119
9. Gynecological Procedures and Operations — 133
10. Bony Pelvis and Fetal Skull — 157
11. Obstetric Cases Performa: Antenatal and Postnatal — 164
12. Induction of Labor — 181
13. Ultrasonography and X-rays — 184
14. Specimens — 203
15. Scores, Tests, FIGO Staging, and Classification — 214
16. Miscellaneous — 225

Course of Practical Exam — 233

Index — *235*

CHAPTER 1

Instruments

SIMS' SPECULUM

It is either single bladed or double bladed metal instrument made up of stainless steel and available in different sizes. In double bladed speculum two blades are of different sizes, bigger blade is used for parous patient while smaller blade is used for nulliparous patient. Blades are rounded at the ends and concave throughout from side to side. It is commonly used to retract posterior vaginal wall, but at times it can be used to retract lateral and anterior vaginal walls also. It is sterilized by boiling or autoclaving.

Duck Bill's speculum is same as single bladed Sims' speculum, but its handle is fenestrated for better griping during manipulations.

Method of Use

It is used in lithotomy or dorsal position with patient at the edge of the table (or in Sims' position—exaggerated left lateral position). Instrument is lubricated with antiseptic solution. Two labia are separated by left index finger and thumb and then speculum is introduced directly posteriorly or first introduced obliquely and then rotated to bring it posteriorly.

Speculum should not be lubricated with antiseptic material when it is used to take cervical or vaginal swab for culture sensitivity or while taking a Pap smear or doing IUI (intrauterine insemination).

Uses

It is a commonly used instrument in obstetrics and gynecology. It is usually used along with anterior vaginal wall retractor.

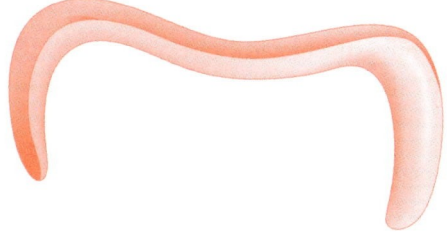

Fig. 1.1: Sims' speculum.

Gynecology

- To do **per speculum (P/S) examination** for inspection of cervix and vagina for diagnosis of vaginitis, cervical erosion, cervicitis, cervical polyp, carcinoma cervix, prolapse, bleeding from uterus.
- To perform **minor procedures over cervix and vagina,** e.g. to take Pap smear, to take cervical swab, to do Schiller's test, to take cervical biopsy, cervical cauterization, cryosurgery, to give vaginal douche with antiseptic solution, e.g. Savlon, Betadine.

- For **minor procedures through cervix**, e.g. endometrial biopsy, insertion and removal of intrauterine contraceptive device (IUCD), hysterosalpingography, intrauterine insemination (IUI).
- In **operations** (minor/major) through vaginal route, e.g. dilatation and curettage, hysteroscopy, vaginal hysterectomy, anterior colporrhaphy, colpoperineorrhaphy polypectomy, conization of cervix.

Obstetrics

- To do **P/S examination** during pregnancy for differential diagnosis (D/D) of leukorrhea in pregnancy, D/D of bleeding per vaginum in pregnancy during first or second trimester or in case of APH and for diagnosis of leaking.
- In **procedures through vaginal route** during pregnancy, e.g. suction evacuation, dilation and evacuation (D&E) operation, cervical cerclage—Mac Donald operation, to put prostaglandin E_2 gel (cerviprime) in the cervix, or introduce Foley's catheter through cervix for inductions of labor, to remove the cervical cerclage stitch.
- At the **time of delivery**, e.g. to confirm leaking, to find out the cause of traumatic postpartum hemorrhage (PPH), i.e. to explore the cervix and vagina, to repair cervical tears.
- **Postpartum**, e.g. for routine checkup, for insertion of IUCD, for examination in case of puerperal sepsis or secondary PPH.

Sim's triad include Sim's speculum, Sim's position and Sim's operation for VVF.

CUSCO'S SPECULUM

It is bivalved instrument having 2 hinged blades. Handles are at right angles to both the blades and arranged in such a way that when the handles are closed, blades will open. There is a screw mechanism on the handles which make the instrument self-retaining. The posterior blade is longer because posterior vaginal fornix is 2 cm deeper than anterior fornix. It is available in different sizes.

Comparison with Sims' speculum

Sims'	Cusco's
Assistant is required to hold the instrument	It is self-retaining
Another instrument is required to retract anterior vaginal wall	Due to presence of anterior blade no other instrument is required
Different sizes are required for different patients	Size is adjustable
It does not obstruct the operative field	It covers vaginal walls and obstructs the operative field at introitus
It can be used for collection of discharges	It cannot, because material spills off

Method of Use

Blades are closed first, then the instrument is lubricated with antiseptic solution or cream and introduced after retracting the two labia by other hand. The blades are then opened by pressing the handles and screw is adjusted.

Uses

It is used in **gyne** side only. It gives better visualization of cervix and upper vagina so used for inspection of cervix for various pathologies, i.e. cervical erosion, polyp, carcinoma, cervicitis, bleeding through OS. It keeps the cervix steady. It is also used for taking swab or smear from the cervix, cervical biopsy and in colposcopy.

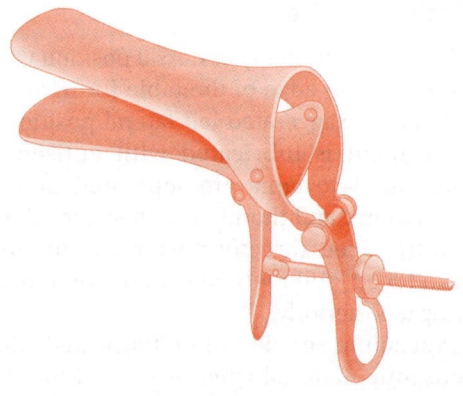

Fig. 1.2: Cusco's speculum.

OTHER SPECULAE

AUVARD'S SPECULUM

It is larger and heavier speculum with a big blade 7.5 cm long. The blade is slightly concave and has two holes on each side for fixing the instrument to the buttocks of the patient by threads. There is a channel in the handle for escape of blood or collection of discharges from vagina. The instrument is made self-retaining by the weight attached to its handle, i.e. detachable lead ball.

Uses

It was used to retract the posterior vaginal wall in operations on anterior vaginal wall, cervix and uterus, e.g. vaginal hysterectomy, anterior colporrhaphy, vesicovaginal fistula repair, etc. It is not used commonly, as it may cause vaginal or perineal tears and postoperative pain.

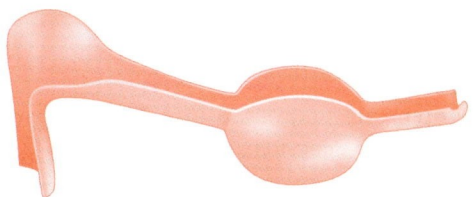

Fig. 1.3: Auvard's speculum.

SOONAWALA'S SPECULUM

It is Z-shaped speculum made up of stainless steel. It has two blades, one short and one long in opposite direction from the handle. It is made self-retaining by the weight attached to the handle. The short blade is 6 cm long, wide and rectangular in shape. The long blade is 11.5 cm long, narrow and with rounded end. The short blade is used to retract the posterior vaginal wall and expose the cervix before opening the pouch of Douglas while the long blade is inserted after opening the pouch. The speculum was especially designed for vaginal sterilization (TL) operation which is **rarely done** now.

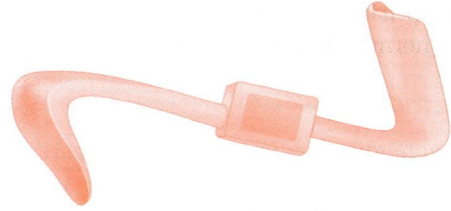

Fig. 1.4: Soonawala's speculum.

SIMS' ANTERIOR VAGINAL WALL RETRACTOR

It is a long narrow, metal instrument with oval fenestrated ends. Two ovals are set at an angles to the shaft. Fenestra is to accommodate laxity of vaginal wall and serrations accommodate rugosity of vaginal wall. Instrument is introduced with angle at the oval facing upwards.

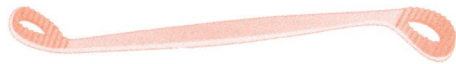

Fig. 1.5: Sim's anterior vaginal wall retractor.

Uses

It is used along with Sims' speculum to retract anterior vaginal wall so its uses are same as those for Sims' speculum for P/S examination. For procedures and operations, it is initially used to visualize the cervix and once the cervix is caught with Vulsellum it is removed. Although used in all cases it is particularly useful in cases of lax vaginal walls or cystocele.

It can also be used as blunt curette while evacuating retained products after second trimester abortion or retained placental bits after delivery. In such cases where the uterus is large, it is more efficient and safe instrument than simple curette.

UTERINE SOUND (SIMPSON'S)

It is 30 cm (12 inches) long metal instrument with handle at the end which is violin shaped. Its tip is olive pointed to prevent injury to the uterus. It is graduated in inches or centimeters with number on it indicating the distance from the tip. It is angulated at 2.5" distance from the tip (normal uterocervical length).

Method of Use

"Before sounding per vaginal examination is must".

First the cervix is exposed and grasped with Vulsellum. The sound is held by the handle like a pen, its tip is immersed in an antiseptic solution and is introduced gently in the direction of the uterine cavity judged by prior per vaginal examination or USG.

Uses

Gynecology

In gynecology it is a dictum "Before intrauterine procedure sounding is must".

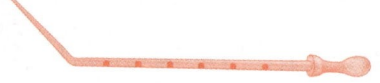

Fig. 1.6: Uterine sound (Simpson's).

Sound is used less commonly in present times as much information is gained by transvaginal sonography (TVS).
- To know the direction and length of uterocervical canal in following conditions:
  – Before dilatation and other intrauterine procedures, e.g. curettage, polypectomy
  – Before inserting an IUCD
  – In cases of prolapse to know cervical (supravaginal) elongation
  – In hysterosalpingography (HSG)
  – For diagnosis of uterine malformation, e.g. bicornuate uterus, hypoplastic uterus. Now sonography (TVS) is used for this purpose
- To check for displaced IUCD: (a) A-P and lateral X-ray of the pelvis are taken with the sound in uterus and checking the relation of IUCD with sound; OR (b) Two A-P X-ray of pelvis are taken, second after manipulating the uterus to one side in the pelvis, any change in the position of IUCD is noted.
- To maneuver the uterus from below in laparoscopy or minilaparotomy. Rubin's cannula or uterine manipulator are better instruments for the purpose.
- To diagnose suspected perforation. One has to be careful while checking as it might cause another perforation.
- To differentiate between inversion of uterus and myomatous polyp. Sound passed in uterus will go to normal uterocervical length in case of polyp, but less in case of inversion USG helps in D/D.
- To know relation of the pelvic mass with the uterus. Now USG and MRI are done.

Obstetrics

It is not used during pregnancy because it damages the normal pregnancy and perforation can occur easily as pregnant uterus is soft.

In terminating the first trimester pregnancy (MTP) it may be used to know the length and direction of cervical canal only, before using metal dilators.

Contraindications

Known or suspected pregnancy, local infection, i.e. cervicitis.

Complications

It does not cause any major complications. If incorrectly used it might cause: (i) false passage and perforation, (ii) hemorrhage due to injury, and (iii) infection. Perforation caused by sound is not much harmful as it usually heals without any sequelae.

Causes of increased uterocervical length (nonobstetric):
- Fibroid
- Adenomyosis
- Pyometra
- Hematometra
- Congenital elongation
- Prolapse
- Subinvolution
- Endometrial carcinoma.

Causes of decreased UCL:
- Menopause
- Hyperinvolution
- Congenital hypoplastic uterus
- Uterine synechiae
- Cervical amputation.

SPONGE HOLDING FORCEPS (SWAB HOLDER)

It is 9" to 9½" long forceps with ring shaped terminal ends having transverse serrations on the inner aspects. Fenestra and serrations are for better accommodation and to obtain better grip of the sponge. There are catches and finger bows on the handles.

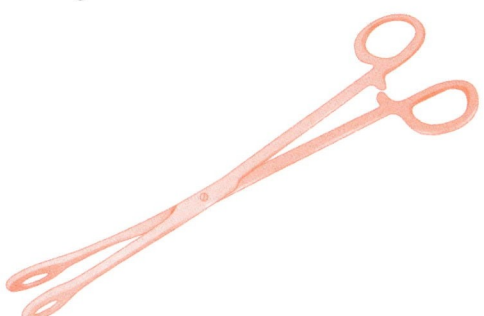

Fig. 1.7: Sponge holding forceps.

Uses

Common

- To apply antiseptic solution at the operative site (painting) before any vaginal or abdominal, major or minor operation.
- To swab out the cavities, i.e. vagina or pelvic cavity or any other operative site during operation.
- To apply pressure with a sponge on deep bleeding points during surgery, for hemostasis.
- For blunt dissection, i.e. pushing down the bladder with its peritoneum after opening the uterovesical pouch in case of abdominal hysterectomy or cesarean section (LSCS).

Gynecology

- In abdominal hysterectomy to retract the bladder while stitches are taken at or near the vaginal vault.
- For packing the vagina to control traumatic or postoperative bleeding.
- For temporary clamping of infundibulopelvic ligaments to control bleeding during conservative operation on uterus like myomectomy. Now, dilute pitressin being commonly used, this is not required.

Obstetrics

- To hold the edges and angles of lower segment incision in LSCS operation. Usually long Allis' forceps are used.
- To catch the cervix for exploration after instrumental delivery or in cases of PPH, or while repairing cervical tear.
- For packing the uterus in cases of atonic PPH.
- McDonald's operation (OS tightening or cervical cerclage) to catch cervical lips.
- It can be used as an ovum forceps to evacuate the products of conception.
- To catch the anterior lip of cervix in all vaginal procedures during pregnancy, i.e. suction evacuation, D&E operation. In practice, Vulsellum is commonly used.

CERVICAL DILATORS

These are metallic instruments for rapid dilatation of cervix. They are made up of stainless steel but nonmetallic (plastic) dilators are also available. They are sterilized by boiling, autoclaving or chemical sterilization.

Commonly Used Dilators

Hegar's Dilator

It is less curved but solid instrument. It is either single ended or double ended. There is number on the instrument which indicates maximum external diameter in mm. Single ended are available in a set of 25 having diameters from 2 mm to 26 mm. Double ended are available in a set of 12 from 1/2 mm to 23/24 mm. The instrument is abruptly tapering at the tip. It is used mainly in gynecological operations. Dilatation with Hegar's dilator is slightly difficult but there are less chances of perforation as only the tip is to be passed beyond the internal os.

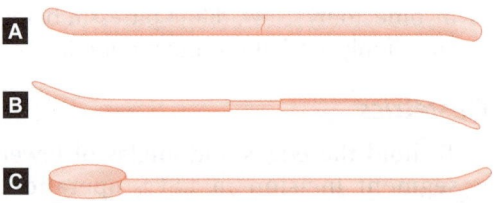

Figs. 1.8A to C: Cervical dilators: (A) Hegar's; (B) Fenton's; (C) Hawkin-Ambler's.

Fenton's Dilator

It is a long double ended instrument. As compared to Hegar's dilator it is a more curved instrument, gradually tapering near the tip, hollow from inside (but closed at the tip), light in weight and always double ended. They are available in set of 12 starting from 3/4 to 25/26 size, number indicating the maximum external diameter in mm, which is at some distance away from the tip.

It is used in gyne as well as obstetrics operation. Because of gradual tapering and more curve, dilatation with this dilator is comparatively easy with less chances of failure. But, there are more chances of injury because (i) it is more curved, (ii) due to gradual increase in diameter sometimes resistance of internal os may not be felt and instrument has to be passed for some length beyond the internal os to obtain maximum dilatation with that dilator.

Hawkin–Ambler's Dilator

It is 17.5 cm long single ended instrument. It is slightly curved and gradually tapering near the tip. There is circular thumb-rest at the nondilating end with number marking on it. Each dilator has a difference of 3 mm from the tip to the maximum dilating portion. They are available in a set of 16 from 3/6 to 18/21 number size. It is mainly used in obstetric operations.

OTHER CERVICAL DILATORS

Hank's Dilator

It is less curved, hollow double-ended instrument gradually tapering near the tip. The difference in the diameters of successive dilators is 0.5 mm instead of 1 mm. It is graduated in number equal to double the diameter of that dilator, e.g. 9/10 number dilator has diameters of 4.5/5 in mm. It is available in sizes from 9/10 to 19/20. Dilatation with this dilator is easy and less traumatic. Due to hollow open central part it can drain the intrauterine contents during dilatation.

Pratt's Dilator

It is solid double-ended instrument. It is less curved like Hegar's but gradually tapering near the tip. Like Hank's dilator difference between the successive dilators is 0.5 mm. and not 1 mm.

Bonney's Improved Cervical Dilator

It is a single ended solid instrument with gradually tapering curved tip. Dilating part has only cervical length, i.e. it is limited by a collar which prevents further entry into the uterine cavity. There is gradual increase in diameter from the tip with total 3 numbers (mm) on each, e.g. 7, 8, 9 up to 18, 19, 20. Purandare's dilator resembles Bonney's dilator.

Method of Use

Before dilatation sounding of the uterus is must to know the length and direction of cervix and uterus (If sound cannot be passed, smallest size Hegar's dilator may be used initially). Dilator is held like holding a sound, i.e. like a pen with index finger and thumb, but from the middle part. Cervix must be held steady by Vulsellum, then gently dilatation is done by to and fro movements with gradually increasing number of dilators till required dilatation is achieved.

Uses

A. Gynecology
1. *Dilatation and some procedures:*
   - D&C (Dilatation and curettage)
   - Dilatation and polypectomy
   - In cervical operations to prevent postoperative stenosis, e.g. cervical amputation (Manchester-Fothergill operation), deep cauterization, cervical repair (trachelorrhaphy), following conization.
   - For diagnostic and operative hysteroscopy.
   - Rarely before IUCD insertion or before doing intrauterine insemination (IUI), if cannula cannot be passed.
   - For manipulating uterus, during laparoscopy or minilaparotomy. Here Rubin's cannula, uterine manipulator or sound are usually used.
2. *Only dilatation:*
   - Drainage of hematometra, pyometra
   - Cervical stenosis (congenital or acquired)

B. Obstetrics
- Suction evacuation (MTP).
- Dilatation and evacuation (missed abortion, incomplete abortion, vesicular mole).
- To dilate the cervix from above, i.e. retrograde in cases of elective cesarean section or hysterotomy.
- Drainage of lochiometra.

Contraindications

- Suspected or known pregnancy (when it is not to be terminated).
- Genital sepsis (exception is drainage of pyometra).

Complications

- Injuries—lacerations or tears of cervix, false passage in the uterine wall, perforation of uterus.
- Hemorrhage—due to injuries.
- Introduction of infection.
- Vasovagal shock—sudden forcible dilatation under inadequate anesthesia.

Late effect: Cervical injury leading to stenosis; OR damage to internal os leading to cervical incompetence.

Other methods of cervical dilatation: Slow dilatation
Commonly used agents are:
- Hygroscopic agents—laminaria tent, Dilex-C.
- Prostaglandin analogues—PGE_2 endocervical gel, PGE_1 misoprostol tablet, PGE_2 vaginal pessary.

HYGROSCOPIC AGENTS

Laminaria Tent

It is made from species of seaweed laminaria japonica and laminaria digitata. The stems of these plants are dried and rounded into stick like shape 5.5 to 6 cm long with blunt ends. It is available in 3 sizes—2-4 mm (small), 5-7 mm (medium), 8-10 mm (large). A white string is looped through one end to facilitate its removal. It is sterilized by gamma radiation.

Dilex-C (Isaptent)

It was developed by Central Drug Research Institute, Lucknow. It is made by using husk of 'Isapgol', made into sticks wrapped in fine gauze. It is available in 2 sizes. There is a black thread, looped through one end to aid its removal. It is available pre-sterilized by gamma radiation.

Mechanism of Action

Both are intensely hygroscopic and they swell up 3-5 times when kept in moist environment, i.e. cervical canal, by absorbing moisture and fluid from the cervix.

Method of Introduction

Tent held in sponge holding forceps or special laminaria tent introducer is introduced into the cervical canal till its distal end passes just beyond the internal os. The string end of the tent remains outside the external os. Vagina is lightly packed with roller gauze after the string of the tent is tied over the gauze. Tent is removed at any time from four hours after insertion to within 24 hours.

Uses

With different prostaglandins now available for cervical dilatation these agents are rarely used and not freely available.

It was used in following conditions for slow dilatation of cervix **before evacuation.** Slow dilatation causes minimum cervical trauma.
- Suction MTP in nulliparous patient. MTP pills are used now before 9 weeks.
- Missed abortion
- Vesicular mole evacuation.

Complications

- Infection
- False passage or perforation of uterus or cervix rarely
- Difficulty in removal because of dumbeling phenomenon
- Occasional upward migration in to the uterine cavity
- Failure – internal os remains undilated
- Uterine cramps and discomfort after insertion in some patients

Lamicel is synthetic dilator. It is polyvinyl alcohol sponge containing 450 mg of magnesium sulphate. As compared to laminaria it caused more rapid and significant dilatation of cervix.

Dilapan-S is also osmotic cervical dilator, made up of aquacryl hydrogel. The rod absorbs fluid and increases in volume causing cervical dilatation.

CURETTES

Simple Curette

Commonly used curette is **Blake's uterine curette** which is double ended-one sharp end and one blunt. Single ended curettes are also available which may be either blunt or sharp (Sim's). Curettes are made of stainless steel and usually 25 cm long. Loops are set at an angle to the central shaft. Blunt loop is slightly wider than the sharp loop. Loops are available from 4 mm to 10 mm sizes. Shaft has got transverse ridges in the middle portion for better gripping. Sharp loop is used for gynecology curettage while blunt loop is used for obstetric curettage.

Method of Use

After sounding of the uterus, cervix is dilated by cervical dilators up to the required number, e.g. for gynecology curettage 8 to 10 number Hegar's dilator is sufficient. If cervix is already dilated, e.g. in some obstetrics cases curette is introduced directly. Curette is held by thumb and middle finger at the middle portion and index finger is extended forward and kept as a guard to a distance of uterocervical length of that patient. Index finger also gives support to the instrument and it is used for pressure while curetting.

Indications

Gynecology: It is used in Dilatation and curettage (D&C) operation. Indications and other details are given in Chapter 9.

Obstetrics: It is used in Dilatation and Evacuation (D&E) operation. Indications and other details, are given in Chapter 8.

Flushing Curette

It is 30 cm hollow instrument open at both ends. Its distal end is spoon shaped blunt curette with vertical slits on it. It was used in the past to wash out uterine cavity and to stimulate the uterine contractions by heat (hot saline between 114°F and 118°F was used) to control: (i) excessive bleeding after D&C operation, (ii) postabortal bleeding, (iii) atonic PPH.

Endometrial Biopsy Curette (EB Curette)

It is a slender tubular blunt ended instrument made up of stainless steel. Two main types are available – simple and suction biopsy curette which is open at proximal end and has stylet. Instrument is slightly curved at the tip, with one or more notches with a cutting edge near the tip. **Sharman's** endometrial biopsy curette has a handle grip at proximal end.

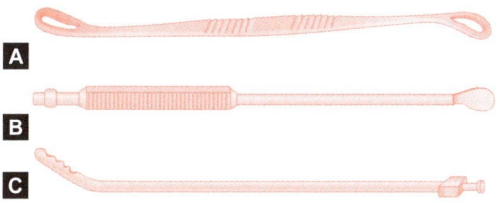

Fig. 1.9: Uterine curettes: (A) Simple curette; (B) Flushing curette; (C) EB curette.

Procedure of taking EB

It is outpatient procedure. Cervical dilatation is not required, so no anesthesia is necessary. With patient in lithotomy position, after all antiseptic precautions cervix is exposed by vaginal speculum and held with a Vulsellum. Sounding of the uterus is done. EB curette is passed and gently a strip of endometrium is scrapped out vertically from the fundus to the isthmus. If necessary a second strip may be scrapped out to obtain satisfactory material. A syringe attached to the outer end in suction type curette, may be used to suck in the curetted material and to wash it out in a suitable container. A stylet can also be used to remove the strip of endometrium from the lumen of the instrument. Material is collected in 10% formalin solution.

Time of Taking EB

It is taken either premenstrually or on the first day of menstruation, taking biopsy on the first day has some advantages: (1) endometrium is in the process of shedding out so it is easy to take biopsy, (2) cervical canal is slightly dilated at the time of menstruation, (3) menstruation has started so pregnancy is out of question, (4) some patients with oligomenorrhea may have prolonged proliferative phase and biopsy taken even after 21st day of cycle thinking it as secretory phase may give wrong result.

The disadvantage of taking EB on first day is, if it is not taken within 12 hours of onset of menstruation histopathological reporting becomes difficult due to advanced necrosis of endometrial tissue.

Indications

It was used in the past for ovulation detection (secretory phase) and corpus luteum insufficiency (24th day of the cycle). It is not done now as noninvasive methods like USG and hormonal assays are available.

It should **not** be used to take biopsy in case of suspected endometrial tuberculosis or malignancy because these pathologies may be focal and may be missed by random biopsy so thorough curettage under anesthesia is necessary.

Ovulation detection methods
- **Clinical evidences:**
  - Regular cycles
  - Primary dysmenorrhea
  - Ovulation spotting
  - Ovulation pain (Mittelschmerz)
  - Ovulation cascade (increased cervical mucous)
  - Premenstrual symptoms, e.g. mastalgia, tension
- **Ultrasonography:** Serial USG at midcycle can diagnose ovulation. In practice this is the **commonly used method** for infertility patients. Ovulation is sonographically characterized by (a) partial or total collapse of mature follicle, (b) appearance of internal echoes inside the follicle or (c) appearance of free fluid in pouch of Douglas. Echogenic endometrium of secretory phase suggests ovulation (progesterone).

- **Basal body temperature (BBT):** Because of thermogenic effect of progesterone, following ovulation there is sudden or gradual rise of temperature by 0.4° to 0.8° F. This may be preceded by a slight fall. Biphasic temperature chart is evidence of ovulation. The patient should record her oral temperature daily before rising from the bed and before eating or drinking anything, preferably at the same time. Special fertility thermometer and BBT charts are available.
- **Hormonal assays:**
  - Plasma progesterone more than 5 ng/mL in 2nd half of cycle.
  - LH peak detected in plasma as well as urine. For urinary detection special kits are available ("I know") testing is done daily in fertile period. Two lines appearing on the strip suggest ovulation.
- **Endometrial changes:** EB taken during the premenstrual phase or on first day of period shows changes of secretory phase, e.g. thick endometrium, vascular and edematous stroma, crockscrew shaped glands, coiled arterioles, etc. Presence of subnuclear vacuoles are diagnostic of secretory phase.
- **Cervical mucous:**
  - Spinnbarkeit phenomenon — under influence of estrogen the cervical glands secrete mucous which can stretch into threads measuring > 6.5 cm and even 10-15 cm at the time of ovulation. During the luteal phase (progesterone effect) the mucous becomes thick, viscid and loses its ability to stretch without breaking.
  - Fern pattern- present in first half of cycle and then absent in 2nd half of cycle confirms ovulation. Fern pattern is due to the deposition of the crystals of NaCl and KCl in a characteristic fashion under estrogen effect.
- **Vaginal cytology:** Progesterone effect— intermediate cell dominance, basophilic cytoplasm, vesicular nuclei, envelop effect, clumping of cells and slide is dirty.
- Laparoscopy is not performed for the purpose but chance finding at laparoscopy of ruptured follicle or corpus luteum suggest ovulation.

In practice, apart from USG and occasionally BBT and LH peak detection other methods are not used for ovulation detection.

VULSELLUM (TEAL'S)

It is a stainless steel instrument with length of 20 cm or more. Its blades are slightly curved near the end. Blades have got vertical teeth at the tip which interlock when the instrument is closed giving firm grip on the cervix. It is applied with concavity facing towards the symphysis pubis, so it does not obstruct the operative field.

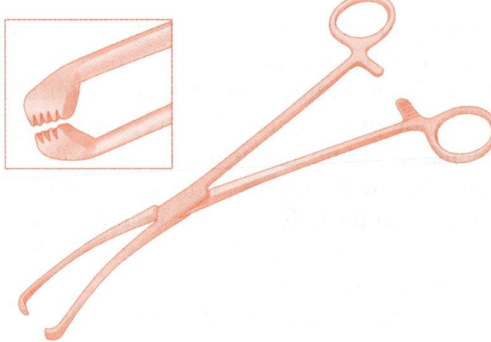

Fig. 1.10: Teal's vulsellum.

Uses

Gynecology

- To catch the anterior lip of cervix for steadying it during (a) various procedures, e.g. sounding of uterus, taking EB, insertion of IUCD and cauterization, (b) minor operations e.g. D&C, polypectomy, etc.
- To test the degree of descent of uterus by traction with Vulsellum in case of prolapse.
- During vaginal hysterectomy to hold the cervix to give traction during hysterectomy.

- To hold the cervix in Manchester or Shirodkar vaginal sling operation for prolapse.
- To catch **posterior lip** of cervix when anterior lip cannot be held because of growth, severe erosion or infection OR when one wants to do some procedure through posterior fornix, e.g. (1) while opening posterior pouch during vaginal hysterectomy, and (2) in vaginal TL operation, (3) colpopuncture (culdocentesis) in suspected ectopic, and (4) colpotomy for drainage of pelvic abscess.
- For grasping or twisting off small fibroids during myomectomy.

Obstetrics

Although meant for gyne use, it is also used to catch cervix in pregnant patient for various procedures during early pregnancy, as it gives firm grip without much trauma, e.g. suction MTP, D&E.

TENACULUM (JARCHO'S)

It is called single toothed vulsellum forceps because of single sharp tooth at the tip. It may be straight or curved. Because, it occupies less space it is better suited for nulliparous cervix and cervix with pinhole os. It is applied transversely just above the anterior lip of cervix when airtight fitting of the cannula is required.

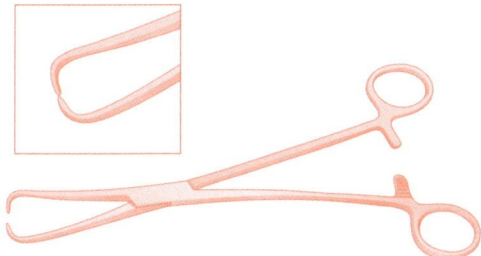

Fig. 1.11: Jarcho's tenaculum.

Uses

It is particularly useful in following conditions:
- For tubal patency tests like hysterosalpingography and chromopertubation during laparoscopy.
- For hydrotubation following tuboplasty (This is not recommended at present)
- Cauterization or cryosurgery of cervix.
- In vaginal hysterectomy it may be used instead of vulsellum to catch both the lips of cervix together to give traction during operation.
- To hold the cervical stump in subtotal abdominal hysterectomy, while it is being sutured.

ARTERY FORCEPS (SPENCER-WELLS HEMOSTAT)

It is a very commonly used instrument in all surgical branches. It is available in three sizes- long, medium and short and it may be straight or curved. It should be called hemostat instead of artery forceps because it catches not only arterial bleeding points but venous and capillaries as well. The blades are gradually tapering towards the blunt tip and there are transverse serrations on the inner aspects of the blades. On the handle there are three catches. When the first catch is approximated it catches the tissue, second one clamps the tissue and when all the three are approximated it crushes the tissue. Long artery forceps with right angled tip called **mixter** is used for working in the depth. Straight ones are used for working on the surface, while curved ones are used for deeper bleeding points and for catching vessels in the walls of a cavity.

Uses (Gynecology and Obstetrics)

- To catch the bleeding points before ligating or cauterizing them.
- To hold the peritoneum while opening or closing the abdomen.
- To preserve one end of a ligature or suture.
- To secure the abdominal pack by catching a long tape stitched to one corner of the pack.
- Stout artery forceps with long blades may be used as pedicle clamps.
- Curved stout artery forceps is used in tubal ligation to crush the base of the loop in modified pomeroy method.

- Small artery forceps with peanut is used for blunt dissection of smaller structures.
- In obstetrics they are used to clamp umbilical cord after delivery of the child.

Criteria for good instrument: (1) It should be light in weight, (2) the joint should be freely mobile, (3) there should not be any side to side movement at the joint, (4) catch should not give way (open) automatically once the forceps is closed, (5) blades should be tapering to facilitate slipping of ligature round it and the tip should be blunt, (6) there should be no gap between the blades when the first catch is approximated.

MOSQUITO FORCEPS

It resembles small artery forceps but it is a very delicate instrument, light in weight and with a fine tip. It may be straight or curved. It is used to catch very fine bleeding points, so used in surgery of small structures and in plastic surgery e.g. tuboplasty, vesicovaginal fistula repair, vaginoplasty etc.

and slightly longer blades. Its transverse serrations are deep and there is one in two teeth at the tip. It may be straight or curved.

Uses

Gynecology:
- To clamp and crush the different pedicles before cutting and ligating them in **abdominal hysterectomy** and **vaginal hysterectomy.**
- To clamp and crush the pedicles of ovarian tumors and pedunculated fibroids.
- In Manchester-Fothergill operation to clamp the cardinal ligaments.
- Straight Kocher's are used to hold the uterus during abdominal hysterectomy after applying one near each cornu of the uterus.

Obstetrics:
- As a pedicle clamp in obstetrics hysterectomy, e.g. cesarean hysterectomy.
- Removal of tubal ectopic pregnancy, e.g. salpingectomy.
- Straight Kocher's may be used for artificial rupture of membranes.
- To clamp the umbilical cord after delivery.

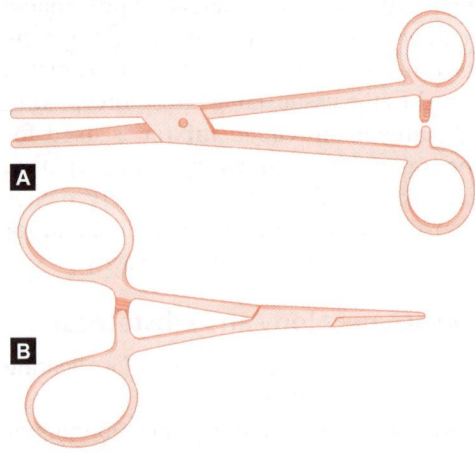

Figs. 1.12A and B: (A) Artery forceps; (B) Mosquito forceps.

PEDICLE CLAMPS

Kocher's Clamp

It resembles Spencer Well's artery forceps in shape but it is a heavier instrument with stouter

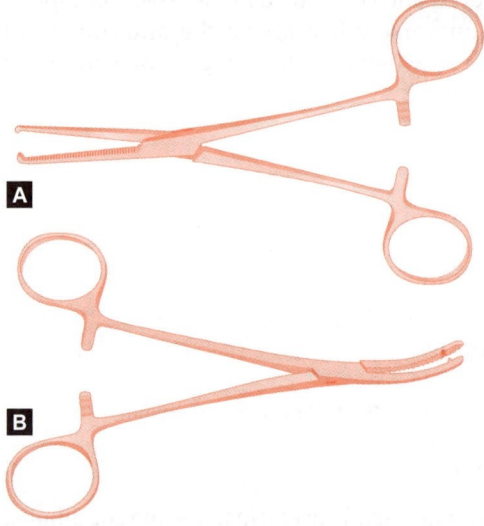

Figs. 1.13A and B: Pedicle clamps: (A) Kocher's clamp; (B) Heaney's clamp.

Heaney's Clamp

It is 20 cm long forceps with a blunt tip, i.e. tip is without tooth. There are oblique serrations on the inner aspects of the blades and a transverse ridge in one blade near the tip which fits into the notch in the other blade.

Comparison with Kocher's clamp

Kocher's clamp	Heaney's clamp
Tip security is better, no slipping of tissues from the tip	Tip is without tooth, so when moved the tissues from tip may slip
Total grip is not very good if tip remains open all the tissues remain loose	Total grip is better than with Kocher's
There are chances of injury to the vessel or viscera by the tooth at the tip	No such possibility. There is always some part of the blade beyond the tooth
More chances of lateral slipping of the structures	Less chances, because serrations are oblique

Uses

As a pedicle clamp during hysterectomy and removal of tumours.

Ochsner's Clamp

It is like Kocher's clamp but is more stout with shorter and broader blades and with vertical serrations. It may be straight or curved. Its uses are same as Kocher's clamp.

Maingot's Clamp

It is curved on flat pedicle clamp. One blade has longitudinal ridge fitting into a longitudinal groove on the other blade. The blades have one in two vertical teeth at the tip. The longitudinal groove and ridge ensures better occlusion of vessels in the pedicle and less lateral slipping of the tissues as compared to transverse serrations.

ALLIS' FORCEPS

It is a tissue forceps made up of stainless steel. The blades are thin and without serrations. They are slightly widened and curved inwards at the tip. The instrument may be short or long. There are three into four or four into five teeth at the tip.

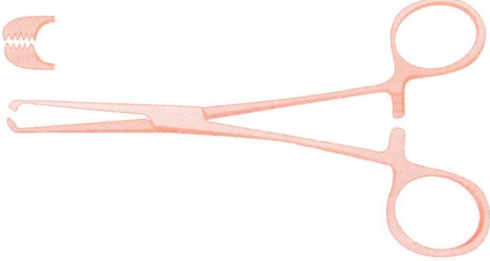

Fig. 1.14: Allis' forceps.

Uses

It is used to catch tough but nonbulky tissues.

Gynecology

- To catch the rectus sheath or its cut edges in any abdominal operations.
- To catch the vaginal walls or its cut edges in different operations, e.g. anterior colporrhaphy, colpoperineorrhaphy, vaginal hysterectomy.
- To catch the anal sphincter (retracted torn ends) in third degree perineal tear repair.
- To hold the vaginal vault from above when it is cut open or when it is sutured during abdominal hysterectomy.
- To catch a small fibroid or cut edges of its fibrous capsule during myomectomy operation.
- To hold the cut edges of uterus during reconstructive surgery (metroplasty) for congenital malformation.
- To hold the skin edge when previous scar is removed.

Obstetrics

- In cesarean section or hysterotomy to catch the edges and angles of incision.
- In McDonald operation-four Allis' forceps are used to catch the cervix.

- To catch the cut edges of rectus sheath in any abdominal obstetrics operation.
- It may be used to catch the apex of episiotomy.
- To hold anal sphincter while suturing third degree or complete perineal tear after delivery.

BABCOCK'S FORCEPS

This is one type of tissue forceps made up of stainless steel. Its blades are fenestrated near the tip, triangular in shape and with grooved jaws. There is a transverse ridge at the tip. It is available in different sizes.

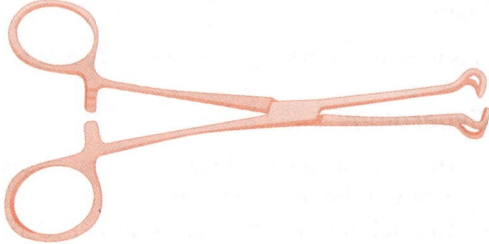

Fig. 1.15: Babcock's forceps.

Uses

It is meant to catch soft and tubular structures like fallopian tube, ureter, appendix, bowel and bladder.

Gynecology

- To catch the fallopian tube in tubal ligation (TL) operations.
- To hold the tube during conservative operations for tubal ectopic pregnancy.
- To hold the tube in tuboplasty operations.
- To hold the ureter in radical gynec surgery.
- To hold the ovary in various conservative operations on it.
- To hold the lymph glands during their dissection in radical hysterectomy.
- To hold the bladder or bowel if they are accidentally injured during gynec surgery. The instrument is used to catch the cut edges of these viscera during repair.

Obstetrics

In tubal ligation operations in obstetrics:
- Postpartum tubal ligation (PPTL)
- Cesarean section with TL
- MTP with abdominal TL
- Hysterotomy with TL

MYOMECTOMY INSTRUMENTS

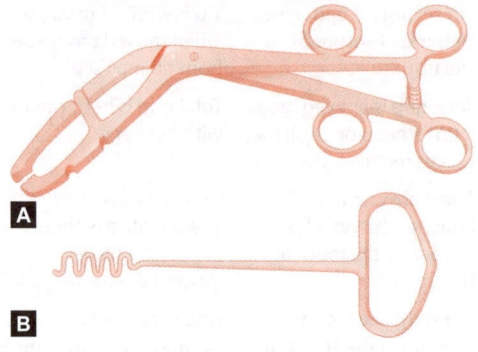

Figs. 1.16A and B: (A) Bonney's myomectomy clamp; (B) Myoma screw.

Bonney's Myomectomy Clamp

The instrument was devised by great **Victor Bonney** of England. It is a long metal clamp with slightly diverging blades which are set at an angle with the handles. There are two transverse overlapping bars which divide the gap between the blades into two compartments. The distal half of the blades are covered with rubber tubes to prevent injury to uterine vessels. Handles have two pairs of finger bows but only proximal pair is provided with catches.

Method of Use

As the name suggests it is used to control hemorrhage during **myomectomy** operation. It may be used for the same purpose in **metroplasty** operation also. In abdominal myomectomy operation, after delivering the uterus from the abdominal incision, the instrument is applied on the uterus from the foot end side, at the level of isthmus, with inclusion of both the round ligaments. Concavity at the joint rests over the symphysis pubis of the patient. No structure is held in the proximal compartment (i.e. one towards the finger bows).

Finger bows at the level of catches are used during application of the clamp. For manipulation during operation, the instrument is held by the distal pair of finger bows so that there is mechanical advantage and fewer chances of giving way (opening) of catches during manipulation.

Functions of the instrument: (1) uterine vessels are clamped so hemostasis is maintained during operation, (2) uterus is held, so it can be manipulated as necessary during the operation, (3) inclusion of the round ligaments keeps the uterus anteverted and prevents downward slipping of the instrument.

Precautions

- Instrument should be released intermittently every 15–20 minutes during the operation. This prevents ischemic damage to the uterus. If not released such damage leads to collection of vasoactive substances, which can cause postoperative shock when liberated in circulation at the end of operation.
- After enucleation of fibroid the instrument should be released just before the cavity of the fibroid is closed to see any bleeding points which otherwise cause postoperative hematoma in the dead space.
- Both infundibulopelvic ligaments are clamped with sponge holding forceps, so blood supply from ovarian vessels is temporarily occluded.
- Before patient is taken for myomectomy operation:
  - Blood is kept cross matched and ready.
  - Husband's semen examination must be done.
  - Other factors for infertility in the patient (i.e. ovarian, tubal) must be ruled out.
  - Written consent for hysterectomy must be taken because during operation, due to severe bleeding or innumerable fibroids, the operator may have to change the decision in favor of hysterectomy. This is rarely required.
- Instead of this clamp usually simple rubber tourniquet is tied at the level of isthmus for hemostasis, by making small holes in the broad ligaments. In case of cervical or isthmic fibroid this instrument cannot be applied so hemostasis can be done by direct manual pressure over uterine vessels.

Medical hemostasis (vasoconstriction) can be done by injecting dilute vasopressin (pitressin) 10 units in 100 mL normal saline in superficial myometrium and serosa overlying the myoma. Half-life of vasopressin is 10 to 20 minutes.
- Use of hypotensive anesthesia, use of GnRH analogues prior to surgery and uterine artery embolization are other methods to decrease blood loos at myomectomy.
- Myomectomy is advised when childbearing is not complete and in young patient of <35 years even, if child-bearing is complete otherwise hysterectomy is indicated.

Myoma Screw (Doyens)

It is stainless steel instrument with shank terminating at one end in the shape of the screw with a pointed tip. At other end shank is attached to a handle which is in the form of solid transverse bar or fenestrated oval. It can be of small or large size.

Uses

- During myomectomy operation (abdominal or vaginal) it is screwed in the center of the myoma to give traction while the myoma is enucleated after cutting its capsule.
- It can also be used to hold and keep steady the big size uterus during abdominal hysterectomy operation.

UTERUS HOLDING FORCEPS

Shirodkar's Uterus Holding Forceps

It is a forceps with diverging rectangular blades and curved transverse bars at the tip. The bars may be covered with rubber caps to prevent trauma to the uterus. The handles have got finger bows and catches.

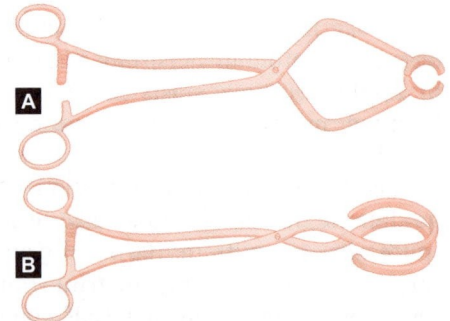

Figs. 1.17A and B: (A) Shirodkar's uterus holding forceps; (B) Dartigue's forceps.

Uses

- It is exclusively used in tuboplasty operations.
- It is also used to hold the uterus in various conservative operations for prolapse, i.e. Shirodkar's sling, Purandare's sling, Khanna's sling operations.
- To hold and lift the uterus in salpingectomy operation for tubal ectopic pregnancy.
- In *Moschcowitz* operation or uterosacral plication from above to prevent enterocele.

Method of Use

In tuboplasty operation after opening the abdomen, the uterus is delivered and the instrument is applied from above, with the body of uterus free inside the blades and the transverse bars at tip clamping the isthmus, so uterocervical canal is occluded at the level of isthmus. Its functions are (1) to lift and steady the uterus and thereby tubes, (2) to check tubal patency under direct vision, i.e. chromopertubation. Methylene blue diluted in normal saline is used for testing. Dye injected from fundus with a syringe and needle will come out from tubes because at the lower end, the uterine cavity is closed. It helps to find out (1) the site of block, i.e. the site for operation, (2) it discolors the endosalpinx so lumen is easily visualized while taking anastomosis stitches. Chromopertubation is also done at the end of tuboplasty operation to see the success of operation (patency) on table.

Different types of tuboplasty operations include:
1. End to end anastomosis (isthmo-isthmic, isthmo-ampullary ampullo-ampullary, cornuo-isthmic, cornuo-ampullary).
2. Cornual implantation.
3. Salpingoneostomy.
4. Fimbrioplasty.
5. Lysis of adhesions.

Dartigues Forceps

This is another uterus holding forceps, the blades of which are shaped like question mark. Both the blades are curved in the opposite directions and are covered with rubber tubes to prevent direct trauma on the uterine wall during its use. Its uses are same as those of Shirodkar's clamp, except that it cannot be used for chromopertubation in tuboplasty operation, as it does not occlude the cervix.

RUBIN'S CANNULA

It is 30 cm long metal cannula with 4 mm diameter. It is slightly curved at the tip which is blunt. There are multiple side apertures near the tip. It has got a movable conical rubber (rubber acorn) near the tip, with fixation screw behind it. There are 2 finger bows for better grip of the cannula.

Uses

- Tubal insufflation test (Rubin's test). It is **not practiced** at present as other better methods of tubal patency are available.
- In chromopertubation during laparoscopy. Dilute methylene blue solution is injected from below and its appearance at fimbrial

ends, seen through laparoscope indicates tubal patency. Other metal cannulae are commonly used.
- To do hysterosalpingography.
- For manipulating the uterus in laparoscopy operations.
- For hydrotubation. It was done postoperatively in cases of tuboplasty. 10 to 20 cc normal saline with 1 ampoule hyalase, 1 bulb of antibiotics and steroid were injected in the uterus between 5th to 10th day through the cannula under aseptic precautions. It is not recommended now.

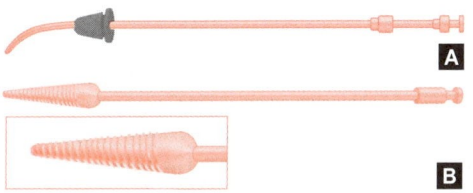

Figs. 1.18A and B: (A) Rubin's cannula; (B) Leech Wilkinson's cannula.

LEECH WILKINSON'S CANNULA

It is a straight metal cannula, 28 cm long with a fixed conical collar at the tip with spiral grooves over it and there is Luer lock mount at the other end. This cannula is better suited for multiparous patient with patulous cervix. It is commonly used for chromopertubation and HSG.

SHIRODKAR'S CANNULA

It resembles Leech Wilkinson's cannula except that it is bent at right angle near its proximal end, terminating in a metal cup with a Luer lock attachment inside and screwcap to close the cup. Shirodkar had devised it especially for hydrotubation, which is not done now.

EPISIOTOMY SCISSORS

It is stainless steel, angle on side scissors with angle at the level of joint. Inner blade is thinner and sharper than outer blade. Angle makes it more convenient to use. Screw joint and nonratcheted finger grips are for better functioning of the scissors. In absence of it bandage scissors or any surgical scissors are used.

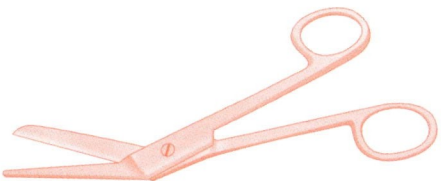

Fig. 1.19: Episiotomy scissors.

Use: It is used to give episiotomy during labor. Episiotomy is discussed in detail in Chapter 8.

Method of giving episiotomy: Episiotomy is given during the second stage of labor at crowning of the head, under adequate local anesthesia and under guidance of 2 fingers of other hand in the vagina protecting the presenting part. Usually 3 to 4 cm long cut is made from fourchette to 60° laterally (mediolateral).

OVUM FORCEPS

It is long straight forceps with spoon shaped ends having longitudinal slits (fenestra) on it. There is **no catch** on the handle. The reason for this is, the instruments which are meant to hold those objects, sizes of which vary, have no catches so the instrument has no crushing action and there is less chance of injury to uterine wall or products being left behind.

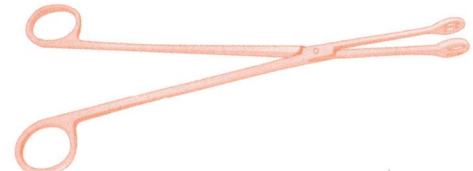

Fig. 1.20: Ovum forceps.

Uses

It is used in obstetrics to evacuate the products of conception in **D&E** operation:
- Inevitable abortion

- Incomplete abortion
- Missed abortion
- Vesicular mole evacuation
- Therapeutic abortion (MTP of 10–12 weeks size uterus)
- Secondary PPH due to retained placental tissues. Here the sponge holding forceps is better and safer alternative to ovum forceps.

Method of Use

In some of the conditions cervix is already dilated but in others it should be adequately dilated before the use of ovum forceps. The finger may be introduced inside the uterus to separate the products before their evacuation.

Introduce the instrument inside the uterus with tips closed, then open the instrument, catch the products, rotate it minimum 90° and then remove it closed. Rotation prevents injury to uterine wall, because if uterine myometrium is held in the instrument, it will not rotate, so instrument is released and less tissue is grasped again. If only decidua is included it will easily tear off with 90° rotation of the instrument.

Complications

They include infection, perforation, hemorrhage and incomplete evacuation.

UTERINE PACKING FORCEPS

It is a long instrument with "s" shaped curve. The curve is to accommodate the angles of uterus and vagina. It is without catch. The blades are with blunt ends and with transverse serrations near the tips.

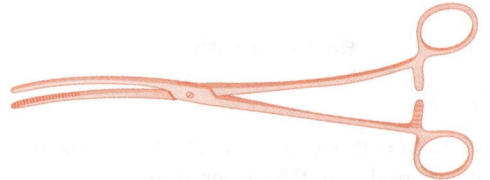

Fig. 1.21: Uterine packing forceps.

Another similar type of instrument is **uterine dressing forceps,** but it has got a catch on the handle. And instead of serrations on them, the blades are smooth or grooved from inside.

Uses

Obstetrics

- To pack the uterus to control the bleeding in cases of: (a) atonic PPH, (b) severe postabortal bleeding.
- For vaginal packing in following conditions:
  - To control traumatic PPH due to vaginal lacerations when suturing is not feasible.
  - After episiotomy hematoma evacuation and repair.
- For cleaning of utero-cervical canal after minor obstetric operations, i.e. suction MTP, D&E operation.

Gynecology

- To pack the vagina in following situations (commonly swab holder is used for the purpose)
  - After vaginal hysterectomy.
  - Before tuboplasty or myomectomy operation vagina is packed to elevate the uterus.
  - To control secondary hemorrhage from the operative site (i.e. cervix or vagina including vault).
- To clean the uterocervical canal after D&C and polypectomy.
- To pack the uterus after polypectomy or operative hysteroscopy, if there is uncontrollable bleeding.
- To remove foreign body from the uterus, e.g. IUCD with thread torn or indrawn.

SUCTION CANNULA

It is made of metal (stainless steel) or plastic. Plastic cannula may be either rigid or flexible (Karman). They may be straight or slightly curved near the tip. They are available in different sizes.

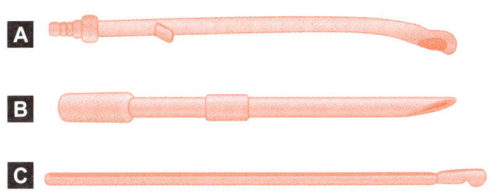

Figs. 1.22A to C: Suction cannula; (A) Metal cannula; (B) Rigid plastic; (C) Flexible plastic.

Metal Cannula

It is 25 cm long cannula slightly curved near the tip. It has a rounded closed tip and one or two subterminal openings. There is a thumb rest near the proximal end with central hole in it, connecting to the lumen of the cannula, so thumb kept over the thumb rest is used to control the vacuum. As it can be sterilized by autoclaving or boiling it can be repeatedly used, an advantage over plastic cannula. Because metal walls are thinner it has a greater internal diameter than that of a plastic cannula of same number. As compared to plastic cannula it is more traumatic instrument.

Rigid Plastic

It may be either straight or curved. The cannula has a rounded tip with single slanted lateral opening at the tip. As it is transparent, the product being sucked during the procedure can be seen through it. There is a centimeter marking on it indicating the depth to which it is introduced. It is available from 8 mm to 12 mm diameter sizes.

Flexible Plastic

It is a transparent, flexible, polyethylene instrument developed by **Harvey Karman**. It has a rounded closed tip with two sharp triangular openings located on opposite sides near the tip. The convex hood which overhangs each opening acts as a curette during procedure. Because of two openings there are fewer chances of blocking and it requires only 180° rotation to cover the whole uterine cavity instead of 360°. They are available in different sizes.

In plastic cannula rarely the tip of the cannula at the level of opening may get arrested at internal os and may break off to be left inside the uterus. It can be removed by uterine dressing forceps or other instrument.

Uses

- Medical termination of pregnancy (MTP) during first trimester by suction evacuation method.
- To complete the inevitable or incomplete abortion during first trimester.
- For evacuation of vesicular mole (11 or 12 no. cannula is used).
- For suction evacuation in case of missed abortion.

In MTP, size of the cannula used is equal to, or one number less than the weeks of gestation. Suction evacuation procedure is described in detail in Chapter 6.

Perforation of uterus:
Common instruments which can cause perforation are:
- Uterine sound
- Cervical dilators
- Curette
- Suction cannula
- Ovum forceps

As such any instrument introduced inside the uterus can cause it.

Diagnosis of perforation:
It is done by one or more of the following evidences:
- Sudden giving way of resistance during the procedure.
- Instrument going inside the uterus for a greater distance than before, without resistance.
- Appearance of fresh bleeding
- Checking by sounding by senior person (Here there is a risk of doing more perforations by sound)

- If perforation is large or suction is being continued, omentum or small bowel may appear through it
- Immediate diagnostic laparoscopy.

Management:
It depends upon the following factors:
- Whether the patient is pregnant or not
- Size of perforation
- Type of instrument which has caused it
- Presence or absence of sepsis
- Associated injury to other abdominal viscera

For perforation in **gynecology case** or by a small instrument in obstetric case, i.e. sound or small dilators, **conservative treatment** is adopted, i.e. stop the procedure, transfer the patient to ward, give her broad spectrum antibiotics and analgescis and keep a close watch on her. It she deteriorates laparoscopy or laparotomy is required. Laparoscopy may be carried out at the time of injury, if doubt exists.

In **obstetrics case** usually at least laparoscopy is done as the uterus is vascular and soft so chances of internal hemorrhage are more and laparotomy with suturing of perforation may be required. If perforation has occurred during MTP, the evacuation may be completed from below under laparoscopy guidance and if there is no bleeding it can be left alone. Suturing can also be done laparoscopically by expert person.

In a septic case and when there is injury to abdominal viscera direct laparotomy is indicated.
- Perforation leads to scar on uterus which in subsequent pregnancy may lead to adherent placenta or rupture uterus.
- If it goes unrecognized at the time of procedure, there are chances of injury to bowel, omentum or mesentery. Severe internal hemorrhage and peritonitis can also occur.

GREEN-ARMYTAGE HEMOSTATIC FORCEPS

This forceps has triangular solid blades near the tip. The base of the triangle is near the tip and there are transverse serrations on the base for better gripping.

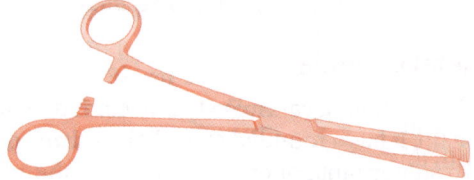

Fig. 1.23: Green-Armytage forceps.

Uses

It is used to catch edges and angles of LSCS incision to hold them for suturing as well as for hemostatic purpose to control the bleeding. Usually four forceps are required one for each angle and one for each, upper and lower edge of the incision.

Advantages

Because of its broad base single instrument catches multiple bleeding points. It is especially useful in highly vascular lower segment incision of placenta praevia. As compared to Allis' forceps it is less traumatic instrument. However applied for a long time it can cause pressure necrosis.

Disadvantages

As the base occupies more space there is mechanical disadvantage in suturing. If the uterine edge is very thick it may cause pressure necrosis resulting in a subsequent weak scar.

It may be used to hold the cervical edges instead of sponge holding forceps while exploring the cervix for any tears or while suturing such tears.

UMBILICAL CORD SCISSORS

It is a short scissors with especially designed short and circular cutting blades. It is used to cut the umbilical cord of the baby after birth. Cord is cut between two clamps, first of which is applied approximately 5 to 6 cm away from the navel of the baby and the second one is applied further 2 to 3 cm away. Because of Wharton's jelly and smooth amnion, cord is slippery and it tends to slip away when it is cut with ordinary scissors. It does not happen with this scissors as the tips are occluded first in this scissors in contrast to other scissors. Like other sharp instruments it should be sterilized by chemical sterilization instead of autoclaving.

As per WHO recent recommendation (2012) delayed cord clamping is to be done, performed approximately 1 to 3 min after birth. This applies to even preterm babies who do not require active resuscitation. Early cord clamping (less than 1 minute) after birth is not recommended unless the neonate is asphyxiated and needs immediate resuscitation.

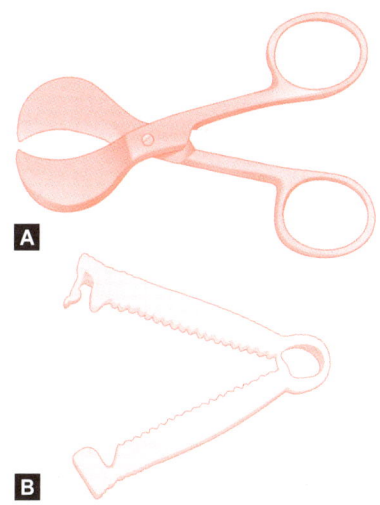

Figs. 1.24A and B: (A) Umbilical cord scissors; (B) Cord clamp.

Umbilical Cord Clamp (Clips)

These are made of plastic. They are supplied sterile in a plastic pack pre-sterilized by gamma irradiation and ideally disposable. They have 2 arms (or 3) with hinge joint between them and inner surface is serrated. Clamp is applied on the cord 3–4 cm. from the umbilicus with arms completely covering it & tips are locked in position with manual pressure or pressure with forceps.

The clamp gets shed of along with the cord falling after 3–6 days of birth. Different clamps used are (1) Kane's cord clamp, (2) K-GAR clamp, (3) Hassetine cord clip, etc.

Instead of clamp sterile silk or cotton thread can be used.

- The cord should be kept long (about 6 inches) in asphyxiated babies, babies of diabetic mother, Rh iso-immunization and exomphalos minor.
- Normal umbilical cord is average 50–60 cm long and 2 cm in diameter. Less than 35 cm is called short cord and > 80 cm is called long cord.
- Normal contents of umbilical cord at term include two umbilical arteries, one umbilical vein (right vein disappears - left is left), Wharton's jelly, remnant of allantois and Vitelline duct at the fetal end, obliterated extra-embryonic coelom and covering of amnion.
- Congenital abnormalities of umbilical cord include unduly long cord, short cord, marginal insertion, single umbilical artery, true or false knots, torsion, stricture and hematoma.
- Cord complications in obstetrics include true knots, cord round the neck, cord entanglement and cord prolapse.

PINARD'S FETAL STETHOSCOPE

It is very simple cone shaped instrument made up of aluminium or wood. Wide-mouthed end is the fetal end and its rim is rounded to avoid injury to the patient's abdominal wall. Aural end is narrow with supporting circular plate.

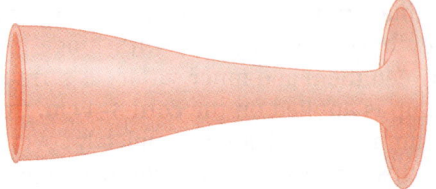

Fig. 1.25: Pinard's fetal stethoscope.

Method of Use

The position of the fetal anterior shoulder (lower most bony part felt on the side of the fetal back) is located by palpation. Fetal heart sounds are best heard on that site. In V1 (LOA) position this site is usually the midpoint of left spinoumbilical line of the mother. Fetal end of the instrument is applied firmly and at right angle to the surface of the abdominal wall at the located site. The ear of the examiner must be firmly closed to the aural end. The instrument should not be touched by the hand while listening as it would dampen the sound passing through the stethoscope. The patient's abdomen may be pressed from the opposite side by the hand for better listening.

- Fetal heart sounds are heard by fetal stethoscope from 24 weeks onwards. The sound resembles the ticking of watch heard through a pillow. Its rate is 110 to 160 per minute. Fetal heart sounds less than 110 is called bradycardia and more than 160 is called tachycardia.
- Causes of bradycardia include hypoxia, maternal drugs (propranolol, local anesthetics), congenital heart block, idiopathic, etc.
- Causes of tachycardia include mild hypoxia, maternal fever, fetal infection, hyperthyroidism, anticholinergic or sympathomimetic drugs, arrhythmia preterm fetus etc.
- Different methods of detecting fetal heart action:
  - Real time USG-6th week
  - Fetal echocardiography -8th week
  - Ultrasound Doppler-10th week
  - Auscultation by stethoscope - 18th week
- **Uterine souffle:** It is soft blowing systolic murmur, synchronus with maternal pulse. It is due to passage of blood through dilated uterine arteries. It is heard low down, at the sides of uterus, after 16 weeks of pregnancy.
- **Funic souffle:** It is faint, rapid blowing murmur, synchronous with fetal heart sound. It is due to passage of blood through compressed umbilical arteries. It is present in only 15% cases and it is of no significance.

BLADDER SOUND

It is long rod shaped instrument with handle at one end. It is usually 25 cm long and available in different sizes. Differences from uterine sound are as follows:

Bladder sound	Uterine sound
Slightly heavier	Less heavy instrument instruments
Blunt tip	Olive pointed tip
There are no markings on it	It is graduated in cm or inches
It is smoothly curved near the tip	It is angulated with or without a knob

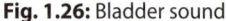

Fig. 1.26: Bladder sound.

Uses

- To define the limits of bladder during operations on anterior vaginal wall, e.g. cystocele repair.
- To determine the relation and position of vesicovaginal fistula in the vagina.
- To diagnose accidental bladder injury during surgery.
- To diagnose a calculus or foreign body in the bladder. USG is now used as it is noninvasive.
- For differential diagnosis of sub-urethral diverticulum or cystocele from anterior vaginal wall cyst.

UTERINE MANIPULATOR

It is a special instrument, devised to manipulate the normal size uterus from vaginal route in laparoscopy. It is a combination of Vulsellum and uterine sound in a single instrument. The sound part is 5.5 cm from the tip of the Vulsellum blade, going either in the direction of the curve of Vulsellum or going in the opposite direction. It effectively manipulates the uterus as per the need of the laparoscopic surgeon. Other type of such manipulator is a combination of a tenaculum and a sound (i.e. **Hulka's manipulator**). For manipulating large size uterus other special manipulator is available.

Uses
- Laparoscopic sterilization.
- Minilaparotomy sterilization operation.
- For better visualization of pelvic structures during diagnostic laparoscopy.

Advantages
- Laparoscopic surgeon himself can maneuver it with one hand.
- Less chances of uterine perforation.

Disadvantages
- As the length of the sound part is fixed (5.5 cm from Vulsellum tip), it may not touch fundus in all cases (particularly in cases of MTP with lap TL due to big uterus) so it may not effectively manipulate the uterus in such case,
- In hyperinvoluted (small) uterus it may cause perforation.

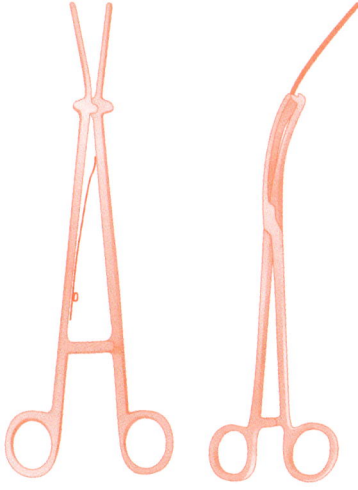

Fig. 1.27: Uterine elevator.

POLYP FORCEPS

It is a long slightly curved forceps with small fenestrated blades at the tip. It is used to remove the endometrial polyps form the uterine cavity.

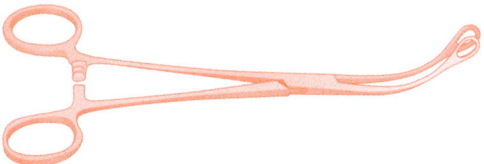

Fig. 1.28: Polyp forceps.

Method of Use

First the cervix is exposed and caught with simple Vulsellum, then the sound part of the manipulator is introduced either anteriorly or posteriorly in the uterocervical canal as the case may be, till the Vulsellum part of the instrument catches the cervix. Original simple Vulsellum is then removed. By moving the handle of the instrument to the **right side** of the patient, uterus is displaced to left side so **right adnexa** are visualized and vice versa. Depressing or elevating the handle makes the uterus anteverted or retroverted.

Method of Use

After adequate cervical dilatation the instrument is introduced inside the uterine cavity. After grasping the polyp, forceps is locked and the polyp is removed by twisting the forceps. Bleeding usually stops by itself or by D&C which is done along with it.

It was recommended that at each curettage uterine cavity should be explored routinely with polyp forceps otherwise an endometrial polyp may be missed by an ordinary curette and patient may have persistent or recurrent bleeding after curettage. Prior USG by TVS probe can readily diagnose polyp.

Different types of polyps:
1. Uterine:
   - Endometrial
   - Adenomyomatous
   - Myomatous
   - Placental.
2. Cervical:
   - Mucous (endocervix)
   - Myomatous

CERVICAL PUNCH BIOPSY FORCEPS

It is 22.5 cm long angulated instrument. The blades have small cup shaped sharp ends with a sharp pin inside one cup, making a shape of a punch. As it is a second type of lever, long handles give the mechanical advantage.

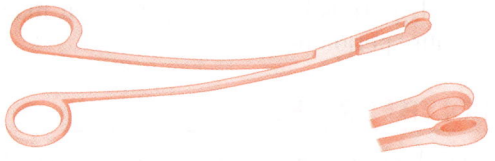

Fig. 1.29: Cervical punch biopsy forceps.

It is used to take cervical biopsy:
- For diagnosis of suspected cervical carcinoma (suspicion may be on clinical grounds, Pap smear report or colposcopy findings).
- In confirmed cases to know the histological type and grade of the tumor.
- In follow-up of cases treated with radiotherapy.

If the lesion is microscopic, i.e. Ca in situ (Ca cervix stage-O) biopsy should be taken after doing Schiller's test (iodine negative area) or colposcopy. Colposcopy is preferred as it is more accurate.

If the lesion is macroscopic, biopsy is taken from the edge of the lesion so that some adjacent normal tissue is removed for study.
- Different types of cervical biopsy are punch biopsy, cone biopsy, ring biopsy, wedge biopsy.
- Different methods to control the bleeding from biopsy site are: (1) pressure with a dry swab or swab moistened with dilute adrenaline solution, (2) tight vaginal packing (3) suturing the biopsy site by mattress sutures, (4) electrocauterization, and (5) Rarely internal iliac ligation.
- Different methods of treating Ca cervix stage-O (Ca in situ) are: (1) cryosurgery, (2) electrocauterization, (3) laser application, (4) conization, (5) large loop excision of transformation zone (LLETZ, Loop electrosurgical excision procedure - LEEP) Last two are excisional methods, so apart from being therapeutic they help in confirmation of diagnosis. It is important to do regular follow-up of all patients with Pap smear examination. Hysterectomy may be advised if child bearing is completed.

NEEDLE HOLDER

It is a stainless steel instrument with short thick blades and blunt tips. The inner surfaces of the blades are serrated in a criss-cross pattern and have a groove to grip the needle. Because of long handles there is mechanical advantage and due to screw joint it can firmly grip the needle. It can be long or short. It may be angulated near the tip.

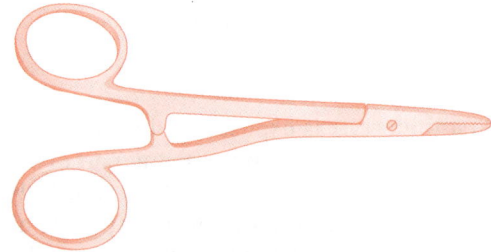

Fig. 1.30: Needle holder.

Uses

It is used to grip the curved needle for suturing. Any suturing at depth is only possible with the needle holder. The needle should be gripped by the needle holder at 2/3rd distance from the tip of the needle. Gripping the needle at this position ensures that the surgeon can pass the needle at the maximum possible distance through the tissues without further adjustments and with the least possible risk of bending or snapping it.

RETRACTORS

Plain

- Abdominal
  - Doyen's retractor
  - Morris's retractor
  - Malleable retractor
  - Deaver's retractor
  - C-retractor
- Vaginal
  - Landon's vaginal retractor.

Self-retaining

- Abdominal
  - Balfour's retractor
- Vaginal
  - Jayle's retractor.

Advantages of Retraction

- It widens the operative field at the surface.
- It gives better exposure and assessment to deeper structures.
- It prevents undue handling and injury to the tissues or organ retracted.
- It causes pressure hemostasis of small bleeders in the tissues retracted.

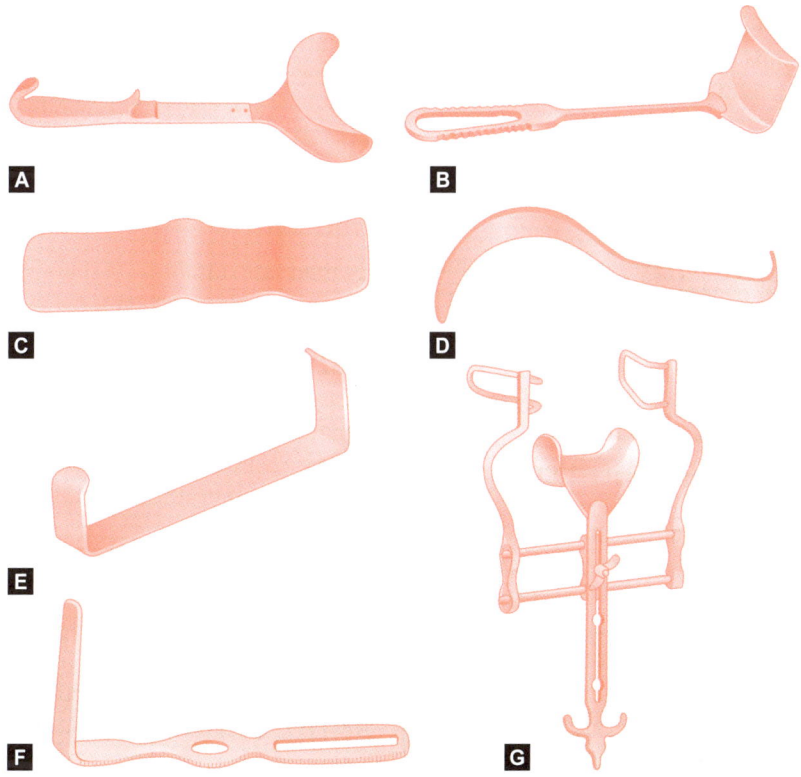

Figs. 1.31A to G: Retractors: (A) Doyen's retractor; (B) Morris's retractor; (C) Malleable retractor; (D) Deaver's retractor; (E) C-retractor; (F) Landon's vaginal retractor; (G) Balfour's retractor.

Advantages of Self-retaining Retractors

- No assistant is required to hold them.
- Uniform retraction is maintained throughout the operation.

Disadvantages (Self-retaining)

- Due to continuous pressure, they may cause pressure necrosis of tissues retracted, if very tight.
- Being fixed it cannot be easily maneuvered to the surgeon's need.
- If improperly placed or if the incision is small it may occupy more space and obstruct during operation.

Doyen's Retractor

It is a short instrument with strong handle and broad transverse blades with concavity towards the handle anteroposteriorly and convexity from side to side. It is available in 3 different sizes of blades 3½", 4" and 4½".

Uses

Gynecology:
- In abdominal hysterectomy
- Any laparotomy in gyne patient, i.e. sling operations, ovarian cystectomy, myomectomy.

Obstetrics:
- LSCS operation
- Any laparotomy operation in obstetric patient, i.e. obstetric hysterectomy, ectopic pregnancy, etc.

After the abdomen is opened, the instrument is used to retract the lower angle, when uterovesical pouch of peritonium is opened and bladder is pushed down, it is included in it so the instrument is also known as bladder retractor.

Morris's Retractor

It is a stainless steel instrument with transverse blade perpendicular to the handle with a lip. It has handle which is fenestrated for better grip. It is available in different sizes. It can be double ended also. It is useful in a medium size laparotomy wound.

Malleable Retractor

It is thin bladed long metal plate made up of copper (because copper is more malleable) with rounded smooth tips. Its shape can be changed and adjusted according to the structures to be retracted. It can be used in small narrow space. It is used to retract small bowels from the pouch of Douglas, during abdominal hysterectomy. Instead, special intestinal depressor is also used.

Deaver's Retractor

It is stainless steel instrument with long blade, bent on its flat with shape resembling question mark "?". Its tip is smoothened to prevent damage to the viscera. In gyne it is used while working in depth, e.g. internal iliac ligation, lymph node dissection in radical gyne surgery. During its use a wet mop should cover its concave surface to prevent damage to the structures retracted.

C-retractor

It is made of stainless steel and shaped like letter "C". Its blade is very narrow so it is used to retract, the small abdominal incision, e.g. abdominal TL operation, minilaparotomy incision. It is also useful in all abdominal operations to retract skin and fat to visualize the angle and edges of cut peritoneum and sheath when they are sutured.

Landon's Vaginal Retractor

It is L shaped chromium plated metal retractor. The handle has fenestration for better gripping. Retracting blade is narrow (2 cm) and straight, so it occupies less space which is required in vaginal surgeries.

Uses

- To retract the bladder through anterior colpotomy incision during vaginal

hysterectomy. First it helps to cut open the peritoneum of uterovesical fold and then it is introduced through the opening of uterovesical pouch to retract the bladder while clamps are placed.
- As lateral vaginal wall retractor.
- To retract posterior colpotomy opening for vaginal TL operation (not done now).

Balfour's Retractor

It is a self-retaining abdominal retractor with three adjustable blades. Two side blades are fenestrated and they retract the edges of abdominal incision. The third blade retracts either the upper or lower angle of the incision and accordingly functions as upper abdominal retractor or supra-pubic retractor. It can be used in all major abdominal gyne operations.

Jayle's Retractor

It is self-retaining vaginal retractor with two L-shaped blades. The right blade is fixed and there is a transverse bar attached to it. Left blade is movable and it slides on and can be fixed in any position along the transverse bar with a screw. It was used to retract the lateral vaginal walls in vaginal operations. It is **not used** now.

DISSECTING FORCEPS

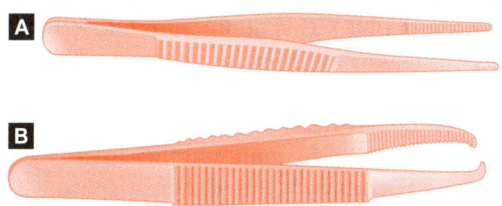

Figs. 1.32A and B: Dissecting forceps: (A) Plain; (B) Toothed.

Two types are available
1. Plain or Toothless or untoothed forceps.
2. Toothed forceps with one in two teeth at the tip.

Both have common features as below:
- The handles have a spring like action.
- There may be few ridges on the central part of the outer surface of the handles to give better grip.
- There are transverse serrations on the inner aspects near the tip (may be absent in toothed forceps) which give better grip on the tissues.

Uses

- Toothless forceps is used to hold soft tissues like peritoneum (parietal and visceral) and muscles while suturing or dissection during surgery.
- Toothed forceps is used to hold tough structures like rectus sheath, skin edges, fascia and vaginal walls while suturing or their dissection during surgery.
- They may be used to hold the needles while tissue bites are taken during suturing.

Toothed forceps inflicts some trauma by the tooth but it gives better grip than toothless forceps where the tissue might slip from the tips.

TOWEL CLIP (DOYEN'S CROSS ACTION TOWEL CLIP)

It is designed in such a way that the blades crossover near the distal end and then curved to end in sharp tapering tips. It resembles number '8'. When the handles are pressed the tips open out, and on release of pressure the tips get approximated with a spring like action. The blades are distally bent at an angle so as to allow them to lie flush with the skin surface without projecting.

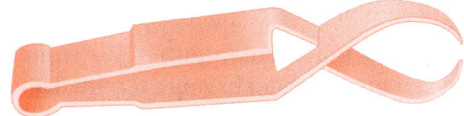

Fig. 1.33: Towel clip.

Uses

In abdominal and vaginal surgery the operative area is drapped with sterile towels after painting. Towel clips are used to fix the towels to the skin and to each other. Isolation of operative field prevents contamination of deeper tissues from the patient's skin.

It may be used to fix a sucker tube or other tubes, cords, wires, etc. in position during operation.

Other instruments used for the purpose are **Backhaus corner clip** and **Moynihan's tetratowel forceps.**

IUCD REMOVING HOOK

This is long instrument resembling Simpson's uterine sound but has hook shaped terminal end. Direction of the hook is toward the angled side of the instrument. It is made of stainless steel.

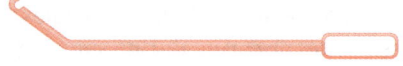

Fig. 1.34: IUCD removing hook.

Uses

- Previously it was required for removal of ring IUCD (Grafenberg ring), which had no threads. Now for Copper IUCDs it is required when threads are missing or torn or IUCD is embedded in uterine cavity.
- To remove intratubal prosthesis from uterine cavity (inserted during cornual implantation).

Complications

It can cause:
- Endometrial trauma
- Pain
- Perforation of uterus.

Shirodkar's hook is another instrument which is more slender having a terminal hook and used for same purpose.

BERKLEY–BONNEY'S ROUND LIGAMENT FORCEPS

It is a long (8 inches) stainless steel instrument. Its blades are long thin, curved on flat with transverse serrations near the tip. There are catches on the handle. It is sterilized by boiling or autoclaving.

Uses

It was basically designed for ventrosuspension (Gilliam's) operation which is **not done** at present.

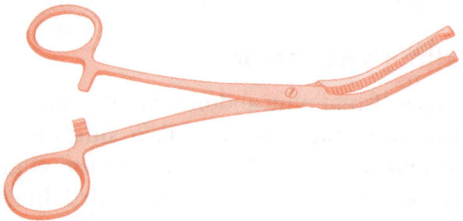

Fig. 1.35: Berkley–Bonney's round ligament forceps.

Now, it can be used in following operation:
- Purandare's cervicopexy operation to catch the strip of rectus sheath while passing it extraperitoneally, in front of the cervix.
- Khanna's sling: To catch and carry Mersilene tape.
- In William Richardson's and Shaw's operation's for correction of vault prolapse, to catch and carry the rectus sheath strip.

In absence of this instrument long curved artery forceps is commonly used for the purpose.

AYRE'S SPATULA

It is a wooden spatula which was introduced by Ayre (1946). It is about 20 cm long. It is used to take Pap smear by scrape method. It is also available in plastic and stainless steel, but wooden one is preferred because of its rough surface maximum number of cells are scraped. Today modified Ayre's spatula is available which has longer endocervical end for better sampling from the endocervix.

Instead of this, simple swab sticks or even ice cream sticks are used. The other smear taking devices include cotton swab, endocervical, cytobrush, etc.

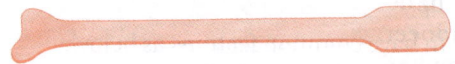

Fig. 1.36: Ayre's spatula.

Pap Smear

It is the most widely used method for screening of premalignant and malignant lesions of cervix. Papanicolaou introduced cytology first in 1928. Then in 1932 the technique was refined by him and traut.

Taking of the Smear

- Materials required are (1) Cusco's (or Sims') speculum, (2) clean glass sides preferably with frosted ends, (3) sampling device (Ayre's spatula), (4) marking pencil, and (5) fixative.
  Fixative can be 95% alcohol or equal parts of 95% alcohol and ether or cytospray.
- Patient preparation include:
  - No sexual relation in last 24 hours
  - No vaginal douche in last 24 hours
  - No use of intravaginal medication in last one week
  - No local infection (it should be treated first)
  - Smear is not taken during menses.

Procedure

- The patient is placed in a dorsal position.
- Prior P/V examination should not be done.
- No lubricants should be used.
- Dry Cusco's bivalve speculum exposes the cervix.
- Ayre's spatula is introduced. Its long narrow end fits into the external os (for endocervical sampling) and board concave end covers the squamocolumnar junction (transformation zone).
- Spatula is rotated 360° with firm pressure.

Sample thus obtained is quickly spread over the glass slide using a circular motion. Slide is immediately fixed with fixative, labelled and sent to the laboratory. Proper requisition form (cytopathology form) completely and accurately filled and signed by authorized person must accompany every slide.

To decrease the false negative results the endocervical brush smear may be taken simultaneously. In case of pregnancy instead of endocervical brush moistened cotton swab is used.

- An adequate smear: A smear is considered adequate if it has adequate cellularity, contains endocervical cells, smear is thin and evenly spread, it is not bloody and there is no air drying artifacts.
  For reporting of Pap smear the original Papanicolaou system (class I to class V) is not used now. Revised Bethesda system (2001) is used.
- Screening of cervical cancer in normal population should start at 30 years of age and subsequent screening is advocated every 3 years if cytology is done alone, but if it is cotest (i.e. Pap smear + HIV test) screening is recommended every 5 years till 65 years of age. In high risk group, it should be started at an early age (20) and should be more frequent (annually).
  Same screening schedule is recommended even in those women who have received HPV vaccination.
- Downstaging of cervical cancer: It is defined as the detection of disease, in an earlier stage when still curable, by nurses and other non-medical health workers using a simple vaginal speculum for visual inspection of cervix.
  This is useful in our country where universal screening is not possible and carcinoma cervix is the most common cancer in females and many cases are detected at an advanced stage.
- For prevention of cervical cancer HPV vaccines are now available (Chapter 7).

RING PESSARY

Ring shaped instrument made up of polyethylene. It has now replaced the older ones made up of rubber or vulcanite. Polyethylene pessary causes much less inflammatory reaction. It is compressible and quite pliable. Available in different diameters (graded according to outer diameter in millimeters).

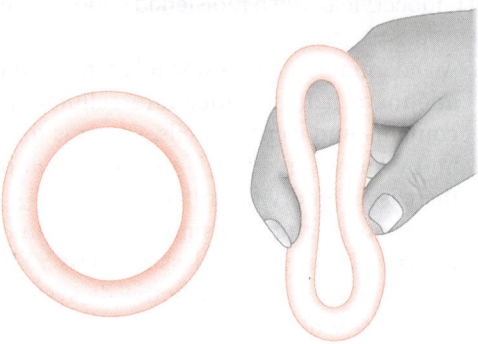

Fig. 1.37: Ring pessary.

Indications

It is used in prolapse as a palliative treatment. In modern day practice its indications are few and decreasing. They are: (1) prolapse of uterus during pregnancy up to first 4 months, (2) immediately postpartum and during lactation, (3) when patient is unfit for surgery, (4) when patient is not willing for surgery, (5) while patient is waiting for surgery, e.g. healing of decubitus ulcer.

Contraindications

- Complete procidentia
- Very patulous vaginal orifice
- Stress incontinence (it is not relieved by pessary, it requires surgery)
- Local infection.

Method of Use

The pessary is first compressed between the thumb and index finger and introduced into the vagina in an anteroposterior sagittal plane after pressing the perineum backwards. It is then rotated until it lies horizontally. The upper end is pushed in the posterior fornix and the lower end lies behind the symphysis pubis.

Correct Size of Pessary

This is determined by trial and error but is governed mainly by the length of the vagina. Distance between the posterior fornix (put on stretch) and lower border of symphysis pubis is measured. 1.25 cm less than this is the correct size. Correct size pessary: (1) it causes no discomfort to the patient, (2) it does not come out when the patient strains or coughs, (3) it is not so tight that it cannot be rotated by examining fingers.

Mechanism of Action

Pessary rests on the upper surface of levator ani-muscles. It distends the upper vagina so wide that it cannot fall through lower vagina and introitus, because its transverse diameter is greater than the transverse diameter of the hiatus urogenitalis. As it stretches only the upper vagina, it does not reduce the low cystocele and rectocele effectively.

Instructions to the Patient

- Daily vaginal douche by dilute antiseptic solutions.
- Follow-up visit after one week to check about the proper placement of the pessary.
- Changing of pessary every 6–12 months, if necessry (larger sizes may be required to control prolapse).
- Stop using pessary if any of the complications occurs.

Complications

- Excessive vaginal discharge
- Local infection, ulceration of vaginal walls.
- Impaction of pessary if kept for very long time.
- Dyspareunia.
- Constipation and dysuria if it is too large and presses on rectum or urethra.

Sterilization

Plastic ones are supplied as pre-sterilized by manufacturers. Otherwise, it may be sterilized by chemical sterilization.

HODGE PESSARY

It is ovoid in shape, with upper end wide and round while lower end is square. It is made up of plastic or vulcanite. Smith modification of Hodge pessary has a less marked profile curve and narrow rounded lower end as compared to Hodge pessary.

It was used in past after correction of mobile retroversion to keep the uterus anteverted. Now, retroversion is considered normal anatomical variation and not responsible for any symptoms, so it is obsolete now.

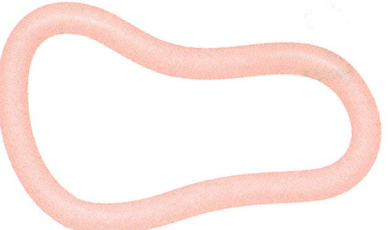

Fig. 1.38: Hodge–Smith pessary.

CHAPTER 2

Catheters

SIMPLE RUBBER CATHETER

It is a long hollow tube made up of rubber (red rubber) with one end closed and other end open. There is a drainage opening on the side just behind the closed end. It is radio-opaque due to its lead oxide content. It is 37.5 cm long and available from 3 to 12 number sizes. **Number 8 is the usual size used in adult.** The external diameter of catheters in mm is N/2 + 1 (N = No. of catheter).

Sterilization

Autoclaving is the best but it damages the rubber. It is usually sterilized by keeping it in boiling water for 30 minutes. Repeated boiling also damages the rubber. Ideal is chemical sterilization, e.g., Savlon, Cidex, Dettol, etc. But this is time consuming and the catheter is to be washed with sterile water before use.

Uses

Gynecology

- Before pelvic examination or any gynec procedure if the patient is not able to evacuate her bladder satisfactorily.
- To measure the amount of residual urine.
- To relieve the retention of urine.
- To collect catheter specimen of urine for culture sensitivity examination in case of chronic urinary tract infection.
- During laparoscopic TL or diagnostic laparoscopy if bladder is found full and uterus and tubes cannot be fully visualized.
- To do three swabs test in differential diagnosis of urinary fistula.
- To do cystourethrography.
- As a rubber tourniquet during myomectomy operation for hemostatic purpose in place of Bonney's myomectomy clamp.

During and immediate postoperative period of major gynec surgery, e.g., hysterectomy Foley's catheter is usually kept.

Obstetrics

- Before an instrumental delivery, i.e., forceps, vacuum extractor.
- During first stage of labor if patient is not able to pass urine (particularly under epidural analgesia).
- Before pelvic examination in obstetric patient if she is not able to evacuate her bladder satisfactorily.
- To evacuate bladder in case of atonic postpartum hemorrhage (PPH).
  - During and immediate postoperative period of major obstetric surgery, e.g., cesarean section Foley's catheter is usually kept.
  - To give oxygen to the mother special tubing or ventimask is now available. Also for suction in eclamptic patient

disposable plastic cannula are now available. Simple rubber catheter was used in past.

Contraindication

Local infection, i.e., urethritis.

Procedure

- Patient is explained the procedure and her confidence is gained.
- Dorsal position.
- Strict asepsis, i.e., thorough scrubbing and wearing sterile gloves, gown, mask and cap. Painting of the local part and draping with sterile towels.
- Vulva is cleaned with Savlon swabs. Sterile anesthetic jelly is applied on the tip of the catheter. Apart from anesthetic effect it works as lubricating agent also.
- Catheter should be sterile, preferably a new one and its patency should be checked.
- With left index finger and thumb labia are separated and external urinary meatus is identified. Catheter is held in right hand and its tip is gently negotiated through the meatus. As soon as it reaches the bladder urine comes out.
- The outer end of the catheter is put in a container (i.e., kidney tray).
- After the bladder is empty the catheter is pinched before it is removed to avoid introduction of air in the bladder.

Ideally the above procedure should be followed in practice but in routine ward side catheterization, minimum touch technique is used as below:

- Hands are washed with soap and water and only sterile gloves are put on.
- No painting and draping but only vulva is cleaned with Savlon swabs.
- Sterile catheter is taken and a loop is made so that no part of it touch the thigh of the patient or the bed, which are unsterile.
- Catheter is held distal to first 4–5 cm and gradually negotiated in urethra as described before.

Measures to be tried before doing catheterization in the ward for self-evacuation: (1) motivation for self-evacuation, providing privacy, change of posture and sound of running tap water, (2) analgesics are given to relieve involuntary spasm of urinary sphincter due to postoperative pain, (3) hot water bag in suprapubic region, (4) parasympathomimetic drugs, i.e., carbachol, neostigmine can be used if there is repeated retention on removal of catheter.

If after introduction of catheter urine does not come out the possibilities are:
- Catheter has not reached the bladder, i.e., false passage, elongated urethra.
- Catheter has reached the bladder but bladder is empty, i.e., anuria.
- Catheter is in the bladder, there is urine in the bladder, but tip of the catheter is above the level of urine, i.e., diverticula, cystocele pouch.
- If none of the above is the cause then the catheter is blocked.

Complications of Simple Rubber Catheterization

- *Infection:* Introduction of new infection or flare up of preexisting infection. Whatever aseptic precautions are taken there is 4% incidence of infection after single simple rubber catheterization.
- *False passage:* It can lead to frank hemorrhage, hematuria, hematoma and extravasation of urine. False passage is diagnosed by (a) resistance to further introduction of the catheter, (b) urine does not come out, (c) patient complains of pain, (d) fresh bleeding occurs.

Risk of false passage is more with metal catheters.
- Repeated simple rubber catheterization can cause urethral stricture.
- Reflex anuria rarely.

PLASTIC URETHRAL CATHETER

- It is made up of PVC—synthetic smooth plastic which is nontoxic and slightly stiffer than rubber catheter.
- It is presterilized by gamma radiation and supplied in plastic pack. Ideally disposable, so it is discarded after single use.
- It is available in sizes 6 FG to 24 FG (K-90 is 14 FG).
- It is 40 cm long with distal end coned for atraumatic introduction.
- It has 2 lateral eyes near the distal end for efficient drainage.
- Proximal (outer) end is fitted with funnel shaped connector for extension. Connectors are color coded for easy identification.
- It contains X-ray opaque line.

Uses

They are same as those of simple rubber catheter. It has now largely replaced simple rubber catheter. Due to connector at proximal end it is better fitted to urine drainage bag and useful for short-term bladder catheterization. As compared to rubber catheter it is less irritant, pyrogen free and transparent.

SELF-RETAINING CATHETERS

Foley's and Malecot's are commonly used.

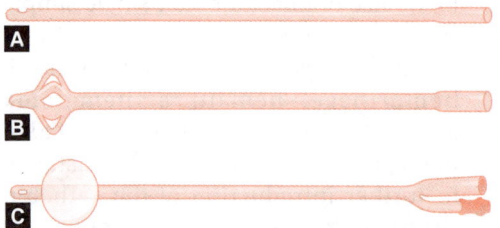

Figs. 2.1A to C: Catheters: (A) Simple rubber; (B) Malecot's; (C) Foley's (Bulb inflated).

FOLEY'S CATHETER

- Made up of latex, it is 40 cm long available in sizes 12, 14, 16....... up to 30 F. Number 16 is commonly used for adult.
- Latex is less tissue toxic and tissue irritant than rubber. Special silicone coated catheters are better tolerated by the patient, as silicone coating reduce urethral irritation so useful for long-term use.
- Presterilized by gamma radiation and supplied in double plastic pack.
- Ideally disposable-discarded after single use.
- Gives faint radio-opaque shadow on X-ray.

Foley's catheter are two types:
1. Self-retaining–2 way Foley's.
2. Foley's oven hemostatic–3 way Foley's.

In normal Foley's 2 tubes at lower end, side one connected to inflatable balloon and main is for drainage of urine. In addition to these 2, in Foley's oven type there is a 3rd tube at lower end which is for introduction of any fluid inside the bladder for irrigation. It is used after surgery on bladder to wash away blood or blood clots.

- Inflatable balloon bulb is near the tip. It is for self-retaining purpose. Its capacity is 30–50 cc usually. Number of catheter in French is written at the lower end of the catheter.
- To calculate external diameter (D) in mm. D=N/3 N=No. of catheter (French) (It indicates circumference).

Introduction

Under all aseptic and antiseptic precautions, the catheter is introduced. Then bulb is inflated by sterile water or saline with the help of a syringe applied to the cuffed outer end of the catheter, where there is one way valve which prevents the fluid from coming out of the bulb. Bulb is inflated much below its maximum capacity but big enough to retain the catheter inside the bladder, i.e., 8 to 10 cc maximum the block and maximum capacity is 30 to 50 cc.

Removal

Direct needle or nozzle of the syringe is applied to cuffed end, so valve gets opened and fluid from bulb comes out under pressure.

When all the fluid has escaped, catheter is gently pulled out.

In case of prolonged use, (i.e., more than a week) before removal of the catheter it should be clamped and released every 2-3 hours for 12-24 hours. This is important to build up the bladder tone for proper functioning after removal. However recent evidence does not support for bladder training when catheter is kept for 14 days or less. The residual urine should be measured after removal of catheter and if it is more than 50 mL the catheter is reinserted.

If the bulb does not get deflated at the time of removal due to block in the side channel, following measures can be done : (1) inject more fluid to overcome the block and rupture the balloon. However block may not allow it, (2) inject $NaHCO_3$. It is organic solvent and may dissolve the block in the side channel, (3) go on cutting the catheter towards the external urethral meatus. If the block is in the outer part of the catheter, i.e., not in 4 cm length from the balloon, it gets deflated and catheter is removed easily, (4) palpate the bulb through anterior vaginal wall (difficult when bladder is distended) and make a blind puncture with needle to deflate the balloon inside the bladder, then pull out the catheter, (5) suprapubic puncture under sonography control.

Uses

Gynecology

- *It is kept postoperatively as follows:*
  - Simple A-P (cystocele-rectocele) repair—48 to 72 hours.
  - Vaginal hysterectomy with repair—48 to 72 hours. In vaginal hysterectomy without repair it may be kept for only 24 hours.
  - Abdominal hysterectomy—48 to 72 hrs.
  - Laparoscopic surgeries—24 to 48 hours if there is no doubt of urinary tract injury.
  - Stress incontinence (SUI) repair—5 to 7 days.
  - Manchester operation—48 to 72 hours.
  - Vesico-vaginal fistula repair—14 to 21 days. For first 3-5 days negative suction is better.
  - Wertheim's hysterectomy—3 to 6 weeks
  - Vaginoplasty—10-14 days.
  - Other surgical bladder operations—7 to 14 days.
- Pre-operatively in VVF to drain the bladder and to make the fistulous tract clean and healthy for operation if opening is small. In fact very small fistula may thus be closed without operation.
- Retention of urine due to impacted mass in pelvis, i.e., ovarian tumor, fibroid.
- Incontinence of urine.
- Pediatric Foley's catheter No. 8 F may be used **intrauterine** (a) to control bleeding after hysteroscopic surgery, (b) to prevent recurrence of adhesions after treatment of Asherman's syndrome, (c) for sonohysterography and sonosalpingography, and (d) sometimes to do HSG.

Obstetric

- *Cesarean section:* Postoperatively to drain the bladder. Catheter is introduced just before operation and kept for 48-72 hours.
- *Eclampsia:* (a) To drain the bladder as the patient is unconscious or sedated; (b) To know the urine output.
- Retroverted gravid uterus with retention of urine at 12-14 weeks of pregnancy.
- Obstetric shock due to any cause, i.e., severe APH, severe PPH, ruptured ectopic, etc. to know the urine output.
- If there are paraurethral tears after normal or instrumental delivery and stitches are taken. If it is not kept, spasm of the external urinary sphincter will lead to retention of urine. It is kept for 1 to 2 days.
- If vagina is packed to control bleeding after delivery by roller pack, catheter is kept in bladder till pack is removed.
- Induction of labor. Foley's catheter is introduced through the cervix. Bulb is

inflated by 30 mL saline and catheter is taped to the patients leg. Catheter is kept for 12 to 24 hours.
- Mid-trimester MTP by intrauterine-extra-amniotic route, i.e., Emcredil instillation.
- *Rupture uterus:* Postoperatively even if rupture has not involved the bladder, as patient may be in low condition unable to pass urine and to keep exact output chart.
- *Obstructed labor:* Postpartum it is kept to prevent VVF, as there may be bladder neck pressure necrosis, which may manifest later. It is kept for 5 to 7 days.

Care of Indwelling Catheter

- Urine bag is kept well below the level of Foley's catheter without causing undue traction to it.
- Patency is to be checked regularly and if it gets blocked, bladder wash may be given or catheter should be changed immediately.
- Adequate fluid intake is must to maintain good urine output to prevent infection. Prophylactic antibiotics should be given. Ideally urine examination must be done at regular intervals in prolonged catheterization.
- Connecting tube is checked for color and density of urine and crystal formation in the wall, indicating infection. If it occurs bladder washes are given and catheter is changed if necessary.
- If urine is acidic, alkaline mixture is given orally to change the pH. In case of infection, dilute betadine wash is also advantageous.
- If bladder is septic and urine alkaline bladder wash with dilute acidic solution should be given at least twice a week to prevent phosphatic encrustation.
- Daily outer surface of the catheter is cleaned with Savlon after gently pulling it out for about 1 cm at external urinary meatus.
- Simple Foley's catheter should be changed at 10–14 days although siliconized catheter can be kept longer (4 weeks).

Advantages of Continuous Catheterization Over Frequent Simple Catheterization

- Minimum number of introductions and removal so less chances of infection and other complications.
- Bladder remains completely empty so there is rest to the operative part, leading to better healing.
- Output of urine can be measured accurately.

Disadvantages

- Ascending infection via the wall of the catheter.
- Discomfort and continuous foreign body or full bladder sensation.
- Relative immobilization. Patient on long-term catheterization can move around holding the urobag in hand.
- As bladder remains completely empty, it may lead to contracted bladder leading to frequency of micturition after catheter is removed, or it may lead to hypotonia and retention of urine.

Complications

- Infection—cystitis, pyelonephritis, bacteriuria.
- False passage at the time of introduction.
- Catheter fever.
- Urethral stricture due to urethral ischemia if catheter is of larger size.
- Stone formation—phosphatic in alkaline urine; oxalate, uric acid and cystine in acidic urine.
- Postcatheterization retention of urine after prolonged catheterization due to decrease in bladder tone.
- Blocking of the catheter—if it goes unrecognized it can lead to damage to operative site.
- Reflex anuria in case of chronic retention of urine if rapid evacuation is done.

MALECOT CATHETER

It is made up of rubber. At distal end just near the tip there is bulging to make it self-retaining. This bulging is not complete, it is longitudinally split with gaps in between the strips. It can be used from both routes in female, suprapubic as well as transurethral. It is not used at present.

Introduction

Requires special introducer or stylet which, when passed through the catheter reaching the tip straightens out the bulb so that catheter is readily introduced in the bladder. Then stylet is removed so near the tip it again becomes bulbous due to elastic recoil of the rubber.

Removal

No instrument is required. It can be simply pulled out.

Disadvantages

(1) Patient may pull it out, (2) at the time of introduction its metal introducer may cause false passage, (3) more chances of infection, (4) more irritant than Foley's catheter.

FEMALE METAL CATHETER

It is 5 to 6 inches long metal catheter with shallow gentle curve near the tip. It has two eyes near the tip and a stylet inside.

As compared to rubber catheter it is more irritant and more traumatic. It can cause urethral laceration or false passage. It is used only when rubber or plastic catheter cannot be passed, i.e., in obstetrics when the head is deeply engaged and the urethra is compressed between the head and the pubis.

It's only advantage is that it can be easily sterilized by boiling and can be used repeatedly.

URO BAG (URINE COLLECTING BAG)

- It is rectangular shape plastic bag, used for collection and measurement of urine output.
- It is presterilized by gamma radiation and supplied in a thin plastic pack.
- On one side, it has printed easy to read scales on it from 25 mL to 2000 mL for measurement.
- On the upper end there are 2 tubings—one shorter tube near the corner with a cap, is drainage outlet for emptying the bag.
- The longer tube near the center (90 to 100 cm long) with plastic cap is meant for attaching it to the catheter after removing the cap.
- Inside the bag end of this long tube there is nonreturn valve to prevent ascending infection. Some urine bags have the drip chamber inside.
- It has one or two strings looped to its upper end for hanging it from the support.
- It is transparent which helps in finding out the color of the urine (concentrated, hematuria) and infection (turbidity, flakes).

Precautions

- Kinking or pressure on the connecting tube should be avoided.
- Urine bag should be kept well below the level of the catheter for better drainage without causing traction on the catheter.
- Leaking bag should be immediately replaced.
- Some air pushed in the bag from drainage outlet helps in free drainage.
- Whenever Foley's catheter is changed for infection or after long use, urine bag should be changed.
- Exact amount of urine shown in the bag may not be correct and sometimes it requires to be rechecked in other container. False measurement is due to different stretchability of different plastic material with different manufacturers.

CHAPTER 3

Suture Materials and Needles

Suture: It is a stitch taken by a strand of material threaded on a needle.
Ligature: It means a thing used for tying of blood vessels or pedicles.
Classification of suture material.

ABSORBABLE

A. **Natural:** Immediate
   - Catgut – Plain or chromic.
   - Collagen
   - Living tissues – Fascia lata (Patient's own), Plantaris tendon.

B. **Synthetic:** Delayed
   - Polyglycolic acid – Dexon
   - Polyglactic acid   – Vicryl
   - Polydioxanone   – PDS
   - Polyglyconate   – Maxon
   - Poliglecaprone   – Monocryl

NONABSORBABLE

A. **Natural:**
   - Silk
   - Silkworm gut
   - Linen
   - cotton

B. **Synthetic:**
   - Polyamides – Nylon
   - Polyesters – Terylene, dacron
   - Polypropylene – Prolene
   - Polybutester – Novafil
   - Polyethylene – Dermalence
   - Metallic wire – Stainless steel, tantalum and silver

In general:
- Natural materials are more tissue irritant then synthetic material.
- Chances of infection are higher with multifilament (braided or twisted) material than monofilament type.
- Tensile strength remains for longer period (more than 6 months) in non-absorbable material.

Tensile strength: It means minimum load (force) required to break that material. It is standardized by measuring breaking load (kilogram force) applied on surgeon's knot.

ABSORBABLE

Commonly used suture materials are described.

CATGUT

The catgut is the commonly used absorbable suture material.

There are two types—plain and chromic.

Plain	Chromic
Tensile strength remains 4–5 days only	Tensile strength remains for 10–15 days
Completely absorbed within 7 days	It is absorbed in 15–20 days
More tissue irritant than chromic one	Less tissue irritant
Light yellow color	Dark brown in color

Plain catgut: Surgical catgut is protein in nature and prepared from connective tissues (submucosal layer) of proximal one-third of small intestine of sheep. In catgut laboratories initially the raw plain catgut is manufactured, which can be used after sterilization.

Chromic catgut: Raw catgut can be chromicized by immersing it in a chromic salt solution bath, for 1 to 96 hours. The color is added for differentiating it from plain catgut. It is then sorted in different standard sizes and cut in to convenient length of 76 cm (2.5 feet) and 152 cm (5 feet).

Chromic catgut is available in eight standard sizes from 6-0 to 2 No.

No. of catgut	Diameter (mm)	No. of catgut	Diameter (mm)
4–0	0.15	0	0.3
3–0	0.2	1	0.4
2–0	0.25	2	0.5

It is sterilized by gamma irradiation or ethylene oxide gas by the manufacturer and supplied in double foil packs containing preserving fluid. Fluid contains 70% alcohol with glycerol and water added to maintain flexibility of catgut.

Uses

Plain Catgut

2-0 and 3-0—ligation of small bleeders and suturing of subcutaneous fat.

Chromic Catgut

For many indications described below chromic catgut is now replaced by delayed absorbable, e.g., vicryl.

No. 0: Suturing of visceral or parietal peritoneum, rectus muscle, vaginal walls, perineal muscles.

No. 1: Suturing of rectus sheath in any laparotomy incision, suturing of uterine muscle in LSCS or hysterotomy, suturing of levator ani muscles in colpoperineorrhaphy.

No. 2: For ligation or transfixation of large pedicles in abdominal or vaginal hysterectomy.

Chromic catgut is also available as atraumatic one, i.e., directly attached to the needle.

Disadvantages of Catgut

- Expensive material as compared to natural nonabsorbable sutures.
- Being foreign animal protein it produces more tissue reaction than synthetic absorbable and most of the nonabsorbable materials.
- It is synergistic with organisms in promotion of wound sepsis. However, as it is absorbed-infection, even if it occurs, can be self-limiting.
- Two-third of tensile strength is lost within 10 days, so it is useless where tensile strength is required for longer time.
- Catgut swells in the tissue, so knot becomes loose and if the ends are cut short it might even slip.
- Handling of catgut is not very good.

POLYGLACTIN 910 (VICRYL)

It is synthetic delayed absorbable material made up of long chain carbohydrate. It is copolymer of glycolic acid and lactic acids. It is slowly absorbed in the tissue by the process of hydrolysis. It is colored violet for ease of identification. It is available from 9-0 to 3 No. sizes. Very little is absorbed before 14 days and it takes about 60–90 days to undergo complete absorption. More than 50% of tensile strength is retained at 14 days.

Advantages

- It is less irritant than other absorbable materials.
- It is much stronger relative to its size than catgut. Its initial strength is also more than silk, nylon and prolene.
- It is stable even in contaminated wound. Moreover, it inhibits bacterial growth because of acidic pH around it.
- It is not affected by moisture or wetting.

Disadvantages

- It is costly suture material.
- It is braided not smooth and may pull and drag the tissue with continuous suture.
- There is difficulty in snugging down the knots (uncoated vicryl).
- It cannot be used when extended approximation of tissues under strain is required.

Uses

It is now increasingly used in place of chromic catgut in hysterectomy and LSCS operations (No. 1-0 and 1). It is used in abdominal wound closure, bladder surgery, gastrointestinal surgery and tuboplasty operations.

Coated Vicryl

There is coating of the braided suture by mixture of polyglactin 370 and Calcium stearate. Coating makes it smoother product that will pass through the tissue with minimal drag. Handling and tying is also better. It is either violet color or natural color (undyed).

Vicryl Rapide

It is braided synthetic absorbable suture. Its initial tensile strength is high but it looses it completely after 14 days. It is completely absorbed in 6 weeks. The rapid absorption characteristics of vicryl rapide are achieved by exposure of suture to gamma irradiation resulting in material with low molecular weight than original vicryl. It is used for suturing episiotomy. It is available in undyed (natural) white color and 3-0 to 1-0 sizes. As compared to catgut patient has less perineal pain and discomfort in postpartum period.

Vicryl Plus

It is a new coated vicryl suture with antimicrobial properties due to addition of triclosan a synthetic broad spectrum antimicrobial agent. Triclosan has been used effectively in consumer products for more than 3 decades. It is very useful in potentially high-risk septic cases.

DEXON

It is synthetic delayed absorbable suture, made up of polyglycolic acid, which is a homopolymer of glycolic acid. **Dexon"s"** is simple while **Dexon Plus** is coated with Poloxamer 188. They are braided sutures. Dexon "s" is also available as monofilament. They are either colored green to enhance visibility in the tissue or undyed with natural beige color. They are available from 8-0 to 2 No. sizes and also as atraumatic.

Advantages

- It is non-antigenic and non-pyrogenic. Tissue reaction is minimal.
- It is smaller in diameter than vicryl of equivalent tensile strength.
- For sizes 6-0 or greater 65% of original tensile strength is retained at 14 days.
- Absorption is by hydrolysis and it is minimal at 7 to 15 days, significant at 30 days and completed between 60 and 90 days.

Disadvantages

- Handling characteristics and knot security of uncoated suture (Dexon "s") is not good.

- It cannot be used where extended approximation of tissues under strain must be maintained. Its safe use in cardiac and major vessels has not been established.

Use: Same as vicryl.

POLYDIOXANONE (PDS)

It is synthetic monofilament delayed absorbable suture. It is violet in color and formed by polymerizing the monomer para-dioxanone in the presence of a catalyst. 50% of tensile strength remains at 4 weeks. Absorption is minimal by 90th day. Complete absorption occurs at 210 days. Absorption is by slow hydrolysis. It is available in silver color pack.

Use: Same as vicryl.

MONOCRYL (POLIGLECAPRONE 25)

It is newer monofilament synthetic absorbable suture material, which is a copolymer of 75% glycolide and 25% caprolactone. It is available in golden color and 5-0 to 1-0 size. Its initial tensile strength is high and after 2 weeks approximately 20–30% tensile strength remains. It is absorbed slowly and completely in 90–120 days. It is smooth and very easy to handle.

Uses: It is used for subcuticular skin stitches, suturing of subcutaneous fat, peritoneal suture and episiotomy.

NONABSORBABLE

SILK

It is natural nonabsorbable material developed from silkworm. It is made by unravelling the cocoon which is spun by silkworm larva. While silkworm gut is monofilament, silk is either braided or twisted. Silk is black in color and available from sizes 6-0 to 4.

Tensile strength remains for quite long period and only half is lost in 6–12 months. It is sterilized by autoclaving and because it contracts on heating it is wound loosely on the spool before autoclaving. It is also supplied in double foil pack in presterilized form.

Advantages
- Fairly cheap material.
- It is very good material to handle.
- Less irritant than other natural nonabsorbable, i.e., cotton, linen.
- It is stronger than catgut size for size.

Disadvantages
- It is more irritant to the tissues than synthetic nonabsorbable material. To reduce its irritant qualities coated silk may be used.
- It is capillary so it may cause spread of infection. Their braided or twisted structure leads to persistence of infection until the suture is discharged or removed. Serum-proofed silk reduces capillary attraction. It can be made noncapillary by wax or silicone.

Uses
- Suturing of skin No. 1 silk.
- Cervical os tightening-No. 2 silk.
- Tension stitches to prevent or to treat burst abdomen No. 2 or thicker.
- Internal iliac ligation-No. 2 silk.
- Purandare's sling (cervicopexy) operation for prolapse No. 2 silk.
- Round ligament plication and uterosacral plication to keep the uterus anteverted, along with sling or other operation No. 1-0 Silk.
- Ligation of umbilical cord after birth No. 1 Silk
- Gastrointestinal surgery No. 3-0 Silk.

NYLON

It is synthetic nonabsorbable material polyamide in nature. It may be monofilament or multifilament braided or twisted. It is either colorless, black or green in color. Monofilament is available in 10-0 to 2 No. while braided is available in 4-0 to 4 No. sizes. 2/3 tensile strength remains up to 6 months.

Advantages

- It is inert material causing minimal tissue response.
- It can be used in presence of infection (particularly monofilament).
- It is stronger than silk size for size.
- It possesses great elasticity.
- It is water resistant.
- It can be autoclaved thrice before it losses its strength.

Disadvantages

- Monofilament is poor in handling.
- It does not knot nicely.
- It tends to slip so it requires multiple throws for security and the ends should be cut 10 mm long.

Uses

- Skin suture—simple, mattress or subcuticular.
- Tension suture or secondary suture of the abdominal wound.
- Cervical OS tightening operation.
- As a splint 2-0 nylon is used in tubal reconstructive surgery, i.e., end to end anastomosis, while 8-0 may be used in the actual anastomosis.

COTTON THREAD

It is natural nonabsorbable material, vegetable in origin made from the seeds of the cotton plant. It is usually twisted rather than braided. It is supplied in sizes 3-0 to 1. Half tensile strength is lost in 3–6 months.

Advantages

- Very cheap
- Good to handle.

Disadvantages

- Weakest suture material, tensile, strength is the least of all sutures.
- It is more irritant to the issues than silk and causes moderate inflammatory reaction.
- It is capillary so more chances of infection.
- Combination of cotton and polyester fiber is available, e.g., ethicot, which is serum proofed and noncapillary.

LINEN THREAD

It is also natural nonabsorbable material. It is also vegetable in origin, made up from linen flax. Its qualities are same as those of cotton thread except that it is more strong and reliable than cotton thread. It is available from 6-0 to 2 No. sizes.

It is commonly used in skin suture, gastrointestinal surgery and radical pelvic surgery.

PROLENE

It is synthetic nonabsorbable material polypropylene in nature. It is available in monofilament form only. It is bright blue in color. It is available in wide range from 10-0 to 2 No. sizes. Thinner ones are available as atraumatic. Its qualities are better than those of monofilament nylon. It is stronger than nylon, tensile strength is retained for longer period than nylon, superior to nylon in handling, and knot slippage is less.

Uses: It is suitable for any instance where a nonabsorbable suture is required. It is widely used in primary or secondary abdominal wound closure (rectus sheath) and various tuboplasty operations.

NOVAFIL

It is synthetic nonabsorbable suture polybutester in nature. It is monofilament and either clear or blue in color. It is available from

Suture Materials and Needles

10-0 to 2 No. sizes and also as atraumatic. It causes transient, minimal acute inflammatory reaction with fibrous connective tissue capsule formation around it. Like other synthetic sutures it requires additional throws for secure knots.

Uses: It is indicated for use in all types of soft tissue approximation including use in cardiovascular and ophthalmic surgery, where a nonabsorbable suture is required.

SUTURE NEEDLES

They are made up of stainless steel and are of different varieties as below:
A. Curved needles:
   1. Round-bodied – With eye/eyeless
   2. Cutting – With eye/eyeless
B. Straight needles:
   1. Round-bodied – With eye/eyeless
   2. Cutting – With eye/eyeless
C. Special variety, e.g., Mayo's needle (Trocar point), taper point, blunt point, micro point, lance point, spatula, etc.

All these are available in different sizes.

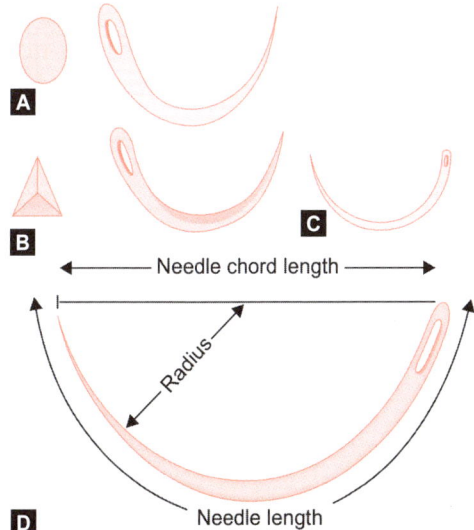

Figs. 3.1A to D: Suture needles: (A) Round bodied; (B) Cutting; (C) Half-circle needle; (D) Anatomy of surgical needle.

Basic Structure of the Needle

All surgical needles have 3 basic components: (i) the tip (point), (ii) the body and (iii) the eye. The eye can be closed eye or swaged (eyeless).

In curved needles curvature of the needle may be 3/8th circle, half-circle or 5/8th circle.

Anatomy of Surgical Needle

Chord length: It is the straight line distance from the tip of a curved needle to the eye (or swage).

Needle length: It is the distance measured along the needle itself from the tip to the eye.

Radius: If the curvature of the needle were continued to make a full circle, its radius is the radius of the needle.

Diameter: It is the gauge or thickness of the needle. It is appreciable on cut section.

- Straight needles are used for working on the surface, while curved needles are used for working in depth. Working in a small space requires small sized needles.

Cutting Needles

They have sharp edges and on cut section they are triangular in shape. In curved cutting needle base of the triangle is on outer (convex) side of the needle, it may be on the inner side in some needles (reverse cutting type). Cutting needles are much traumatic and cut a track as they pass through the tissues.

Uses: They are used in tough or thick tissues, i.e., skin, rectus sheath and vaginal walls.

Round Bodied Needles

They have smooth edges and are round on cut section so they do not cut the tissue but only puncture it while passing through it. The hole made by them very easily closes afterwards.

Uses: They are used in soft and delicate tissues, i.e., peritoneum, fat, muscles, bladder fascia, fallopian tubes.

Eyeless Needles

There is no eye and catgut or other suture material is fused at its proximal end. This avoids double thickness of material which is present when it has been threaded through a needle eye. Almost any type and shape of needles are available as eyeless needles, i.e., atraumatic.

Uses: They are used for suturing of viscera, blood vessels, very small structures and in plastic surgery (e.g., tuboplasty).

- Mayo's suture needle is a very strong needle with a large square eye. There are two varieties-round bodied and trocar point. They are available as eyeless needles also. They are extensively used for suturing of the pedicles (hysterectomy operations).
- Blunt point needle is especially used for operation on HIV or HbsAg positive patients and in friable tissues.
- **Sterilization:** They are available as pre-sterilized. Nondisposable needles are resterilized by autoclaving after putting them in proper envelops. Cutting needles should be examined regularly for their sharpness and should be replaced by new ones when required.

CHAPTER 4

Obstetric Forceps and Vacuum Extractor

Obstetric forceps were invented by doctors of Chamberlen family in England during the 17th century. It was kept as a family secret for almost three generations. More than 600 types of forceps have been invented up till now.

SIMPLE CLASSIFICATION

- *Conventional traction forceps:*
  Short: Wrigley's, Simpson's short, Elliot.
  Long: Without axis traction, e.g.,
  - Simpson's long
  - Elliot's long
  - Das' forceps
  With axis traction, e.g.,
  - Milne-Murray's
  - Barnes-Neville's
  - Haigh-Ferguson's
- *Rotational forceps:*
  - Kielland
  - Moolgaoker
  - Barton
- *Special forceps:*
  - Piper's for after coming head of breech
  - Hale forceps for LSCS
  - New rubberized forceps (Greenberg.)

Only **short forceps** are used at present.

Description

All forceps have same fundamental components. Each has 2 metal branches called blades articulated by a lock.

Each blade consists of following parts:

BLADE PROPER

It is usually fenestrated but may be solid. Solid blade is better for rotation of head but it causes more compression and makes the instrument heavy, while forceps with fenestrated blades is light and is better for traction because it obtains good grip, only disadvantage of it is rare chance of inclusion of cord or fetal limb in the fenestra. Each blade has 2 curves.

Cephalic Curve

It is the curve on the flat. It fits over the fetal head. Its radius is 11.25 cm in Simpson's long forceps. Due to shallow cephalic curve Simpson's forceps is meant for molded fetal heads. While in Elliot type cephalic curve is more accentuated for unmolded head.

Pelvic Curve

It is the curve on the edge. It fits the curve of maternal pelvis. Its radius is 17.5 cm. It may be absent in some short forceps, i.e., Simpson's short forceps.

The blade which lies on the right side of maternal pelvis is called the **right blade** and that which lies on the left side is called the **left blade.** When articulated, the maximum distance between the 2 blades in a standard forceps is 8.5 cm while between their tips (Toes), it is 1.5 cm (Elliot short) to 3.5 cm (Simpson's long).

SHANK

It is the portion between the blade and the lock. It may be parallel or overlapping. It is 6.25 cm long in Simpson's long forceps.

Lock: Common types are as below:
- *English:* Double slot lock, a slot in each blade fitting with each other, the slot in the left blade faces anteriorly: (1) it is easy to lock, (2) causes less compression of head, and (3) one can readily relax the blades in between contractions.
- *French:* Pivot on left blade fitting with the notch in the right one.
- *German:* Combination of both types.

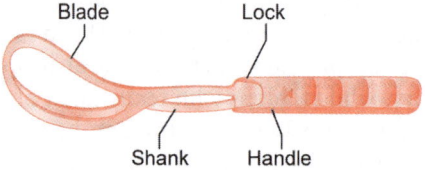

Fig. 4.1: Parts of forceps.

SLIDING LOCK-KIELLAND FORCEPS

Handle: It is a long metal rod, 12.5 cm long in Simpson's long forceps. It may have finger grips or rests which flare outside.

Fixation screw: When present, they are placed on the handles. It is for fixing and keeping the blades together during traction.

In addition some long forceps may have facility for axis traction mechanism, i.e., axis traction rods and traction handle.

Cephalic curve radius	– 11.25 cm
Pelvic curve radius	– 17.5 cm
Distance between 2 blades	
maximum	– 8.5 cm
minimum	– 1.5–3.5 cm
Shank	– 6.25 cm
Handle	– 12.5 cm

WRIGLEY'S FORCEPS

It is a simple and delicate instrument invented by Wrigley in 1935. It is a type of short forceps with total length of 27.5 cm. It is very light in weight, about one-third the weight of an ordinary long curved forceps. Handles and shank are short. Shank is only 2.5 cm long instead of usual 6.25 cm blades have got marked cephalic curve and slight pelvic curve. It is meant to apply on the head low in pelvis. It can be applied under minimum of anesthesia with ease. As it is not possible to exert strong traction with it, there are less chances of injury to mother or fetus.

TYPES OF FORCEPS OPERATION

American College of Obstetricians and Gynecologists (ACOG 1988, revised 2002) classified forceps application as follows:

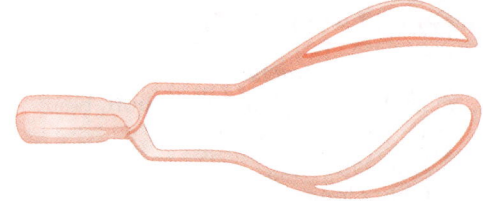

Fig. 4.2: Wrigley's forceps.

Outlet Forceps

- Scalp is visible at introitus without separating the labia.
- Fetal skull has reached the perineal floor.
- Sagittal suture in the anterior-posterior diameter or in the right or left occiput anterior or posterior position.
- Fetal head is at or on the perineum.
- Rotation does not exceed 45°.

Low Forceps

The leading point of the fetal skull is at station >/+ 2 cm and not on pelvic floor. Rotation are divided into 45° or less and more than 45° in anterior or posterior positions.

Midforceps

Station above +2 cm but head is engaged. Here the station is +3 or more.

High not included in classification.

Functions of Forceps

- **Traction:** It is the most important function. With each individual traction, average force required is usually 16–18 kg in weight for primigravida and 12–13 kg for parous patient.
- **Rotation:** Kielland forceps is best for the purpose but even simple long forceps may be used for rotation, i.e., by Scanzoni maneuver. Rotational forceps are NOT done in modern obstetrics due to lack of skill and training and high safety of cesarean section.
- **Compression:** Because forceps is a first type of lever with fulcrum in the middle, compression even if unwanted is unavoidable. Compression just enough to ensure a safe grip (to prevent slipping) is needed. When correctly applied only such is obtained.
- **Stimulation of uterine action:** Traction should be given only in the presence of uterine contraction. But in uterine inertia slight initial traction stimulates uterine contractions reflexly.

Indications

Fetal Indications

- Fetal distress in second stage of labor.
- Failure to progress in second stage of labor.
- Prolonged second stage of labor due to fetal cause like malrotation or large size fetus. More than 2 hours in primi and > 1 hr in parous patient is considered as prolonged (one hour extra is allowed in both if epidural is given for labor analgesia).
- Postmaturity—some cases.
- Cord prolapse with full dilatation of cervix (rarely).
- Aftercoming head of breech

Maternal Indications

- Prolonged second stage of labor due to rigid perineum, weak uterine action or pendulous abdomen.
- Inability to bear down due to frank exhaustion, excessive sedation, epidural analgesia.
- To give less strain to mother in certain medical and obstetric disorders.

Obstetric: Pregnancy induced hypertension, eclampsia.

Medical: Valvular heart disease, pulmonary tuberculosis and other lung diseases, acute or chronic liver diseases, acute or chronic kidney diseases, general debility, anemia, diabetes etc.

Others

- Prophylactic forceps (discussed later).
- Trial forceps in borderline CPD cases.
- To end successful trial of labor.
- Previous one LSCS–to give less strain to the scar.
- During cesarean section–outlet forceps or its one blade can be used to deliver the head.

Common indications: Fetal distress, prolonged second stage of labor and to give less strain to mother in certain medical and obstetric disorders.

Contraindications

- Incompletely dilated cervix
- Floating head
- Moderate or severe degree contracted pelvis
- Malpresentation—brow, face-mentoposterior
- Contraction ring dystocia
- Pelvic tumors.

Pre-requisites

- **The pelvis must be adequate.** There should not be cephalopelvic disproportion

(Forceps done in borderline CPD is trial forceps).
- **Cervix must be fully dilated (10 cm)** and fully effaced in between pains. Forceps in less than fully dilated cervix (1) cause injury to cervix, (2) can produce neurogenic shock, and (3) damage paracervical ligaments.
- **Membranes must be ruptured,** because (1) forceps might slip if applied on intact membranes, (2) sometimes rupture of membranes improves uterine contractions leading to normal delivery, and (3) unruptured membranes when pulled might detach the placenta.
- **Bladder should be empty,** because full bladder: (1) inhibit uterine contractions (2) may get injured during forceps delivery.
- **Head must be engaged,** preferably deeply engaged.
- **Presentation must be favorable,** i.e., vertex, face mentoanterior and aftercoming head of breech.
- Position must be precisely known.
- **Anesthesia must be adequate.**
  For outlet forceps—minimum perineal infiltration.
  For low forceps—minimum pudendal block.
  For mid forceps (or Kielland): S/A, E/A or G/A is required.
- Episiotomy at proper time should be given, although in multipara it is not must.
- Baby resuscitation facilities should be available.
- Operator must be properly trained in operative vaginal delivery.

Steps of Operation

- Consent
- Lithotomy position, painting and draping.
- Anesthesia—perineal infiltration or pudendal block is given.
- Evacuation of bladder by simple catheter.
- Pervaginal examination.
- One vein is kept patent (i.e., simple or oxytocin drip if indicated is started).
- Articulate blades in front of the patient, to decide right and left blades. Lubricate the blade before introduction, by dilute Savlon.
- Left blade is to be introduced first because of peculiarity of English lock (Slot in left blade faces anteriorly). It is held in left hand vertically, 2 fingers or whole of right hand is introduced in the vagina and posterior vaginal wall is depressed. Blade is introduced posteriorly in the hollow of the sacrum, pushing it by the thumb of right hand keeping flush contact with fetal head, till the blade becomes almost horizontal, then under guidance of internal fingers the blade is rotated to left side of the maternal pelvis.
- Hands are changed and right blade is introduced by holding it in right hand in the same manner, passing in front of the left blade.
- In occipito-anterior position after application **right blade** remains on **right side of maternal pelvis,** applied on **right parietal bone of fetus** and handle is in **right hand** of the **obstetrician.**
- Blades are depressed and then locked, if application is proper there should not be difficulty in locking.

Criteria for Proper Application

- Sagittal suture throughout its length should be perpendicular to the plane of the shanks.
- Lowermost part of the head should be within one inch reach from the shank OR the fenestration in advance of the head should not admit more than tip of one finger.
- Posterior fontanelle should not be more than one finger breadth away from the plane of the shank and should be equidistant from the side of the blades.
- **Traction:** It is given with following principles:
  1. Before starting traction criteria for proper application should be checked.

Easy application and easy locking usually suggests proper application.
2. Head is to be extracted slowly, and traction should be given during and up to the uterine contraction only.
3. In between traction separate the handles slightly, i.e., relax the blades, without actually unlocking them.
4. Traction should be given in axis of pelvis. For midforceps and low forceps first downward and backward, then horizontally downward, then downward and forward as occiput fixes under the symphysis pubis and lastly forward and upward to deliver the head by extension. For outlet forceps horizontally downward, downward and forward and then forward and upward.
   In practice this can be easily accomplished by giving traction posterior to direction of handles.
5. The operator should be in a comfortable position, with fixed forearms slightly below the level of delivery table. Ideally the power of elbow muscles of one hand only, is to be used. If both hands are used, the flexed elbow should not cross the waist line of the operator.
6. Placing of folded towel or finger in between shanks prevents undue compression of fetus.

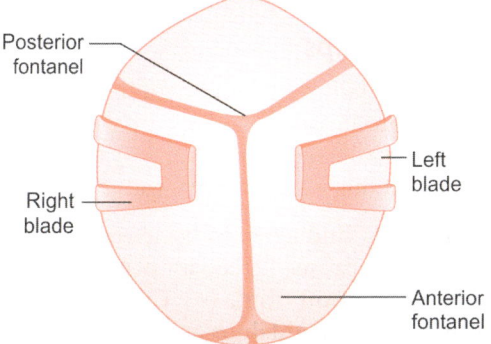

Fig. 4.3: Blades in relation to fetal head.

- Episiotomy is given before starting traction or after one or two pulls when perineum gets stretched (In outlet forceps it can be given before introduction of blades).
- As soon as the head is delivered, blades are removed first right and then left. Upper respiratory passages of the fetus are cleaned out. Suction is not must if liquor is clear.
- Placenta and membranes are delivered by controlled cord traction.
- Cervix is explored to check for tears if there is active bleeding.
- Episiotomy wound is sutured in layers.
- Outlet forceps are carried out in labor room, but mid and low forceps deliveries should be done in operation theater.

Complications

Maternal

1. **Injuries:**
   Birth canal:
   - Extension of episiotomy
   - Vaginal lacerations
   - Perineal tears
   - Paraurethral tears
   - Cervical tear, lacerations, rarely annular detachment
   - Rupture or laceration of lower uterine segment
   - Undue stretching of ligaments leading to prolapse in later life.

   Bowel: Injury to anal sphincter, anal canal or lower rectum, i.e., third or fourth degree perineal tear.

   Bladder: **Not common**—they were found with high forceps. But urethral injuries may occur.

   Bones: **Very rare** at present-fracture of coccyx, dislocation of sacrococcygeal joint, injury to symphysis pubis.

2. **Hemorrhage:** External (PPH)—traumatic, atonic or both.
   - *Internal:* Vulva or vaginal hematoma, broad ligament hematoma, intraperitoneal hemorrhage (uncommon).

3. **Infection:** If proper aseptic precautions are not observed, puerperal sepsis including thrombophlebitis of pelvic veins can occur.

4. **Obstetric shock:** Hypovolemic—if there is severe bleeding.
   - Neurogenic—if done on incompletely dilated cervix.
5. Anesthetic complications.

Fetal Complications

- Birth asphyxia—due to compression of brain or intracranial injuries.
- Intracranial hemorrhage—it can be subependymal, subdural or subarachnoid.
- Scalp injuries—lacerations, pressure necrosis.
- Cephalohematoma (blood collection under the periosteum)
- Linear or depressed fracture of skull bones (rare—occurs only when excessive force is used).

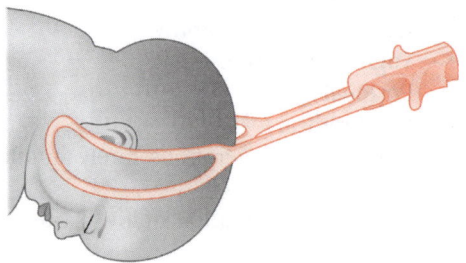

Fig. 4.4: True cephalic (biparietal, bimalar) application.

Axis Traction Forceps

Three types:
1. Milne–Murray's forceps—axis traction mechanism is at the heel of the fenestra.
2. Haig-Ferguson forceps—axis traction attachment is upon the shank.
3. Barnes–Neville's forceps—axis traction device is applied at the handle.

Advantages of Axis Traction

(1) Force-arm of the lever is lengthened so there is mechanical advantage-less force is required, (2) traction with axis traction happens to coincide with axis of pelvis so no force is wasted, and (3) rotation of head during its descent is not interfered with.

Axis traction is required when head is high in pelvis, so **not done** in modern obstetrics.

Trial Forceps

In case of borderline cephalopelvic disproportion (CPD), forceps attempted with full preparation ready for LSCS if it becomes necessary, is called "Trial forceps" (It is usually a midforceps operation). It is done as routine with normal force of traction. With 3 pulls if head does not descend even a little, the procedure is abandoned in favor of LSCS. With "Trial of forceps" many LSCS have been prevented, at the same time traumatic and failed forceps are also avoided.

Prophylactic Forceps

The concept of prophylactic forceps was introduced by De Lee in 1920. It is always a low forceps delivery and it is used to shorten the second stage of labor when maternal and fetal complications are anticipated. Common indications of it are—very painful second stage of labor, heart disease, eclampsia, severe pre-eclampsia, postcesarean section labor, patient under epidural analgesia. It reduces injury to fetal head as there is no sudden release of pressure on the fetal head. It also prevents perineal muscle relaxation and laceration. And lastly it has greatly reduced the apprehension of birth.

Failed Forceps

It may be failure in application or failure in traction. It usually means a vigorous but unsuccessful attempt of delivery by forceps. It is very traumatic experience for all concerned.

Causes: (1) Undiagnosed occipitoposterior-commonest causes, (2) cervix not fully dilated, (3) constriction ring, (4) Cephalopelvic disproportion, (5) Malpresentation, i.e., brow, and (6) soft tissue obstruction-lower segment fibroid, ovarian tumor.

For failure in application treatment consists of removal of the blades and reassessment of the case. Reapplication may be done once if everything is normal. For failure in traction no further attempt should be done and LSCS is safer alternative.

Forceps in Abnormal Presentation

Occipito-posterior

Forceps rotation is described later on. Here it means face to pubis forceps delivery. Forceps bladers are applied as routine. Horizontal traction should be applied until the root of the nose is under the symphysis. Then forward pull is given to deliver the vertex and occiput by flexion and finally backward pull to deliver the face by extension. Generous episiotomy is a must.

Face Presentation

Presentation must be mentoanterior with chin completely rotated to the front and there should be no disproportion. Forceps is applied as in vertex anterior position. The handles should be kept some what forward so that blades remain in occipito-mental diameter. First downward and backward pull is given, this will extend the face fully till chin comes well below the symphysis pubis. Then handles are lifted upwards and delivery is completed by flexion.

Aftercoming Head of Breech

Long forceps is used. **Piper's forceps** with long shanks having perineal curve ("S" shape) is especially designed for this. Forceps is applied from the ventral aspect of the fetus. At first the child is allowed to hang unsupported so that its head descends down until occiput lies up against the back of the symphysis pubis. Assistant should hold the trunk upwards. Forceps are applied as routine first left blade and then right blade from beneath the trunk. Traction is given first downwards and backwards till the chin appears. Then, it is carried forward and upward to deliver the head by flexion.

Advantages of forceps for aftercoming head of breech:
(1) Controlled delivery of head is done, (2) flexion is maintained, (3) traction is directly applied over the fetal head contrary to other manual methods where it is applied via the vertebral column, and (4) baby can take respiration.

It is also the most reliable method, but due to lack or experience and required skill it is not commonly done.

Kielland Forceps

It is long rotational forceps with overlapping shanks. It has sliding lock for correction of asynclitism of fetal head. There are **small knobs** (buttons) over the handles. Slight pelvic curve of the blades is on the side of knobs. The blades are 15 cm long, 4 cm broad and slightly thicker than usual forceps with beveled edges. The **blades are anterior and posterior** rather than left and right. It is decided by articulating the forceps in front of the patient, keeping knobs on the side of occiput, the blade remaining anterior is anterior blade. The objective of Kielland's forceps was a biparietal application to the fetal head in any position.

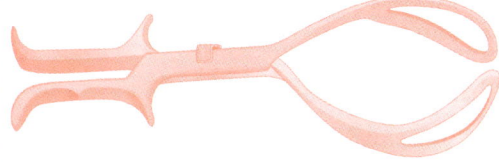

Fig. 4.5: Kielland forceps.

Indications: (1) deep transverse arrest, (2) persistent occipito-posterior.

Method: Anterior blade is always introduced first. There are three methods for it.
1. *Wandering method:* Most frequently used. Blade is introduced laterally over the face side or posteriorly in the hollow of sacrum and then wandered over the face side to bring it anteriorly.

2. *Direct method:* Used when head is very low in the pelvis or very small. Blade is introduced directly anteriorly and correctly over the fetal head.
3. *Classical or inversion method:* Obsolete.

In any of the above method posterior blade is applied directly posteriorly.
- Blades are articulated by sliding lock. Asynclitism is corrected.
- Generous episiotomy is must.
- Rotation is done in relaxation phase while traction is given during uterine contractions.

Risk: If injudiciously used it can cause injury to lower uterine segment, cervical tears, injuries at vaginal vault and spiral tears of vagina.

THE VACUUM EXTRACTOR (VENTOUSE)

It was introduced by **Malmstrom's** in 1954.

Original unit consisted of **suction cups** (made of steel, in 4 sizes 30, 40, 50 and 60 mm diameter with 20 mm depth), **traction chain** (metal chain from the metal plate to traction bar), **traction bar** (handle with lockpin) connected by rubber tube to **vacuum flask** (glass bottle with a rubber stopper) and vacuum pump.

Bird's Modifications

Bird modified the original Malmstrom cup by making the traction chain and vacuum tube separate. While traction chain is still kept in the center, vacuum tube is placed eccentrically in Bird's anterior cup (used for occipito-anterior position) and shifted to the side wall of the cup in Bird's posterior cup (used for occipito-transverse and occipito-posterior positions).

Silastic cup was introduced by Kobayashi in 1973. It is now commonly used instead of metal cups, because flexibility and cone shape further simplifies the use of ventouse. The cup is available in 2 sizes 60 mm and 65 mm. The cup is attached to about 20 cm long plastic shaft which is perpendicular to the axis of the cup and with the handle at the end. Silastic cup is reusable after chemical sterilization.

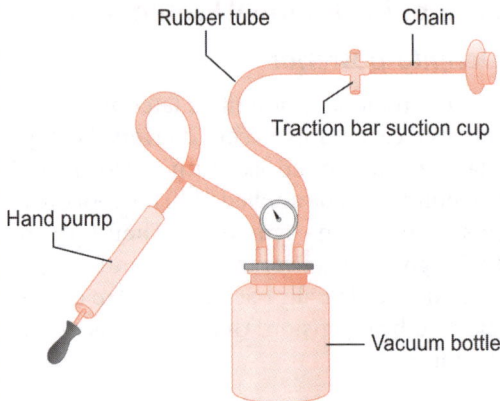

Fig. 4.6: Vacuum extractor.

Mityvac vacuum assisted delivery system comprises of hand operated vacuum pump which is reusable pump and different plastic cups (from 50 to 70 mm diameter) for use in vaginal delivery as well as cesarean section. M style mushroom cup of 50 mm diameter is commonly used. Ideally the cup is disposable.

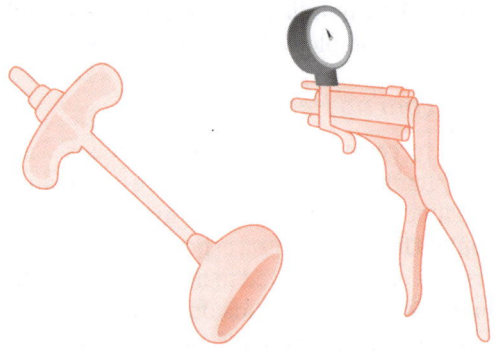

Fig. 4.7: Mityvac vacuum.

Kiwi Omni is another complete vacuum delivery system with hand operated pump. There is ease of insertion due to low profile cup and flexible stem leads to application over the flexion point of fetal head. Traction force indicator in the system measures the force exerted during traction. Like Mityvac cup it is to be disposed after single use.

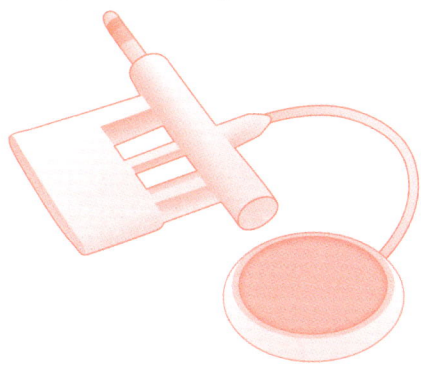

Fig. 4.8: Kiwi Omni.

Odon device is a new device which was developed by Jorge Odon from Argentina for instrumental vaginal delivery. It is permitted for clinical trial by WHO. It is low cost device and claimed to be safer and easier to apply than forceps or vacuum. It consists of plastic sleeve that is inflated around the baby's head and used to gently pull it out. Results of initial clinical trials are encouraging.

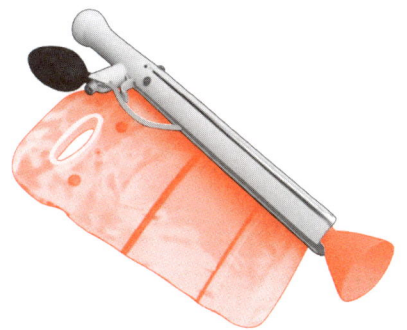

Fig. 4.9: Odon device.

Indications

Maternal

- Prolonged second stage of labor due to rigid perineum, frank exhaustion, excessive sedation, epidural analgesia, etc.
- To give less strain to the mother in conditions like PIH, cardiac disease, lung disease, previous LSCS or maternal distress due to any cause.
- To end successful trial of labor.

Fetal

- Prolonged 2nd stage of labor.
- Occipito-posterior position.
- Fetal distress in 2nd stage of labor (parous patient)
- At cesarean section.
  Rarely, it is useful to deliver second baby of twin (high cephalic).

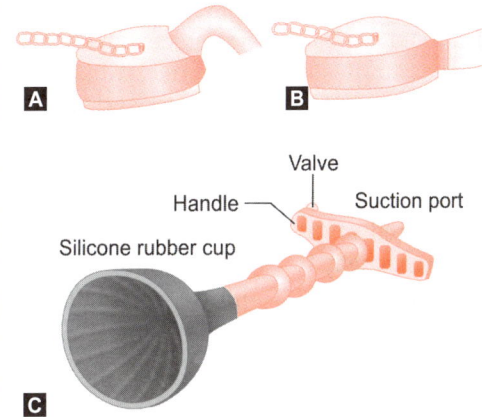

Figs. 4.10A to C: (A) Bird's anterior cup; (B) Bird's posterior cup; (C) Kobayashi silastic cup.

Contraindications

All those described under forceps + face presentation, breech presentation (i.e., aftercoming head), congenital fetal head anomalies, prior fetal scalp trauma (scalp 34 wks blood sampling, scalp electrodes), prematurity,

Intrauterine death, large caput, general anesthesia and severe fetal distress are relative contraindications.

Prerequisites

- Same as those for forceps.
- Presence of uterine contractions is helpful but not essential.

Steps of Operation

- Consent, lithotomy position, aseptic precautions, emptying of bladder
- L/A, i.e., perineal infiltration or pudendal block depending upon the station of fetal head.
- Per-vaginal examination.
- 5 and 6 cm metal cups were are used. 6 to 6.5 cm silastic cups have now replaced metal cups.
- Vacuum flask is prechecked for leaking.
- Cup is introduced inside the vagina after depressing the perineum. Cup should be applied as near the occiput as possible, to maintain flexion. In practice, it happens to be applied to the most dependent and accessible part of the scalp.
- Check before creating vacuum that the cervical lip or vaginal wall is not included in the cup. Create vacuum 0.2 kg/cm slowly in 2 minutes initially. After checking correct application vacuum is then created rapidly to the required level of 0.8 kg/cm.

Principles of Traction

- Before starting see that sufficient pressure is created. Check again that maternal soft tissues are not included in the cup.
- Traction is given during uterine contractions only. There is no difference in outcome whether traction is maintained in between contractions or not.
- Traction is given perpendicular to the cup.
- Traction should be given in pelvic axis to get maximum advantage.
  It is difficult to practice both, points 3 and 4 simultaneously, so 10° off-center traction may be given.
  >10° direction will lead to leakage of vacuum and slipping of cup.
- With the left forefinger and thumb the cup (upper part) is pressed backward over the fetal head during traction.
- Episiotomy is given when the head is bulging the perineum.

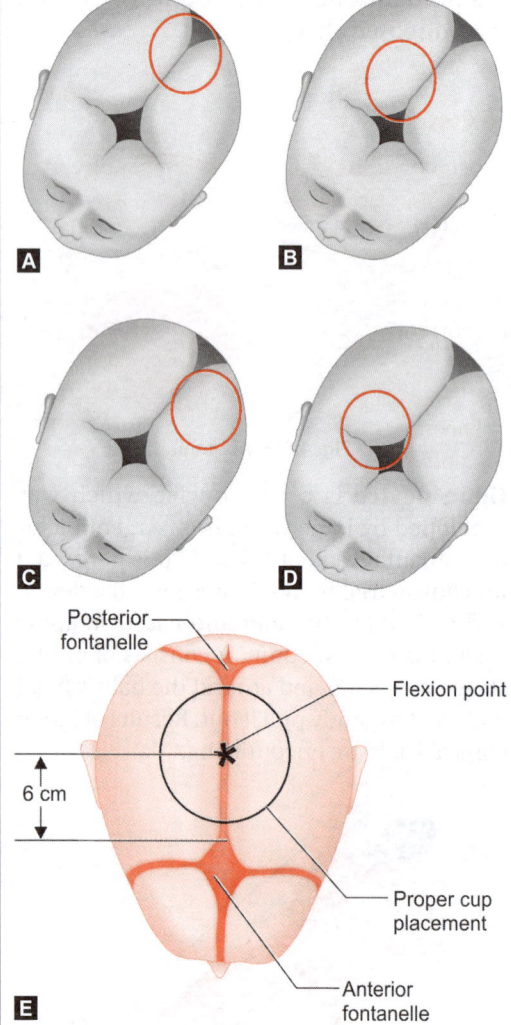

Figs. 4.11A to E: (A) Flexing median; (B) Deflexing median; (C) Flexing paramedian; (D) Deflexing paramedian; (E) Flexion point.

- Safety rules as suggested by bird should be observed:
  - Head should be delivered in not more than 3 pulls. With first pull head and not just the scalp must begin to move. By second pull the head must be on the pelvic floor. The head must be completely or almost completely delivered by the third pull.
  - The cup should not be applied more than twice in one patient.

- Applications—delivery interval should not exceed 20 minutes (except in dead fetus).

Complications

If correctly performed, they are minimal.

Maternal

They are comparable to spontaneous vaginal delivery. Injury to cervix, vagina or perineum if incorrectly used.

Fetal

- Laceration, abrasion or necrosis of scalp
- Cephalohematoma
- Intracranial hemorrhage
- Subaponeurotic hemorrhage
- Hyperbilirubinemia
- Alopecia
- Retinal or subconjunctival hemorrhage
- Depressed fractures of skull.

Advantages of Vacuum Extractor Over Forceps

- Easy to use
- Much less increase in intracranial pressure during traction
- Does not interfere with internal rotation of head (autorotation)
- No trauma to maternal soft tissues if correctly applied
- Minimum anesthesia is required
- Safety factor, because at some pressure (20 kg) vacuum will break and cup will pop off.
- Ability to rotate fetal head without the instrument impinging upon the maternal soft tissues.

Failure

Failure rate varies from 4% to 27% in different studies reported.

Causes of Failure

- **Faults in the instrument:** Leak in the instrument, pump not working properly, loose traction chain.
- **Faults in the technique:** Wrong size of the cup, deflexing and paramedian application, wrong direction of pull, pulling too hard or too less, vacuum pressure too low, cervix or vaginal walls trapped in the cup.
- **Adverse obstetric factors:** Disproportion, brow presentation, very large caput.

Important

- If advancement is not evident after 2 pulls stop the procedure and reevaluate the case.
- If cervix or vagina is included, hissing leak will be heard when traction is applied.
- **Application distance:** As by bird the distance between the leading edge of the cup and the anterior fontanelle is called the application distance. For **flexing** application it should be ≥ 3 cm.

    It the center of the cup is situated more than 1 cm to either side of the sagittal suture the application is described as **paramedian.**
- For flexing application the center of the cup should overlie the flexion point. **Flexion point** (or **pivotal point**) lies 6 cm from anterior fontanelle on sagittal suture.

    Both above points implies the same thing.

    Deflexing and paramedian application lead to failure as mentioned earlier.
- It allows the head to come the way it wants to, even sometimes face to pubis, (i.e., posterior rotation).
- Artificial caput produced by vacuum is called **Chignon.**
- Sequential delivery (first apply vacuum and then forceps) is not advocated due to bad results.
- As per recent Cochrane database of systematic review (2010) which included 32 studies involving 6597 women, forceps produced more maternal trauma than vacuum while vacuum (metal cup) caused more newborn scalp injury and cephalohematoma than forceps.

CHAPTER 5

Contraception

METHODS OF CONTRACEPTION

Contraception method of two types:
A. Temporary, B. Permanent

Temporary Contraception

- **Natural family planning methods**:
  - Total abstinence
  - *Coitus interruptus*: During sexual intercourse (coitus) penis is withdrawn from vagina just before ejaculation.
  - *Lactational amenorrhea method (LAM)*: Criteria for this method include
    - Exclusive breastfeeding
    - Menstruation has not started
    - Up to 6 months postpartum

    It is effective in preventing pregnancy by 98%.
  - Methods based on fertility awareness:
    - Calendar or rhythm method: Record the number of days for previous six menstrual cycles. Subtract 18 from the length of her shortest cycle. This is first day of her fertile period. Then subtract 11 days from the length of her longest cycle. This is the last day of her fertile period. Sexual intercourse is avoided during this period.
    - Basal body temperature method (BBT): Daily morning temperature is recorded before getting up from the bed. With ovulation temperature rises to 0.4°F or more due to progesterone effect. Fertile period ends three days after the temperature rise. In this method preovulatory safe period is not detected. Couple has to abstain from intercourse for a longer period, i.e. onset of menses to end of fertile period.
    - Cervical mucous (billings method): Here the fertile period starts from the first day of any cervical secretions or feeling of vaginal wetness until the 4th day after the peak day of slippery secretions. Its typical use failure rate is up to 22%.
    - Symptothermal method: At least 2 indicators are used to identify fertile period, i.e. BBT+ Cervical mucous or BBT + calendar rhythm for calculating fertile period.
    - High tech hormonal monitoring: Here small electronic devices detect urinary metabolites of LH and estrogen, estrone-3-glucuronide (E_3G). Threshold level of estrogen determines the beginning of the fertile period and 4 days past a threshold level of LH marks the end of fertile period. "Persona" is such personal device with test strips. The

strips are daily dipped into urine and then fed into the monitor. A green light displayed on the device means a woman is not fertile, a red light indicates that a woman is at or near ovulation and woman should then abstain from intercourse. It is 94% reliable.
- **Barrier contraceptives:**
  - *Mechanical*:
    - Male: Condom
    - Female: Female condom, diaphragm, Cervical cap, dumas cap, etc.
  - Chemical: Spermicidal substances in the form of foam tablets, creams, jellies, suppositories.
  - Combined: Mechanical + chemical.
- Intrauterine contraceptive devices (IUCD): TCu 380A, multiload 250/375, Mirena, etc.
- Steroidal contraceptives: Oral contraceptives (OCs), injectables, implants, vaginal rings, skin patch.
- Emergency contraception: Postcoital contraception.
- Uterotubal junction devices – Silastic or ceramic plugs, Essure coils.
- Miscellaneous: Male pill - gossypol immunological (under research).

Permanent Contraception

- Male: Vasectomy operation.
- Female: Different sterilization operations (See Chapter 9)

Commonly used temporary methods are discussed.

BARRIER CONTRACEPTIVES

They are especially suitable for the following couples:
- Those who have contraindications to OCs and IUCDs
- Those who cannot tolerate OCs and IUCDs
- Those who have intercourse infrequently
- Those who take a break, for a period of time from OCs and IUCDs
- Those who are sexually active with a number of partners
- Those who for personal reasons prefer not to use OCs or IUCDs.

CONDOM

It is male barrier contraceptive. The origin of word "Condom" is believed to have come from the latin word "Condom" meaning a receptacle. Its invention is also attributed to physician Dr Condom who recommended it to King Charles II to prevent illegal offsprings. It is made up of fine latex material and is disposable one. Thick rubber washable (reusable) condoms, used in past, are now outdated. The natural (animal) membrane (lambskin) condoms are also rarely used. They are costly and as they contain tiny pores transmission of HIV and other STIs is not prevented unlike other condoms.

Latex condoms are available in different sizes from 160–180 mm length, 49–52 mm in flat width and thickness varying from 0.04 to 0.07 mm. It may be plain or there is teat at the tip for collection of semen during ejaculation. It is available in different colors and also as flavored condoms, warming condoms, glow in the dark condoms, etc. It is always checked by manufacturer for tear or leaks, so there is no need for retesting by the user. It can be prelubricated type, e.g. Deluxe Nirodh, Durex, Kamasutra or spermicidal ones, e.g. Rakshak, Share. According to WHO spermicidally lubricated condoms should no longer be promoted.

Method of Use

- It should be applied on erect penis and prelubricated one is preferred.
- If there is no teat, some space pressed empty of air, is left at the end.
- During sexual act, after ejaculation is over one should be sure that condom does not get dislodged from the penis, i.e. penis should be withdrawn while still erect and

condom should be held firmly at the root of the penis by fingers.
- Chemical contraceptive (spermicidally jelly) used along with it gives extra protection and lubrication.
- Do not use oil based lubricants with condom, it might break the condom.
- Store condoms in a cool, dark place. Heat, light and humidity damage condoms.
- Handle condoms carefully. Fingernails and rings can tear them.
- Do not unroll condoms before use. This may weaken them. Also, an unrolled condom is difficult to put on.
- Check the condom for tear before throwing it away and if it has torn, use one of the emergency contraceptive methods.
- Do not reuse the condom. Do not use double condoms.

New polyurethane condoms are nonlatex condoms available as "Avanti, on", etc. Polyurethane is resistant to deterioration. They are thinner, stronger and less elastic than latex. It is useful for those who are sensitive or allergic to latex. Tactylon is a new condom made up of synthetic material styrene ethylene butylene styrene (SEBS). Polyisoprene condoms (SKYN) are also new nonlatex condoms. As compared to polyurethane condoms they are softer, stretchier and more resistant to breakage.

The newer condoms are claimed to have less odor, fit more comfortably and are less constricting. However, they brake or slip more often during intercourse than latex condoms yet the failure rate is almost same.

Advantages

- Easy to use
- Relatively cheap
- Freely available without medical supervision prescription
- Failure rate is low as compared to physiological and chemical methods
- Protects against common vaginal infections, i.e. trichomoniasis and moniliasis as well as sexually transmitted diseases like syphilis, gonorrhea, nongonoccocal urethritis, chlamydia, herpes virus, human papilloma virus, hepatitis B virus and human immunodeficiency virus (HIV) infection.
- Protects against Ca cervix. Because Ca cervix is caused by highly oncogenic strains (e.g. 16, 18) of human papilloma virus which is sexually transmitted.
- Safe. No hormonal side effects.
- Can be used at any age.
- Often helps in preventing premature ejaculation.
- Can be used where pills and IUCD are contraindicated, i.e. follow-up of vesicular mole, diabetes, valvular heart disease.

Disadvantages

- Failure rate is high as compared to IUCD and pills.
- Because it prevents full genital contact, it may decrease sensation making sex less enjoyable for either partner.
- Couple require some time to put the condom on the erect penis before sex. It must be readily available.
- In male partner rarely it causes psychological disturbances and even impotence.
- Disposal is a social problem. It may embarrass some couples to buy condoms.
- Hypersensitivity reaction to either of the partners.

Failure rate: 3–18/100 women years observation (3–8/HWY if used with chemical contraceptive). It is known as **Pearl index.**

Pearl Index

The **Pearl index** is defined as the number of contraceptive failures per 100 women-years of exposure so the formula would be:

Pearl index

$$= \frac{\text{No. of Pregnancies} \times 12}{\text{No. of women} \times \text{No. of months}} \times 100$$

There are two types of failure rates described.
1. **Typical use failure rate:** Failure rate occurring with that contraceptive method used in real life scenario. It takes into account human error.
2. **Perfect use failure rate**: Failure rate occurring with correct and consistent use of that contraceptive method. It happens in clinical trial.

Usually the typical use failure rate for any contraceptive method is higher than perfect use failure rate except LARC (long acting reversible contraception) methods.

Causes of Failure

- Incorrect use
- Inconsistent use. Not used with each sexual act, e.g. patient under effect of alcohol
- Defect in condom
- Used without chemical contraceptive
- Tearing or bursting of condom during sexual act (4%).

Other Uses of Condom

- In **transvaginal sonography:** It is applied over the vaginal probe to prevent cross infection
- In obstetrics condom is used to create **condom balloon tamponade** in treatment of **atonic PPH.** It is done aseptically by tying condom to simple rubber catheter or Foley's catheter, passing it into the uterine cavity and inflating it by 250–500 mL normal saline as per need. It is kept for 12–24 hours and then gradually deflated at convenient hour.
- For preparation of **mould for vaginoplasty.**
- Immunological cervical factor in infertility. Husband should use it for 3 to 6 months so that antibody level against the sperms in cervical mucous decreases. Then chances of pregnancy might increase.
- Threatened abortion: After 4 to 6 weeks if couple resumes sexual relations, male partner should use condom, because semen contains prostaglandins which may cause abortion.

Female Condom (Fem Shield)

It is a female barrier contraceptive. It has combined features of diaphragm and condom. It consists of two flexible polyurethane rings located at the either end of a 15 cm soft loose fitting polyurethane sheath. The inner ring is placed high in vagina, while outer ring covers the labia and base of penis. It is prelubricated with silicone based lubricant. It is available with different names, e.g. Reality, Femidom, Femshield. New FC2 female condom is made from synthetic nitrile, which is softer than polyurethane (FC1) and less costly.

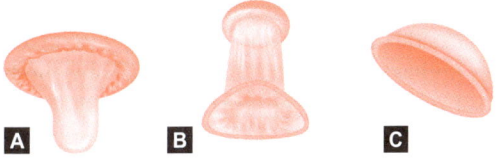

Figs. 5.1A to C: (A) Male condom; (B) Female condom; (C) Diaphragm.

Advantages

- Controlled by woman
- It prevents STDs more effectively than condom as it covers some perineal area also.
- No allergic reactions as it is made up of polyurethane.
- More convenient than male condom as it can be inserted precoitus.
- Less chances of breakage.

Disadvantages

- Expensive.
- Some women have difficulties in insertion.

It is meant for single time use however WHO recommends reuse for maximum 5 times with proper care for disinfection, washing and drying. Its perfect use failure rate is 5% while typical use failure rate is 21%.

VAGINAL DIAPHRAGM (DUTCH CAP)

It is female barrier contraceptive. It is saucer shaped device made up of latex or silicone with flexible metal spring in its rim. Spring can be of different types, i.e. arcing spring coil spring or flat spring. It is available in 5-10 cm diameters with 2.5-5 mm increments. Its rim fits firmly across the vagina from upper end in the posterior fornix to lower end at the back of symphysis pubis (at least one finger breadth above external urinary meatus). Its typical use failure rate is 12%.

Method of Use

Patient should be able to feel her cervix by self-examination. Spermicidal jelly is smeared on both sides of diaphragm and some jelly is taken in hollow. It also lubricates the instrument. It is inserted before the sexual act in a squatting position or sitting at the edge of the table. Before use check for its intactness by filling it with clean water. Diaphragm is compressed between fingers and thumb, introduced in A-P diameter and upper end is pushed by index finger high up in posterior fornix. It should be kept for minimum 6 hours after sexual act. It remains in position by tension of the spring and elasticity of vaginal wall.
- Douching is unnecessary but if it is done it should be done before the diaphragm is removed.
- Refitting is advisable after pelvic surgery, delivery, annually or after rapid and large alterations in weight (10 kg or more).
- Changed yearly as wear and tear process may occur.

Contraindications

These include uterine or vaginal wall prolapse. Severe retroversion, local infection and allergy to rubber.

Failure rate: 4-12/100 women years.

Failure can be due to wrong size, improper insertion, lack of spermicidal jelly, defect in the diaphragm or displacement during coitus.

Advantages

- Relatively cheap.
- Effective as compared to physiological and chemical methods.
- Used by female so cooperation of male partner is not required.
- It does not interfere with natural coitus or orgasm of either of the partners.
- It also gives some protection against PID.

Disadvantages

- In sensitive patients it may cause embarrassment and some women may consider diaphragm unesthetic. Use of spermicide is messy.
- Failure rate is high as compared to IUCD and pills.
- High degree of motivation of the patient is required for its use.
- Allergic reactions to rubber may occur.
- Vaginitis, UTI and rarely toxic shock syndrome are reported.

Preservation: After use wash it with mild soap and warm water, then it is kept in its container or wrapped in clean cloth.

Other female barrier contraceptives are cervical cap, dumas cap (Vault cap), vimule cap. Contra cap is cervical cap with one way valve, which is said to permit the passage of cervical secretions and menstrual fluid down in the vagina but not sperms upwards.

Today

Today is vaginal contraceptive sponge containing 100 mg of Nonoxynol-9. It is effective for 24 hours. It is made wet with clean water before insertion. One should wait for 6 hours after last intercourse before removing the sponge. Sponge should not be kept in vagina for > 30 hours. One should not reuse the sponge. Today is also available as small pessary form containing Nonxynol-9.

Nonoxynol has bactericidal and virucidal activity, however it does not effectively prevent HIV infection or other STIs. Usually, there are no major side effects. It may produce allergic type reactions and vaginal or penile irritation. Patient may have vaginal discomfort like soreness, itching, stinging. Rarely toxic shock syndrome can occur.

INTRAUTERINE CONTRACEPTIVE DEVICES (IUCD)

Grafenberg's ring, a silver coiled wire ring was the first popular IUCD widely used in the past. It was introduced by Grafenberg of Germany in 1929. Since then many different types of devices are invented. They are divided into two groups: **first generation** or inert or unmedicated devices, e.g. Lippes loop, Saf-T-coil, **second generation** or bioactive or medicated devices containing metals like copper (Cu-T, Cu-7,) zinc, silver or containing hormones, e.g. Mirena, Progestasert.

Hormone containing IUCDs are also called as **third generation** IUCDs.

Various IUCDs were used in past, e.g. Grafenberg's ring, Chinese ring, Ota ring, Birnberg bow, Margulies coil, soonawala loop, Saf-t-coil, Dalkon shield, Hall-stone ring, Antigon-F, Dana super.

Copper-T was invented by Howard Tatum (USA) and Jaime Zipper (Chile).

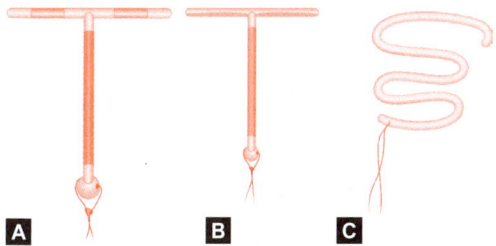

Figs. 5.2A to C: (A) T Cu 380 A; (B) Cu-T 200; (C) Lippes loop.

TCu 380A

TCu 380A is a T-shaped IUCD made from low density polyethylene with barium sulfate added for X-ray opacity. The device is 32 mm wide and 36 mm long with plastic ball at the bottom of vertical stem to prevent cervical penetration. Copper wire (surface area 310 mm^2) is wound tightly around the vertical stem. There are 2 solid copper sleeves on transverse arms. (each has surface area 35 mm^2). Thus total surface area is 380 mm^2. It has 2 monofilament polyethylene white threads tied through a hole in the ball at lower end. The diameter of vertical stem is 1.5 mm and that of horizontal arm is 1.6 mm. Its applicator, made up of synthetic plastic consists of cannula with guard and a plunger rod. Guard is blue and mobile. Cu-T along with its applicator is supplied in a plastic pack presterilized by gamma radiation.

Specifications:
- Length - 36 mm
- Width - 32 mm
- Weight - 310 mg
- Surface area of copper - 380 sq mm
- Diameter - 0.25 mm

The Cu-T 380S (slim line) has the copper wire on vertical stem as usual but copper sleeves are the ends of horizontal arms (as against middle of each arm in 380A) embedded into the arms. In TCu-380 Ag (silver line) copper wire on the vertical stem has a silver core. The silver core prevents fragmentation of copper and lengthens the effective life of the device.

Copper T (Cu-T 200)

Previously Cu-T 200 was used. Its dimensions are same as Cu-T 380, but it has only copper wire on vertical stem (surface area 200 mm^2) and no copper sleeves on transverse arms. Cu-T 200 B has a small ball at its lower end.

Lippes Loop

It was serpentine device made up of polyethylene or polypropylene. It was barium sulfate impregnated device. It was available in 4 sizes: A, B, C, and D with difference in length, width, and color of 2 nylon threads. Its guard was white and fixed. With Cu-T available since decades lippes loop is not used or available now.

Time of Insertion

- During menstrual period from 2nd day onwards or within 10 days of menstruation. (During menses it is easy to insert and bleeding related to insertion is masked). It can be inserted even after 10 days if patient is sure of not pregnant.
- Immediately after first trimester MTP or spontaneous abortion or within 7 days.
- Postpartum
  - Postplacental
  - Within 48 hours
  - After 4 weeks

  Postplacental insertion is done within 10 minutes of placental delivery vaginally (If required by using long sponge holding forceps). At cesarean section it is inserted manually before the uterus is closed. Long nylon threads are passed down the cervical canal in the vagina and cut short in follow-up.
- Postcoital - within 5 days of unprotected intercourse in a fertile period, i.e. as emergency contraception.

Life Span

- Cu-T 380A is for 10 years. Its effectively decreases afterwards.
- There is no time limit for non-medicated device, i.e. loop. It can remain for several years without causing any harm.

Contraindications

Absolute
As per WHO Medical Eligibility Criteria (discussed under steroidal contraceptives) 2015 following conditions are **category 4** for copper IUDS:

- Suspected pregnancy.
- Postabortal or puerperal sepsis.
- Unexplained abnormal vaginal bleeding.
- Cervical or uterine cancer
- STI
- Pelvic tuberculosis.
- Uterine abnormalities
- H/O pelvic infection in past 3 months.

Category 3
- Postpartum between 48 hours and 4 weeks.
- Benign gestational trophoblastic disease
- Ovarian cancer.
- AIDS.

Method of Insertion

- Patient is explained about the type, principles, side effects and failure rate, etc. of the device.
- Informed consent is taken.
- Detailed history is elicited and complete pelvic examination is done to rule out contraindications.
- Full aseptic and antiseptic precautions are observed.
- Sounding is done to know the direction and the length of utero-cervical canal.

For TCu380A Withdrawal Technique

Loaded applicator is introduced with guard adjusted at the total utero-cervical length of that patient, so that when the guard is at external OS, tip of the applicator with Cu-T is at fundus. Now plunger is fixed by one hand and cannula is withdrawn over it, so Cu-T is released high up at fundus without being pushed. Then plunger is withdrawn, cannula is withdrawn and threads are cut for 2-3 cm from external so that patient can easily feel it by self-examination.

Method of Removal

Per-speculum examination is done, threads are visualized, caught by any simple instrument, i.e. artery forceps and the device is pulled out. It should be checked for its intactness.

Contraception

Advice to the patient
- Patient is taught to feel the thread by self-examination and should regularly check the thread and particularly after the first menstrual period.
- She is informed about possible initial reactions increased bleeding, pain for first 2–3 months, etc. They are treated symptomatically. They gradually disappear with time.
- She should come for follow-up after first menstrual period and then yearly.
- She should consult the doctor immediately if she misses a period, it she develops any complications, or if she does not feel the thread.
- The device should be replaced, when time limit is over.

Mechanism of Action

Exact mechanism of action for Cu-T is not yet established. It works primarily by preventing fertilization.
- Presence of device with its nylon thread causes mechanical obstruction to ascent of sperms.
- Nylon threads cause changes in the cervical mucous and make it hostile to sperms.
- IgM levels in serum is increased so antifertility action is in part to their ability to produce antibodies.
- Actions of copper:
  - Directly damages sperms and fertilized ovum.
  - Biochemical changes in cervical mucous and renders it hostile. Sperm motility and capacitation are affected.
  - Changes in the endometrium: (1) enzymatic inhibition, i.e. carbonic anhydrase (copper replaces zinc), alkaline phosphatase, glycogen synthase, etc., (2) intense leukocytic infiltration, (3) changes in DNA constituent of endometrial cells, (4) decrease in glycogen content of cells, (5) increase in fibrinolytic activity of endometrium, and (6) endometrial vasoconstriction and ischemic damage.
- Increase in tubal motility so fertilized ovum, before it is mature enough for implantation, reaches the uterus which is also unprepared.
- Increase in uterine contractions which result in expulsion of newly implanted ovum.
- Device causes low-grade tissue reaction (i.e. inflammatory) in the endometrium making it unreceptable for implantation. It attracts macrophages which engulf the sperms as well as fertilized ovum by phagocytosis.

Indications for Removal of Cu-T
- If patient develops complications
- Time is over
- Patient has entered in menopause
- Displaced device
- Patient wants to become pregnant
- Failure - pregnancy
- Sterilization operation of patient or her husband

Failure rate: Both typical use failure rate and perfect use failure rate is < 1%.

Side-effects and Complications
- Menstrual problems: Spotting, heavy periods and prolonged periods frequently occur in first 2–3 months
- Cramps like pain in lower abdomen. Removal due to excessive bleeding and pain occurs in 5–15/100 users
- Dysmenorrhea: Spasmodic type, with infection there can be congestive type also
- Leukorrhea
- Pelvic infection: Risk is more in first month of insertion. It occurs if IUD is inserted without proper aseptic precautions or it is inserted in presence of an undiagnosed pelvic infections. If may also develop later in women at risk of STIs. If infection is diagnosed treat it with proper antibiotics.

There is no need to remove IUD if woman wishes to continue its use.
- Displacement - Device may penetrate the uterine wall or cause perforation of uterus and migrate into pelvis or upper abdomen. Perforation commonly occurs at the time of insertion. Common sites of perforation are fundal and isthmic region. Incidence of perforations is 1 to 3 per 1000 insertions.
- Spontaneous expulsion - During first menstrual period or within the first year of insertion. Women who had dysmenorrhea or heavy menstrual flows are more likely to expel IUDS. The rate is 5–15/1000 insertions.
- Failure, i.e. pregnancy (discussed later).
- Ectopic pregnancy: 3–4% of pregnancies with IUCDs are ectopic, but as the failure rate is very low, overall there is protection against ectopic pregnancy as compared to no contraception used.
- Fracture or breaking of IUCD and embedding in the endometrium resulting in decreased efficacy and difficulty in removal.
- Rarely fainting and collapse at the time of insertion if patient is not properly motivated.

Advantages of IUCD over Other Methods

- Simplicity in insertion
- No loss of time
- Return of fertility is immediate on removal of device
- Cheap (supplied free by Government)
- Does not interfere with sexual act
- No systemic side effects
- Less failure rate (except pills)
- Long-term - TCu 380 A lasts for 10 years
- No effect on breast milk, can be inserted immediately after child birth.

Disadvantages

- Side effects: As mentioned before
- Does not prevent HIV/STDs
- Patient cannot use on her own or stop on her own. Some medical help required for insertion and removal
- May get expelled out without woman's knowledge
- Male partner may feel the strings during sexual act.

Other Uses of Cu-T

- After breaking of adhesions in a case of uterine synechia (Asherman syndrome) to prevent refusion of walls. Cu-T after removal of copper wire is kept.
- After strassman operation - to prevent fusion of anterior and posterior walls.

Management of a Patient who does not feel the Threads

Possibilities Mistake of the Patient

- Indrawing of threads inside the uterine cavity or cervix, or it is torn and expelled out.
- Perforation of uterus and migration in the peritoneal cavity.
- Spontaneous expulsion.
    - Do per speculum examination, if the thread is seen everything is alright and make the patient to palpate it.
    - If thread is not seen, USG (TVS) is done, if the device is inside the uterus it is easily seen on USG. But, if it has migrated in the peritoneal cavity it is **not seen on USG. Take simple X-ray abdomen,** if device is not seen anywhere in the X-ray, it is expelled out.
    - But, if it is seen in the X-ray it is displaced device.
    - IUCD whether it is intra-uterine or extra-uterine was in past checked by one of the following:
      1. A-P and lateral X-ray,
      2. A-P X-ray and X-ray with sounding after moving the uterus
      3. HSG.

Treatment

Any displaced IUCD requires removal either by laparoscopy or laparotomy. Medical devices cause adhesions and intestinal obstruction. In such situations patients is also psychologically disturbed.

If it is intrauterine it can be removed by different instruments like simple curette, long artery forceps, uterine dressing forceps, Shirodkar hook or with the help of hysteroscope. It may be badly embedded.

Management of Patient having Pregnancy with Cu-T in situ

Advice should be termination with removal of Cu-T because of following risks:

Increased risk of abortion, septic abortion, premature rupture of membranes, premature labor, IUGR, accidental hemorrhage, puerperal sepsis and ectopic pregnancy. However, it does not produce any congenital malformation.

With all risks explained, if patient is keen to continue her pregnancy at least Cu-T should be removed- if uterus is less than 12 weeks, if threads are seen and if device can be removed easily without disturbing the pregnancy. Otherwise leave it. Cu-T may be retrieved at the time of delivery.

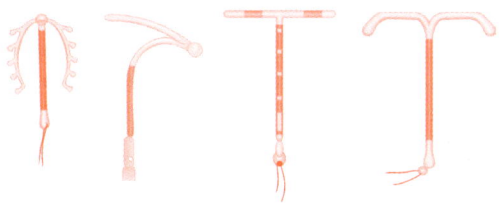

Fig. 5.3: From left to right multiload, Cu-7, TCu-220, and Nova T.

Other IUCDs

Multiload-Cu 250 (or Multiload-Cu 375)

It is made up of mixture of high density polypropylene and ethylene vinyl acetate copolymer impregnated with barium sulfate. Its shape is different from Cu-T, i.e. side arms of T are bent with small outer projections (Serrated fins) which help to hold the device in place without stretching the uterine cavity. Copper wire with 250 sq mm (or 375 sq mm) surface area is wrapped around vertical arm. Both are 36 mm long and 21 mm wide, but multiload Cu-375 has copper wire of 0.4 mm diameter effective life for Cu-250 is 3 years while that of Cu-375 is 5 years. Its inserter has **no plunger** and it is introduced by **withdrawal technique.** It has 2 nylon threads at its lower end, perforation and expulsion is less with multiload as compared to Cu-T.

Cu-7 (Gravigard)

It is "7" shaped device made up of polypropylene impregnated with barium sulfate. Copper wire is wrapped around vertical arm. Surface area of copper wire is 200 sq mm. It is 36 mm long and 26 mm wide. It has only one (instead of usual two) polypropylene thread blue in colour. Its life span is 3 years. It is inserted by withdrawal technique.

T Cu-220

It is T shaped device with 7 solid copper sleeves, 2 on transverse arm and 5 on vertical stem. Total exposed surface area of copper is 220 sq mm. It is developed by Population Council and its effective life is estimated to be 15–20 years. It has 2 threads and it is introduced by withdrawal technique.

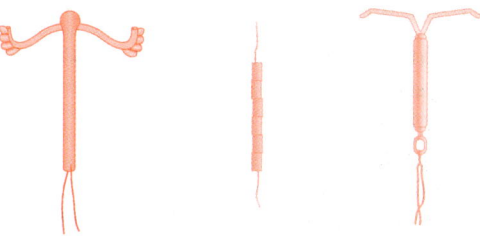

Fig. 5.4: From left to right Zicoid, Flexigard, LNG-20 (Mirena).

Nova-TCu-200 and 200 Ag

It is T-shaped device made up of polyethylene with barium sulfate impregnated. The fine copper wire is wrapped around the vertical stem. The surface area of copper is 200 sq mm. In 200 Ag variety a silver core has been added to the copper wire to reduce its fragmentation. It has 2 white threads and it is inserted by withdrawal technique. As compared to other copper devices, it is slightly short (32 mm long instead of 36 mm).

Zicoid

It is T shaped device with flexible and resilient side arms with small projection on the inside of the side arms. This prevents irritation of the cervical canal during insertion. It's surface area is 350 sq mm and copper wire is placed in the upper part of the stem. Diameter of wire is 0.5 mm. Plunger with special stop at proximal end ensures high fundal placement of the device. It is effective for 5 years.

Gynefix

It is a frameless IUD. Originally developed frameless IUDs like flexiguard and Cu-Fix are now discarded due to complexity in insertion technique Gynefix consists of six 5 mm long copper sleeves on a polypropylene thread. It is inserted through vaginal route with a special applicator that sutures the thread to the fundus of the uterus. If is effective for 5 years.

Progesterone Containing Devices

a. **LNG 20 (Mirena, LNG – Intra-uterine system):** T-shaped device with flexible arms. The shape is that of Nova -T, but it has capsule on the stem. The core of the capsule contains a mixture of silicone rubber and 52 mg levonorgestrel, which is released at 20 µg/day. It is 32 mm long and 32 mm wide. It has a different type of inserter and it is inserted by special withdrawal technique. It is effective for 5 to 7 years. As contraceptive it has dual mechanism of action, i.e. that of IUCD as well as hormonal contraceptive. Apart from **contraception** it helps in treatment of **AUB, fibroids, adenomyosis** and **endometriosis**. It is also useful for protection from **endometrial hyperplasia** during estrogen replacement therapy. Failure rate is 0.1 to 0.2 per 100 women in the first year of use. Side effects due to hormone can occur, e.g. nausea, vomiting, headache, acne, dizziness, breast tenderness, weight gain, ovarian cysts and bleeding disturbances in first 3 months.

Progestasert was the first hormone containing IUD developed in 1976. But due to its short life span of 1 year, it did not become popular and replaced by Mirena containing levonorgestrel instead of progesterone.

Skyla and Liletta are other LNG releasing IUDs effective for up to three years available in western countries.

b. **Fibroplant:** It is derived from Gynefix, so it is frameless. It is levonorgestrel releasing IUD. LNG is released frame fibrous delivery system which is attached to the anchoring thread by means of a stainless steel clip. It is effective for 5 years.

STEROIDAL CONTRACEPTIVES

They contain synthetic female hormones (estrogen and progesterone) which are steroid in nature.

Types:
1. Oral: Commonly known as **Pills - OC pills.**
2. Injectable: Intramuscular.
3. Newer sustained release systems.

Oral Pills (OCs)

Types

1. Combined
2. Phasic
3. Minipill
4. Newer pills

Combined Oral Pill

- Combination of estrogen and progesterone-21 such tablets. As the dose of estrogen and progesterone remain constant they are called monophasic pills.
- Supplied as 21 tablets or in a pack of 28 tablets, where last 7 tablets are placebo containing iron and vitamins, to complete the menstrual cycle.
- Commonly used estrogen is ethinyl estradiol (EE) 30 µg or 20 µg.
- Commonly used progesterone are norethisterone, DL norgestrel, levonorgestrel, desogestrel etc.
- It is started from any of the first 5 days of the cycle (usually 5th day). It is taken daily one preferably at bedtime for 21 days. Second pack is started after 7 day irrespective of onset or stoppage of menstruation.
- In a family planning program it is supplied free of charge by Government: Mala D, Mala N.
- Composition of few OC pills preparations mentioned below:

Preparation	Estrogen (EE)	Progestogens
Mala D	30 µg	Norgestrel 0.3 mg
Mala N	30 µg	Norethisterone 1.0 mg
Ovral	50 µg	Norgestrel 0.5 mg
Ovral L	30 µg	Levonorgestrel 0.15 mg
Duoluton-L	30 µg	Levonorgestrel 0.25 mg
Novelon Intimacy Plus 3	30 µg	Desogestrel 0.15 mg
Femilon Intimacy Plus 2	20 µg	Desogestrel 0.15 mg

PHASIC PILLS

Biphasic, Triphasic or Quadriphasic
- Biphasic: All 21 tablets contain E + P, but dose of progesterone is doubled after first 10 days, dose of estrogen remaining constant (ethinyl estradiol 35 µg, Norethindrone 50 µg and 100 µg). It has slightly high failure rate and not available in India.

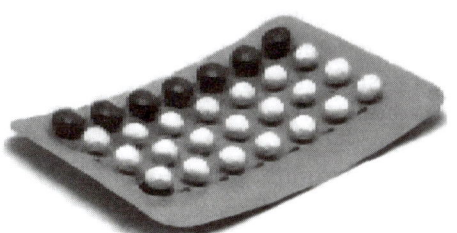

Fig. 5.5: Combined oral pills.

- Triphasic: All 21 tablets contain E + P, but dose vary in 3 phases, e.g.
  a. **Triquilar:**

EE	Levonorgestrel	Days
30 µg	50 µg	1–6
40 µg	75 µg	7–11
30 µg	125 µg	12–21

Triquilar is started from the 5th day of cycle while second pack is started after 7 days of pack free interval.

  b. **"Cyclessa"** contains ethinyl estradiol 25 µg and triphasic desogestrel and **"Ortho-tricyclen"** contains EE 25 µg and triphasic norgestimate. They are not yet available in India.

- Quadriphasic pills provide 4 different doses of estrogen and progestogen both, estradiol valerate and dienogest. It is considered more physiological as it simulates natural cycle, so side effects are reduced. However there are more chances of pill taking errors and high cost. It is available in foreign countries as **Natazia** and **Qlaria.**

Mini Pill

- As they contain only synthetic progestogen (not estrogen) they are called mini pill or progestogen only pill (POP).
- Two are currently available **Cerazette** containing Desogestrel 75 µg and Micronor or Noriday containing Norethisterone 350 µg. Only cerazette is available in India.
- It is available as 28 tablets pack, all active tablets (No placebo).
- It is to be started from the first day of period for first 7 days backup method (condom) should be used.

- Daily one tablet is taken at the same time (3 hours window) throughout the cycle.
- One should started the second pack immediately after the first pack is completed.
- It acts by inhibiting ovulation and also acts locally by making endometrium unreceptable for implantation and renders cervical mucous hostile to sperms.
- Its typical use failure rate is 9% while perfect use failure rate is only 0.3%.
- It avoids undesirable side effects of estrogen found with combined pills and sickle cell patients or lactating mothers can take it.
- Menstrual irregularities and amenorrhea are common with its use.
- Side effects contributed to progesterone content can occur, i.e. alopecia, loss of libido, weight gain, breast tenderness, bloating, nervous irritability. Androgenic side effects are less with cerazette.

Newer Pills

- **Intimacy plus 2, Femilon:** They contain only 20 µg ethinyl estradiol (as compared 30 µg in intimacy plus 3, Novelon) and 150 µg Desogestrel. Due to lowest dose of estrogen, estrogen related side effects like nausea, breast tenderness and headache are quite less.

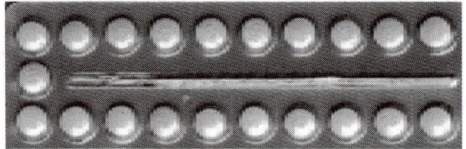

Fig. 5.6: Anti-androgenic pills.

Desogestrel a newer progestogen which has minimal androgenic side effects: reduces the risk of cardiovascular disease and cures acne and hirsutism.
- **Post-coital pill:** Discussed in detail under emergency contraception.
- **Once a month pill:** Each pill contains 3 mg of Quinestrol (long acting estrogen) and 12 mg megestrol acetate (Progesterone). It is not available in India.
- **Pill with antiandrogenic effects:** It contains ethinyl estradiol (35 µg) + cyproterone acetate (2 mg) e.g. **MY Pill, Diane 35, Krimson 35.**

    Dronis, Rasmin and Yasmin contains EE (30 µg) + Drospirenone (3 mg) (aldosterone derivative).

    Freedase is recently introduced pill. Here 21 tablets contain ethinly estradiol 30 µg and dienogest (newer progestogen) 2 mg.

    Due to antiandrogenic effects they are useful in patients with PCOS, acne and hirsutism and androgenic alopecia. Cyproterone is considered most potent anti-androgen progestin. Drospirenone due to its antimineralocorticoid activity also decreases BP and weight in the users. It has favorable effect on lipid metabolism also. Dienogest has minimal effect in thyroid and glucose metabolism. Due to high selectivity as a progestogen it has favorable safety profile and tolerability as compared to other progestins.

- **Pills with extended cycle length (continuous use OC):** Seasonale contains 150 µg of the progestin LNG and 30 µg of estrogen EE. This monophasic pill is taken continuously for 84 days and then hormone free pill for 7 days. It leads to only 4 periods in a year and also reduces the side effects associated with monthly hormone withdrawal, e.g. migraine, headache, mood changes. However breakthrough bleeding is more than conventional OCs which diminishes after 3 courses, i.e. 9 months.

    Lybrel was another continuous OC pill approved by FDA. It contains 365 tables of 90 µg LNG and 20 µg EE. The Pill completely stops a women's period for full one year. Lybrel is discontinued by the manufacturer due to license issue and now it is available as generic under brand names **Amethyst, Lutera** and others.

Mechanism of Action

Pills containing estrogen and progesterone work in following ways:
- Their main action is inhibition of ovulation. They act at hypothalamic level inhibiting release of gonadotropin releasing hormone (GnRH). Secretion of FSH and LH from pituitary are thus suppressed, so there is no follicular growth. As there is no LH surge, ovulation is suppressed. It is also suggested that they directly inhibit pituitary as there is no response to exogenous GnRH administration in Pill users.
- They alter the maturation of endometrium making it unsuitable for implantation. Under the effect of progesterone there is stromal edema with glandular exhaustion and atrophy.
- Progesterone makes cervical mucous thick viscid, scanty and impermeable to sperms.
- Effect on tubal motility by progesterone is also suggested.

Patient Selection

- Before prescribing the pills to any patient complete clinical history and thorough examination is carried out to rule out contraindications (WHO-MEC).
- Weight and blood pressure are recorded and Pap smear is taken.
- Diabetes should be ruled out and liver function tests are carried out if necessary.
- Patients are informed about initial side effects and assured that they usually disappear spontaneously in course of time or with treatment.

Follow-up

- First at the end of 3 months and then annually. History regarding symptoms of thromboembolic disease is elicited.
- Pelvic examination, breasts examination, cervical smear, BP and weight recording are done and urine is tested for glycosuria.
- It is advisable to stop the pills after 50 years (35 years in smokers) and to keep breaks for 3–6 months every 3–5 years.
- Recent evidence shows that modern pill can be taken for 10 or even more years in a row without increased risk.

Contraindications

WHO published **medical eligibility criteria** (WHOMEC, 2004) for initiating and continuing use of contraceptives on the basis of latest clinical and epidemiological information taking into account health risks and benefits. The criteria are revised and updated in 2015. There are four categories for use of any contraceptive method as follows:
- **Category I:** No restriction for the use of the contraceptive method.
- **Category II:** Advantages generally outweigh the theoretical or proven risks (The method is used with precautions).
- **Category III:** Theoretical or proven risks usually outweigh the advantages (The contraceptive method generally should not be used. An alternative method is preferred. However health personnel may make an exception in individual case with her informed consent).
- **Category IV:** A method that represents an unacceptable health risk (It should not be used).

WHO (2015) has come out with **WHOMEC wheel** for starting use of contraceptive methods. The wheel includes recommendations on initiating use of nine common type of contraceptive methods, i.e. COC pills, progesterone only pills, patch, vaginal ring, combined injectables, progesterone only injectables, progesterone only implants, copper bearing IUDS and LNG-IUD.

WHO has recently launched an App for contraceptive use. This digital tool will help healthcare workers in recommending safe, effective and acceptable contraceptive methods for women with different medical conditions.

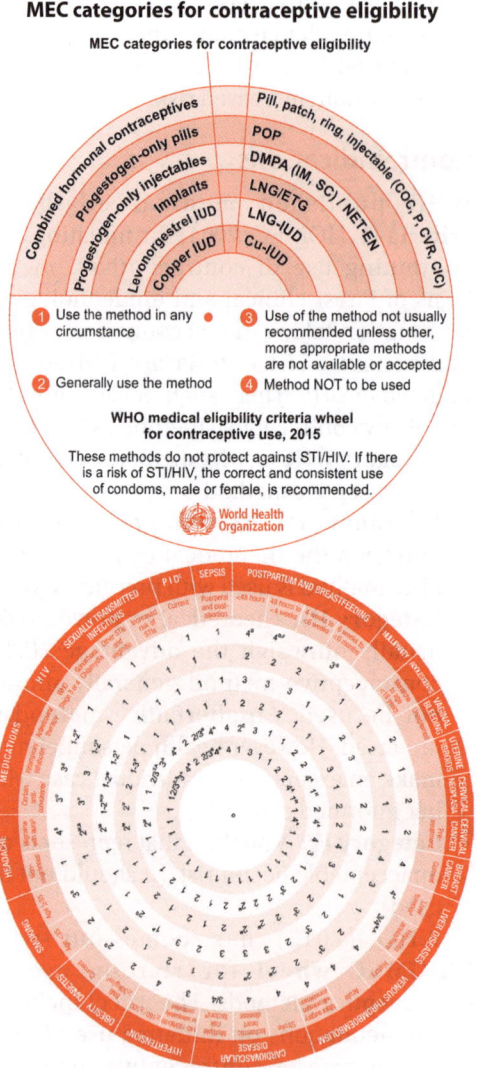

Fig. 5.7: WHOMEC wheel.

Side Effects and Complications

1. **Nausea and vomiting:** It is very common side effect. It is related to the estrogen content of the pill. It is managed by (a) reassurance that it subsides as therapy continues, (b) taking the pill after food or with cup of milk, (c) taking the pill at bedtime so that the individual is sleeping during peak concentrations of drug in the blood, (d) changing over to another compound with lower dose of estrogen.

2. **Break through bleeding:** It occurs in almost half of all patients at some time. It may be due to failure to take the pill at the same time each day. It is more common with low dose pill. However with newer pills cycle control is good. It diminishes after first 3-4 pill cycles.
   Management: (a) Switching to another low dose compound or (b) increase in the estrogen dose of the pill temporarily or taking short course of additional estrogen temporarily, (c) a search for pathological causes of bleeding must be made.

3. **Absence of withdrawal bleeding (Pill amenorrhea):**
   Management: After ruling out the pregnancy either of the following options is given to the patient (a) reassuring the patient the likelihood of regular menstruation when the pills are discontinued and second pack is started from the seventh day of last pill, (b) if withdrawal bleeding is desired switching to a pill with higher estrogen activity or adding tablet of estrogen, i.e. EE 0.02 mg last 7 days for few cycles is advised. Amenorrhea and oligomenorrhea are less common with triphasic pills.

4. **Hypertension:** It is 3 times more common in pill users. Both systolic and diastolic BP rises. It is minimal with triphasic pills.

5. **Cardiovascular diseases:** Venous thromboembolism—deep vein thrombosis is 5–6 times more common in users, while superficial vein thrombosis is 2–3 times more common in users. It is due to estrogen and it is dose dependent. OC pills containing drospirenone has increased chances of venous thromboembolism.
   Myocardial infarction—It is 2–3 times more common in pill users. It is due to

both estrogen as well as progesterone. The incidence is now decreasing with greater care in selecting the patients and due to low dose pills.

Cerebrovascular stroke: Cerebral thrombosis is more common than cerebral hemorrhage. It is not dose dependent so the incidence is not decreased with low dose pills.

6. **Weight gain, fluid retention:** 5–50% of women gain weight. Tendency is more in first 6 months of use. Weight gain is negligible with newer low dose pills.
7. **Breasts:** Pain, tenderness, encouragement are common side effects.
8. **Carbohydrate metabolism:** Glucose tolerance is impaired in pill user. Latent diabetic patients may become symptomatic. This is less found with low dose pill.
9. **Liver and gallbladder:** Altered liver functions are noted in pill users. Cholestasis jaundice can also occur. Gallstones and infection of gallbladder are found in young women on pills.
10. **Post pill amenorrhea:** It is found in 3–5/1000 users. It is not related to duration of use and it is common in women having oligomenorrhea before starting the pill.
11. **Neoplasia:** Cervix—there is higher incidence of dysplasia and Ca in situ-cervix reported in pill users. Little increase in the risk of cervical cancer is reported in women who use OCs for > 5 years and in those infected with human papilloma virus.
Breast-risk of breast cancer is not convincingly proved. It is very slightly increased only in young women, nulliparous patient, in current and recent users, after prolonged use and with positive family history.
Liver-for hepatic adenoma (benign) there is unequivocal evidence. The risk is rare (3–4/lakhs) but condition may be fatal due to severe, intraperitoneal hemorrhage. With long-term use (8 years or more) there is increased risk of hepatocellular carcinoma.
Malignant melanoma-controversial.
12. **Teratogenicity:** If pregnancy occurs during the course of pill, i.e. pill failure, there is a small but definite risk to the fetus.
13. **Miscellaneous:** These include, melasma, headache, giddiness, leukorrhea, acne, change in libido, mental depression, alopecia, leg cramps and some ophthalmic complications like retinal vascular disease, corneal edema or diseases of eyelids and conjunctiva.

Failure rate: Perfect use failure rate is 0.3% while typical use failure rate is high (5–9%).

Causes of failure:
- Irregular taking
- In very first cycle, if it is not started from the first day
- Malabsorption disorders.
- Taken along with some drugs like Rifampicin, Penicillin, Tetracycline, Ampicillin, Barbiturates, Phenytoin, Sulfonamides.

Missing a Pill: It patient forgets to take one tablet white (hormonal) she should take it as soon as she remembers and 2nd pill is taken as usual. If she misses for consecutive two days, then for 7 days she should avoid sex or use condoms. If 7 or more white tablets are left in the pack, she should take all the rest of the pills as usual. But, if < 7 tablets are left in that pack, take rest of the white pills as usual, Don't take brown tablets and start a new pack after the last white tablet of previous pack. She may miss a period. This is okay.

Missing of 1 or more brown pills is of no importance, take the rest of the pills as usual, one each day.

Missing a Minipill: If patient misses one tablet she should take the missed pill as soon as she remembers and take other pills as usual at regular time. If she is more than 3 hours late in taking missed pill, she should use backup method, i.e. condom for next 48 hours or do not have sex.

Other Uses of Pills

- Regularization of cycles
- Abnormal uterine bleeding (AUB)
- Endometriosis (Taken continuously for 6–9 months and not cyclical as in other uses)
- Postponement of menstrual period
- Amenorrhea to test for withdrawal bleeding
- Primary dysmenorrhea.
- Suppression of functional ovarian cysts. Recent reports do not support this.
- Polycystic ovarian disease.
- Treatment of acne and hirsutism.
- Adenomyosis.

Beneficial Side Effects

- **Menstrual comforts:** Regularization of cycle, blood loss is controlled (cure of anemia), relief from primary dysmenorrhea and premenstrual tension.
- **Prevents pelvic inflammatory diseases:** Cervical mucous is thickened, menstrual blood loss is reduced, uterine contractions are inhibited (so spread of infection to tubes prevented). Prevents pregnancy and abortion which provide opportunity for infection.
- **Prevents ectopic:** As it is highly effective contraceptive method and also as it prevents pelvic inflammatory disease.
- **Lowers risk of endometrial cancer:** Because of progesterone component. Up to 50% reduction in risk of endometrial cancer and protection persists up to 20 years after discontinuation.
- **Lowers risk of ovarian cancer:** Because of suppression of pituitary secretion of gonadotropins and ovulation. There is 40% decrease in risk of ovarian cancer among users compared to never users. Protection lasts for 15 to 20 years after discontinuation. There is 80% reduction in risk for both ovarian and endometrial cancer with pill use for more than 10 years.
- Protection against benign breast diseases. 30–50% decrease in the incidence in current and recent long-term users.
- Protection against functional ovarian cysts, i.e. follicular cysts and lutein cysts due to suppression of ovulation.
- Studies have shown reduced risk of uterine fibroids, colorectal cancer (30–40% reduction), rheumatoid arthritis and benign thyroid conditions.
- Improvement in bone mineral density also occurs.

Indications for Stopping Pills

- Pregnancy (pill failure)
- Uncontrollable side effects
- Development of complications
- If patient wants to become pregnant
- Age >35 years in smokers otherwise at 50 years of age
- Six weeks before elective surgery

Important

- Risk of mortality from circulatory system diseases in pill users is increased only in women more than 35 years of age and in women who smoke.
- Return of fertility may be delayed for 1–2 months after stopping pills, but at the end of 3 months there is no difference.
- Pregnancy should be postponed for at least 2 months after stopping the pills to avoid teratogenic effect.
- Drugs like Rifampicin, Barbiturates, Phenytoin, Ampicillin decrease the contraceptive effect of pills.
- Pills increase the requirement of insulin and oral antidiabetic drugs, anticoagulants, thyroid hormone and folic acid in respective individuals.

Centchroman (Ormeloxifene)

It is non-steroidal oral contraceptive pill. It is one of the selective estrogen receptor modulators (SERMs) which exhibits weak estrogenic and potent antiestrogenic (5 times) activity. It is started in a dose of 30 mg (1 tablet) on the first day of menstruation, given twice a week for the first 3 months and then once weekly. It is safe and reliable and with correct use its failure rate (1.6 HWY) is comparable to OC pills. It is available as **Sevista, Novex DS, Centron, Saheli.**

It has no effect on HPO axis, so it does not inhibit ovulation. The contraceptive mechanism is local either by defective implantation of blastocyst due to abnormal decidualization or blastocyst abnormality itself. Added effects are antiestrogenic effects on tubal motility and poor cervical mucous sperm penetration. Return of fertility is reported within 6 months of discontinuation.

As it is non-steroidal all the major side effects of steroidal contraceptives are avoided. Menstrual disturbances like oligomenorrhea, amenorrhea and ovarian cysts are found in >1/3rd users. Because of these side effects it could not gain much acceptance.

Now, it is being successfully used in treatment of **AUB**. Clinical trials are on for its use in treatment of breast cancer and for HRT. Dose for AUB is 60 mg twice a week for first 3 months, followed by once a week for next 3 months. USG (TVS) is recommended every 2 months too detect ovarian cyst or endometrial hyperplasia (typical cystic).

Injectable Contraception

A. Long acting progestins:
- Depotmedroxyprogesterone acetate (**DMPA**) —150 mg every 3 months (Depo provera).
- Norethisterone enanthate (**NET-EN**) - 200 mg every 2 months (Noristerat).

B. Combined injectables (oest + prog): Not available in India.
- DMPA 25 mg + estradiol cypionate 5 mg (Cyclofen) - monthly.
- NET-EN 50 mg + estradiol valerate 5 mg (Mesigyna) - monthly.
- Dihydroxyprogesterone acetophenide 150 mg + estradiol enanthate 10 mg (Deladroxate) - monthly.

Combined injectables disturb vaginal bleeding patterns less and allow earlier return to ovulation after women discontinue use (6 wks). Discontinuation rates are lower than those for only progestin injectables. Failure rate is 0.1–0.4 HWY. The disadvantage is it cannot be used in nursing mothers and it requires monthly injections.

DMPA

- It is highly effective, long acting, safe, reversible and easy to administer.
- It is given as 150 mg I/M every 3 months with a grace period of 2 weeks late or early.
- It should be given deep I/M in gluteus or deltoid muscle with all aseptic precautions. Injection into the fat (decreases absorption) or rubbing the injection site (increases absorption) changes the efficacy.
- Time: It is given within 7 days of menstrual cycle. It can also be given immediately after abortion and MTP. In postpartum patient it can be given immediately within 7 days, however in breastfeeding patient one can wait for 6 weeks postpartum.
- Failure rate: Perfect use failure rate is 0.3% while typical use failure rate is 3%.
- Mechanism of action is same as that of OC pills and it also hinders the rate of ovum transport.
- Return of fertility after DMPA is about 9 to 10 months after the last injection. There is no long-term impairment of fertility.

Advantages
- Very effective
- Long - term - 3 months injections
- Does not interfere with sex
- Reduces the incidence of PID and candidal vulvovaginitis
- Flexibility in return visit due to 2 wks grace period
- No estrogen related side effects
- Makes sickle cells crisis less frequent and less painful
- Decreases seizure frequency in epileptics

- Can be used in nursing mothers. It increases milk production.
- Decreases primary dysmenorrhea and symptoms of endometriosis.
- Helps in preventing endometrial cancer and uterine fibroids.

Disadvantages
- Delayed return of fertility – 7 to 9 months after last injection.
- Menstrual irregularity and ammenorrhoea occurs in 10 to 15% of women.
- Weight gain of 1–2 kg each year may occur.
- Decrease in HDL and increase in LDL cholesterol is reported so women with severe vascular disease should not use it.
- May cause headache, breast tenderness, mood changes, nausea, hair loss, less sex drive.
- Recent studies have shown decrease in bone mineral density (BMD) in current users of DMPA. Studies have also shown that BMD changes are reversible after discontinuation. For this reason it is not advisable to use DMPA in adolescents and perimenopausal patients.
- DMPA subcutaneous is a new formulation approved by US-FDA. It is by the name **Depo-sub Q provera 104.** It allows for a 30% lower dose of progestin (104 mg instead of 150 mg) with the same duration of effect, i.e. 3 months. It is supplied in single-use, prefilled nonreusable syringe. Being SC injection it requires less training for health providers than conventional DMPA injections.

Sustained Release Systems
- Subdermal polysiloxane capsules (Norplant)
- Biodegradable implants
- Silastic vaginal rings.
- Contraceptive patch.

Norplant
- It is a long acting, low-dose, progestin only contraceptive system. It is highly effective and highly reversible.
- **Norplant-2** rod system **(Jadelle)** comprises 2 silastic rods containing a total of 150 mg of levonorgestrel (75 mg/rod). **Sino-implant II** from China is same, i.e. 2 rods containing 75 mg LNG/rod, but it is less costly than Jadelle. The rods are implanted subdermally in the women's arm employing a minor surgical technique.
- **Time:** Within 7 days after the onset of menstruation or immediately after abortion or first trimester MTP. The implants become effective within 24 hours of placement.
- Mechanism of action is mainly local on cervical mucous and endometrium, but it also inhibits ovulation in about 50% of the cycles.
- **Failure rate:** Less than 0.5/HWY.
- **Contraindications:** Anticoagulant therapy, undiagnosed abnormal uterine bleeding, known or suspected pregnancy, hemorrhagic diathesis and liver diseases.
- **Side effects:** Bleeding disorders, amenorrhea, nausea, loss of appetite, dizziness, headache, changes in libido, depression, acne, infection at implant site.
- **Removal:** Implants work up to 5 years, after that they should be removed employing a minor surgical technique.

Implanon
- It consists of an ethyl vinyl acetate copolymer device (single rod 4 cm long, 2 mm diameter) containing 68 mg of **progestogen 3-ketodesogestrel** also known at **etonogestrel.**
- It is much easier to insert or remove implanon as compared to Norplant, however specific training is essential.
- It releases 30 to 40 µg of drug/day. It is effective for 3 years. As compared to other implants implanon users have few if any ovulatory cycles. It's failure rate (typical as well as perfect use) is 0.05%.
- There is no effect on BMD as against DMPA.
- It is a good choice for women with high blood pressure, anemia, adolescent girls and breastfeeding women.

- Other single rod device is **Nestorone** (segesterone acetate) for 2 years.

Biodegradable

They deliver progesterone from a carrier that gradually dissolves and disappears. Compared with norplant they are easier to insert and need not be removed.

Two were used - **Capronor** (40 mm rod) containing levonorgestrel (effective for 1.5 years) and **Norethindrone** pellets (1 year).

Silastic Vaginal Rings

These have advantage over previous methods that women can insert and remove themselves and they are immediately reversible. Progesterone is slowly released from the ring and can be absorbed through the vaginal epithelium. Most rings are between 50 mm and 60 mm in outer diameter and 7.5–9.5 mm thick. They are pliable and similar to the inert pessaries used for prolapse. The ring containing levonorgestrel 5 mg releases 20 µg per day and can be left in place for 3 months. If necessary the ring can be removed for up to 3 hours for comfort during sexual intercourse or for cleaning. Progestin only rings are less effective overall than rings containing both estro + prog, but they are useful in breastfeeding women.

The ring containing estro + prog (**Nuva ring**) releases 120 µg of etonogestrel and 15 µg of ethinyl estradiol per day. It is effective after 7 days of insertions. Like OCs the women use Nuva ring for 3 weeks and then remove it for one week, during which they have withdrawal bleeding. A new Nuva ring is needed for each 4 weeks cycle. Failure rate is less (1.8/HWY) but break through bleeding is a problem. Nonhormonal side effects include vaginitis, irritations and vaginal discharge.

Contraceptive Patch

Combined estrogen + progesterone patch available as **Evra** and **Xulane**. Evra is a square patch 4–4.5 cm long. It delivers in the blood stream 20 µg of ethinyl estradiol and 150 µg norelgestromin. Every week new patch is worn. After 3 weeks no patch is worn for 1 week. The patch contains 3 layers - an outer protective layer of polyester, a medicated adhesive middle layer and a clear polyester release liner which is removed just before application. It may be applied over abdomen, buttocks, thighs or upper outer arms or upper back.

The patch is applied to a new location each week. Skin irritation or rash at the site of application may occur in 20% users. It takes 2 days to achieve therapeutic level. Perfect use failure rate is 0.3% while typical use failure rate is 9%.

LARC Methods

LARC means long acting reversible contraception. It includes intrauterine devices (IUDS), subdermal implants and injectables. Long acting means it works for minimum one month (to many years).

Two main advantages of LARC methods:
1. As it is long acting, almost no user action required.
2. Highly effective: Typical use failure rate and perfect use failure rate are same. It is almost comparable to sterilization failure rate.

EMERGENCY CONTRACEPTION

Emergency contraception means a particular type of contraception that is used as an emergency procedure to prevent pregnancy following an unprotected but possibly fertile intercourse.

Indications for emergency contraception include unprotected intercourse, failure of barrier method, unsuccessful withdrawal (coitus interruptus), missed oral contraceptive pills and sexual assault.

Emergency contraceptive methods are effective, safe and simple to use.

Method

1. **Progesterone only Pill:** It is now commonly used. Single dose of levonorgestrel 1.5 mg is taken in 72 hours, e.g. Unwanted, I pill. Previously 2 doses of 0.75 mg 12 hours apart were recommended.

   There are no major side effects. Nausea, abdominal pain, fatigue, headache and menstrual changes can occur in some women.

   If it is taken in first 12 hours, failure rate is only 1%, but if taken later and within 72 hours failure rate is 2%.

2. **Yuzpe method:** It was introduced by a Canadian Physician Albert Yuzpe. Combined pills containing OC 50 µg and norgestrel 500 µg (or levonorgestrel 250 µg) are taken: 2 pills as early as possible and 2 after 12 hours of first dose. The treatment is most effective if first dose is taken within 12 hours of intercourse, but it can be taken up to 72 hours.

   OC pills containing lower dose of estrogen (30 µg) should be taken as 2 doses of 4 pills 12 hours apart.

3. **IUCD:** Insertion of copper IUCD within 5 days intercourse (later than hormonal method). It can be kept inserted if couple wants to continue with it as method of temporary contraception.

4. **Ulipristal acetate (UPA):** It is recommended as single dose of 30 mg taken in 72 hours. With UPA pregnancy rate of 1.2% is reported.

5. **Antiprogesterone:** Mifepristone (RU-486) 600 mg oral single dose within 72 hours after unprotected intercourse. Doses as low as 50, 25 and even 10 mg are also found effective.

Failure rate reported for different hormonal methods are < 2% while for IUCD it is 0.1%. As per recent Cochrane review (2019) UPA and mifepristone are more effective than levonorgestrel.

Women should come for follow-up if she misses a period or has scanty period. If there is failure and she is pregnant proper counseling should be done. Most women will prefer MTP, but if they wish to continue pregnancy after failure of EC, she can continue pregnancy as there is no harmful effect on pregnancy. In IUCD failure device should be removed if she continues pregnancy.

Emergency contraceptive should be used for indications mentioned before and not as regular contraception (i.e. after regular unprotected intercourse).

CHAPTER 6

Medical Termination of Pregnancy

INTRODUCTION

The Medical Termination of Pregnancy (MTP) Act, 1971 was passed by Indian Parliament in August 1971 and came into force from April, 1972. Implementing rules and regulations were revised in 1975, so as to make services more readily available.

Some important aspects of the act are as under:

- **Indications:** Indications (conditions under which the pregnancy can be terminated).
  - Medical grounds: Where continuation of pregnancy might—(1) endanger the life of the woman, (2) cause grave injury to her physical and mental health.
  - Eugenic grounds: Where there is substantial risk that if the child is born it would suffer from such physical and mental abnormalities as to be seriously handicapped in life.
  - Humanitarian grounds: Where pregnancy has resulted from rape.
  - Social grounds: (1) Where actual or reasonably foreseeable environment (whether social or economic) would lead to risk of injury to the health of the mother, (2) failure of contraceptive measures.

  The MTP Act allows abortion up to 20 weeks of pregnancy. As some of the major fetal malformations may not be diagnosed by 20 weeks, the government is currently considering the amendment to increase the MTP limit up to 24 weeks (The MTP amendment Bill, 2017). Up to 12 weeks opinion of only one registered medical practitioner (RMP) is required, pregnancy between 12-20 weeks requires opinions of two RMPs. The actual termination may then be carried out by one RMP.
  - *Consent*: Written consent of the patient only, is required. If patient is under 18 years of age or in mentally ill persons even if they are older than 18 years, consent of guardian is necessary.
- **The person:** The Person who can perform MTP—The Chief Medical Officer (The Civil Surgeon) has the powers to certify the doctor for MTP provided he/she possess any of the following training or experience:
  - Postgraduate degree or diploma holder in obstetrics and gynecology.
  - Six months training as house surgeon (resident) in **Obstetrics** and gynecology.
  - Experience for one year in **Obstetrics** and gynecology Department of any hospital.
  - Assisted a registered medical practitioner in 25 cases of MTP. Out of which at least five have been performed independently.

- **The place:** The place where MTP can be performed– no MTP shall be carried out in any place other than (1) a hospital established or maintained by Government, or (2) the place approved for the purpose by Chief Medical Officer/Civil Surgeon of the District.
- **Records:** Every head of the hospital or approved place shall maintain a register in Form III for recording the admissions of women for MTPs serially. The admission register shall be a secret document and the information contained there is as to the name and other particulars of pregnant women shall not be disclosed to any person. Records are to be maintained for 5 years.
- **Penalty:** The person who contravenes the provisions of the act is punishable with rigorous imprisonment for a term not less than 2 years and up to 7 years rigorous imprisonment. It is a cognizable offence, i.e., police officer can arrest a doctor without warrant.

METHODS

First Trimester

Up to 12 weeks

- Anti-progestin RU486 – Mifepristone orally + misoprostol (MTP pills)
- Suction evacuation
- Manual vacuum aspiration (MVA)
- Dilatation and evacuation.

Second Trimester

From >12–20 weeks

(A) medical methods, (B) surgical methods.
- **Medical:**
  - **Prostaglandins:**
    - I/M Carboprost [15 (S) 15 M ethyl PGF2α] 250 µg 3 to 4 hourly
    - Vaginal pessary (PG E1 analogue misoprostol) 200 µg 3 hourly
    - Oral - Mifepristone + misoprostol
  - Extra-amniotic injections (Intrauterine transvaginally):
    - Ethacridine lactate (not available now)
  - Intra-amniotic injections (Trans-abdominal):
    - Hypertonic solutions
    - 20% saline (not used now).
- **Surgical:**
  - Hysterotomy (rarely done)
  - Aspirotomy (not done)

MIFEPRISTONE:
RU 486 (ROUSSEL-UCLAF 486)

Mifepristone is an antiprogesterone compound which blocks progesterone receptors in the myometrial, endometrial and decidual cells leading to local withdrawal of progesterone. This leads to detachment of trophoblastic cells, breakdown of endometrium and detachment of embryo. It can initiate myometrial contractility, softening and dilatation of cervix and even expulsion of embryo. It also sensitizes the uterus to the actions of prostaglandins.

Protocol for First Trimester MTP

Drug controller in India has permitted its use for MTP up to only 63 days from LMP:

Day 1: Confirm intrauterine pregnancy and its gestational age (if necessary by USG).
200 mg mifepristone orally.

Day 3: 400 µg misoprostol orally or vaginally, followed by 200 µg after 4 hours and again 200 µg after another 4 hours if required.
Recent studies suggest that misoprostol can be given as early as 6 hours after mifepristone on the same day.

Day 14: Follow-up to check for complete abortion (USG preferred).

- Ectopic pregnancy should be ruled out before its use.

- If it fails, woman is advised MTP due to teratogenic effects of the drug.
- Side effects include nausea, vomiting and abdominal cramps. Risk of heavy bleeding requiring emergency curettage is up to 5%.
- The failure rate is 2–5%.

Advantages

- Noninvasive
- No risk of anesthesia
- Can be performed in very early pregnancy (suction not suitable in such case)
- Orally effective drugs
- Privacy of the patient is maintained.

Disadvantages of Medical Abortion

- Painful cramps may last for few hours
- Bleeding more than surgical method
- Time of actual abortion unpredictable
- 2–5% failure requiring surgical curettage. True failure is considered when cardiac activity is present on day 14. It is less than 1%. Incomplete abortion with retrained products of conception (RPOC) is more common
- Officially permitted only up to 63 days from LMP, i.e., 9 weeks
- It is a prolonged method.

Other Uses of Mifepristone

Obstetrics:
- Evacuation of missed abortion
- Cervical priming before surgical evacuation (1st trimester)
- Cervical priming before 2nd trimester MTP by other methods (200 mg on day before)
- Induction of labor (200 mg orally for 2 days)

Gynecology:
- *Emergency contraception*: 600 mg single dose in 72 hours
- *Endometriosis*: 50–100 mg for 3 to 6 months
- *Fibroid*: Same as endometriosis.

Others: Under research– (1) meningioma, (2) breast cancer, (3) Cushing syndrome, (4) ovarian cancer.

SUCTION EVACUATION

- Done up to 12 weeks gestation
- After 12 weeks placenta is well-formed and fetus is cartilaginous so there are problems of excessive bleeding and incomplete evacuation. It requires more cervical dilatation which is traumatic.

Advantages Over Conventional (D&E)

- Less time is required
- Blood loss is reduced
- Substantially lesser dilatation of the cervix is needed
- Less incidence of incomplete evacuation
- Less painful than curettage
- Danger of uterine damage, i.e., perforation is less
- Less risk of Rh iso-immunization.

Instruments

Routine D&C instrument-set, suction cannula, suction tube with electric operated suction machine.

Anesthesia: Any of the following is given:
- Paracervical block with premedication (atropine or glycopyrrolate + narcotics or sedatives)
- G/A Propofol 2–3 mg/kg body wt or by I/V Pentothal 5 mg/kg body wt following premedication. Ketamine 2–3 mg/kg body wt. Fentanyl 50 to 100 µg or midazolam 2–4 mg produce good sedation.
- S/A, if TL operation is also to be done simultaneously.

Procedure

- Preoperative preparations, with emptying of the bladder
- Lithotomy position
- Painting and draping is done
- G/A is given at this step, while S/A is given before lithotomy position and paracervical block (L/A) is given after cervix is caught with Vulsellum

- P/V examination: (1) To confirm the size of uterus, (2) to detect the position of uterus (3) to check that there is no abnormal adnexal mass in the fornices
- Sim's speculum is introduced, anterior vaginal wall is retracted and cervix is exposed. Cervix is swabbed with sterile swab and anterior lip is caught by Vulsellum
- Sounding of the uterus is controversial and not routinely done
- No. of suction cannula used is equal to gestational age in weeks
- Dilatation with metal dilators is gradually done up to half to 1 mm more than the size of the uterus in weeks
- PGE-1 (misoprostol) tablet kept in vagina 4–6 hours back leads to easy dilatation
- Suction cannula is checked for its patency and tight fitting and then introduced in the direction of the uterus
- It is passed up to the fundus and then withdrawn up to middle of the cavity. Negative pressure created by switching on the suction machine (i.e. 600–700 mm of Hg or 0.5 to 0.7 kg/cm^2 surface area in bottle). Then cannula is moved up and down slowly from the fundus to the internal os and gradually rotated
- Whole of the cavity is aspirated by going clockwise or anticlockwise.

Endpoints of Suction

- Gripping of the instrument
- No active bleeding
- Gritty feeling (also called grating sensation) of the uterine walls
- No products coming when suction is on or at the most air bubbles are seen if cannula is transparent
  - Check curettage with sharp curette is always done which (1) can remove some adherent products or products particularly at the region of Cornu, and (2) to ensure that evacuation is complete
  - Injection Methylergometrine is given
  - Uterine cavity is cleaned by sterile gauze piece taken on uterine dressing forceps.

If patient is motivated for IUCD and has given consent, Cu-T can be inserted at this step.
- Instruments are removed and Vulsellum bite site is checked for bleeding
- P/V is done to confirm that uterus has contracted and size is decreased to near normal.

Special Points

- Oxytocin drip is not given routinely. It can be helpful in cases where G/A is given for 2 reasons: (1) Bleeding is less, (2) there is some degree of tension in uterine wall so perforation is made less likely.
- Sounding: Information gained by routine sounding is not worth the risk of perforation and hemorrhage with it. Sounding of cervical canal only is helpful for dilatation.
- If mother is Rh-negative anti-D is given 50 μg I/M in pregnancy beyond 6 weeks
- Products removed should be checked that amount matches with weeks of pregnancy
- If no products comes the possibilities are:
  - False passage or perforation
  - Patient not pregnant
  - Ectopic pregnancy
  - Very early intrauterine pregnancy and uterine anomalies, i.e., bicornuate or septate uterus.

Complications

- Cervical injury
- Incomplete evacuation
- Perforation of uterus
- Failure: Continuation of pregnancy
- Excessive blood loss
- Anesthetic complications
- Infection: If proper aseptic precautions are not taken or there is incomplete evacuation.
- If perforation goes unrecognized there are chances of damage to bowel, bladder, omentum and mesentery.

Delayed

- Infertility: Due to tubal block or uterine synechiae

Medical Termination of Pregnancy

- Repeated abortions or premature births: Due to cervical incompetence
- Chronic PID
- Ectopic pregnancy.

MANUAL VACUUM ASPIRATION (MVA)

- It has evolved from menstrual regulation
- MVA offers a simple, safe and easily maintained modality which could be used by peripheral medical staff with basic training
- In contrast of MR syringe here there is double valve syringe which easily connects to 4 to 12 mm size cannula, so it is applicable to all cases of first trimester MTP
- MVA syringe has a capacity of 60 CC. It consists of a barrel, plunger with a bush, circular slot for 'O' ring on the plunger, double valve adaptor with internal 'O' ring and two pinch valves and a collar stop
- Cannulae are also made of high density polypropylene with less molecular weight. The cannulae and the adaptors are color coded to fit into the double valve adaptor.

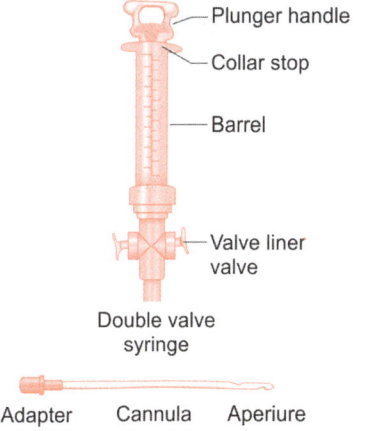

Fig. 6.1: MVA equipment.

Steps of the Procedure

- Create the vacuum in the syringe (charge the syringe)
- Check the uterine size by bimanual examination
- Antiseptic precautions
- Catch the cervix
- Administer local anesthetic
- Select size of cannula as per uterine size. Required dilatation may be carried out by increasing No. of cannula from the set
- Insert the cannula through the os towards the fundus
- Attach the "charged" syringe
- Release the pinch valves and allow the vacuum to get transferred into uterine cavity
- Use rotatory or back and forth movements.
- Evacuate the contents of the uterus.
- Inspect the evacuated material for chorionic villi.
  - Inspect the syringe and cannula before use to check for any crack and check the vacuum capability before use
  - If the cannula gets clogged remove it from the uterus. Displace the clog with instrument and do not touch the tip of the cannula with your fingers
  - If the vacuum is lost, recharge the syringe, reattach to the cannula and complete the procedure.

Comparison

Manual vacuum aspiration (MVA)	Suction (Electrical) evacuation
Portable and economical	Heavy expensive, noisy apparatus
Not dependent on electricity so useful for rural settings	Electricity dependent
Takes 1 second to create 26" (660 mm Hg) vacuum	Takes 1-1.5 min to create 26" of Hg vacuum
Rotation possible to 360° because of easy maneuverability	Rotation possible on either side 180° only because of kinking of tubing
Pre-created transfer of vacuum helps to find cleavage between sac and the endometrial lining. So sac gets sucked into the cannula as a mass, causing minimum bleeding	Since vacuum takes time to reach 26" of mm Hg it is not possible to the create cleavage easily and therefore, material comes in pieces causing more bleeding

Manual vacuum aspiration (MVA)	Suction (Electrical) evacuation
In case of perforation the vacuum drops to < 10 mm Hg and therefore, prevents sucking in of mesentery or intestines	In case of uterine perforation, the vacuum continues endangering pulling in of mesentery or intestines if plugged into the aperture of cannula
Cannula act as dilators causing minimum discomfort and pain	Metal dilators to be used which cause pain and damage to internal os

Menstrual regulation: It was done up to 14 days after period, i.e., 6 wks gestation. It was done with Karman 50 cc plastic syringe and 4, 5 or 6 mm size Karman flexible plastic cannulas.

MR did not become popular due to restriction up to 6 wks and higher failure rate.

ETHACRIDINE LACTATE

It is yellow dye with antiseptic action (acridine derivative). It was available under the trade names Emcredil, Abortil, Vecredil (0.1% solution of ethacridine lactate in 50–100 mL bulbs).

It is commonly used by extra-amniotic route.

Procedure

- Premedication-injection Atropine.
- Lithotomy position. Painting and draping. Vaginal cleaning
- Cervix is exposed by speculum, anterior lip of cervix is held with sponge holding forceps or Vulsellum
- Foley's catheter No. 14 or 16 is inserted beyond the internal os between the uterine wall and membranes
- The bulb of the catheter is inflated by 15-20 cc sterile solution
- Emcredil is injected by 20 mL syringe through the catheter
- Total 100 to 150 cc is injected at a time
- Lower end of catheter is tied to prevent escape of drug from the uterus. Excess of catheter is pushed in vagina and vagina may be packed with roller gauze; OR outer end of the catheter may remain outside and may be fixed to the back of the thigh of the patient by sticking plaster
- Catheter can be removed immediately or at any time afterwards up to its spontaneous expulsion. Additional bulb (50mL) may be injected 4 to 6 hours after initial injection.
- Prophylactic antibiotics are started
- Oxytocin drip may be started after contractions establishes, to shorten the induction abortion interval.

Mechanism of Action

- Ethacridine itself has oxytocic effect on human myometrial strips
- Excessive detachment of membranes and mechanical stimulation of uterus
- Catheter left in situ also causes mechanical stimulation of uterus
- Decidual lysosomes are damaged leading to synthesis and release of PGs which cause uterine contractions.

Advantages

- Safe-minimum lethal dose is 50 mg/kg so, even if intravasation occurs there is no danger
- Can be used when PG and saline are contraindicated, i.e., impaired cardiac and renal function
- Drug itself has potent and wide-spread bactericidal properties. So, it minimizes the risk of infection.

Disadvantages

- Induction-abortion interval is slightly more than other methods (36–48 hours)
- Failure rate slightly higher than other methods (5–15%)
- Higher incidence of incomplete abortion
- Fetus may be aborted alive.

Precaution

If blood comes out of catheter during its introduction or membranes rupture, procedure is abandoned.

Failure is considered when contractions do not start within 72 hours and is treated by oxytocin drip or repeat extra-amniotic emcredil injection or intramuscular prostaglandin or hysterotomy.

INTRA-AMNIOTIC HYPERTONIC SALINE

It was used for termination of 15–20 weeks pregnancy in which sterile hypertonic saline is instilled through the abdominal route.

Advantages

- Cheap
- Easily available
- Success rate is high
- Procedure is relatively easy
- Fetus is delivered dead
- It can be stored at any temperature

Contraindications

- Hypertension
- Cardiac disease
- Renal disease
- Diabetes
- Sickle cell anemia
- Scar on uterus (relative)
- Suspected low implantation
- Dead fetus.

Procedure

Premedication: Injection atropine 0.6 mg 1/2 hour before operation.
- Emptying of bladder
- Abdomen is prepared as for any surgical procedure
- Prior USG for localization of placental site is must so as to avoid it in needle insertion
- Skin site is first infiltrated with 2–3 cc 1% xylocaine and some amount is injected in subsequent abdominal wall layers
- No. 18. gauze sterile spinal needle with stylet is introduced vertically. Important resistances are those of rectus sheath and uterine wall. With loss of resistance, stylet is removed
- With 20 cc syringe first few cc of amniotic fluid is removed to check that flow is free and liquor is clear
- Calculated amount of 20% sterile hypertonic saline is injected gradually, with syringe or with IV set in a drip form.

Formula: Amount of 20% saline = No. of gestational weeks x 10. Maximum amount is 200 cc.
- After injection stylet is again pushed in situ and needle is withdrawn
- Puncture site is cleaned with spirit and sterile dressing is applied
- Prophylactic antibiotics are given.

Side Effects and Complications

- Failure of technique (i.e., dry tap, bloody tap)
- Nausea, vomiting, pyrexia.
- Symptoms of systemic infusion, i.e. hypernatremia. Intense thirst, feeling of warmth or burning sensation, sudden onset of headache, constant abdominal pain, flushing, anxiety.
- Incomplete abortion – less than with ethacridine
- Severe hemorrhage
- Cervical tear, uterine rupture
- Coagulation disorder–DIC
- Renal failure
- Infection–septicemia

Deaths have been reported rarely. It may be due to cardiac failure, renal failure, CV stroke, DIC, septicemia or amniotic fluid embolism. Due to this **intra-amniotic saline** is **NOT used** now.

PROSTAGLANDINS (PG)

- PGs are local hormones involved in a variety of physiological processes. Unlike classic hormones they are synthesized and released at the site of demand and get rapidly inactivated

- Von Euler of Sweden first found out PG in 1935. In the belief that this active acidic lipid found in human semen, is a secretion of the prostate gland he named it as prostaglandin
- They are 20 carbon atoms unsaturated hydroxy fatty acids (acidic lipids) containing a cyclopentane ring (five carbon ring) and two side chains and they are based on parent saturated acid called prostanoic acid.
- There are at least 14 naturally occurring PGs. They are synthesized in the body from essential fatty acids such as arachidonic acid.
- PGS are named A to I depending upon the structure of the five carbon ring. There are one or more double bonds in the side chains, they are expressed by the numerical subscript e.g. PGE1, PGE2, PGE2.
- A series of PG analogues are prepared and tried in an attempt to improve potency and prolong the duration of action (as they are less rapidly metabolized).
- PGE2 is 5–10 times potent oxytocic weight by weight than PGF2α.
- 15 methyl analogues are at least 10 times more potent than parent PGs.

Uses

- 1st trimester:
  - Preoperative cervical dilatation in MTP
  - First trimester MTP
- 2nd trimester:
  - For MTP
  - Hydatidiform mole evacuation
  - Missed abortion evacuation
- 3rd trimester:
  - Cervical ripening
  - Induction of labor
  - Augmentation of labor
  - Prevention of atonic PPH
  - Treatment of PPH

Uses other than MTP are discussed in the Chapter 7.

FIRST TRIMESTER MTP

Preoperative Cervical Dilatation

PG analogues have been tried successfully both locally and systemically for obtaining cervical dilatation prior to suction MTP. It has many advantages: (1) priming of cervix avoids pain and injury of rapid mechanical dilatation, (2) further dilatation if required is easier, (3) much reduced blood loss, and (4) less chances of perforation as uterus is firm under the effect of PG.

For MTP

In recent years PGs are extensively used and found very successful and safe for first trimester MTP. Following PGE analogues are used:
- **Misoprostol** – PGE1 analogues oral or vaginal route 200–800 ug.
  For first trimester MTP, it is given orally after prior treatment with RU 486 (Mifepristone)
- Gemeprost – PGE1 analogue 1 mg vaginal pessary
- Metenprost – PGE2 analogue 10 mg vaginal pessary.
  Success rate is more than 90%.
  Gemeprost and metenprost are not yet available in India.

SECOND TRIMESTER MTP

PGE1 PG analogues (misoprostol) are extensively used or this indication. Synthetic analogue of PGF2 OC is available. Chemically, it is tromethamine salt of 15(S) –15 methyl PGF2 OC. The generic name is **Carboprost** tromethamine.

ROUTES OF ADMINISTRATION

- Vaginal route: Misoprostol – 200 µg 3 hourly
  - Induction abortion interval is around 12 hours
  - It is noninvasive, side effects are less and it can be removed in case of hyperstimulation.

- Oral: Misoprostol 400 µg 3 hourly administered buccally or sublingually. Pretreatment with mifepristone 200 mg 24–48 hours prior increases success rate. Maximum 5 doses of misoprostol are recommended.
- Intramuscular: Carboprost (Prostodin Endoprost, Deviprost) 250 µg 3 to 4 hourly.
    - Natural PGs are locally irritating and causes pain and erythema so they are unacceptable for clinical use
    - Mean induction abortion interval is 16 hours
    - Success rate—85 to 90%
    - GI tract side effects are more as compared to other methods
    - This route is useful when other methods of MTP or other routes of PG have failed.

CONTRAINDICATIONS

- Hypersensitivity to any of the component of the product
- Acute PID
- Cardiac diseases
- Pulmonary diseases
- Renal diseases
- Liver diseases
- Glaucoma
- Relative contraindications are epilepsy and scar on uterus.

SIDE EFFECTS AND COMPLICATIONS

- Nausea, vomiting, diarrhea
- Cervical tear-bucket handle type
- Headache, flushing, fever
- Uterine rupture
- Bronchospasm
- Hemorrhage
- Hyperventilation
- Infection
- Seizures
    - PG failures are treated with hysterotomy
    - To reduce induction abortion interval oxytocin drip may be used along with PG.

DISADVANTAGES OF I/M PG

- Costlier drug
- Must be stored in cool place to maintain potency
- Troublesome side effects requiring antiemetics and antidiarrheals in almost every case, 1-2 hours before each injection
- Fetus may be aborted alive
- Before full dose sensitivity testing is necessary in I/M use
- Though abortion may be quicker, hemorrhage and cervical lacerations common

MISOPROSTOL

It is PGE1, analogue approved by FDA for the treatment and prevention of peptic ulcer associated with the use of NSAIDs.
- It is well absorbed from upper GI tract, vaginal mucosa and rectum.
- It is cheap, effective and does not require special storage conditions.

Uses

- Combined with mifepristone it is used in first trimester MTP (MTP pill)
- Preoperative cervical ripening before suction evacuation
- 2nd trimester MTP: 200–400 µg vaginally, every 3 hourly
- Induction of labor: 25 to 50 µg vaginally every 4 to 6 hourly
- Prevention and treatment of PPH: 600 to 800 µg orally or rectally
- Treatment of incomplete abortion and missed abortion
- It is useful preoperatively for cervical softening in gynecology in hysteroscopy and laparoscopic procedures
    - It is contraindicated in case of previous cesarean section
    - When used in 50 µg doses for induction or augmentation of labor one should be careful as it may cause fetal distress, meconium stained liquor, cervical lacerations and PPH.

HYSTEROTOMY

- Hysterotomy is not done as primary method for 2nd trimester MTP as medical methods are quite successful and with less complications
- Currently the indications are failure of medical method, if concurrent TL is to be done, MTP in case of 2 or more previous cesarean sections, for low lying placenta covering the os and scar ectopic pregnancy
- Preoperative preparation should be as like for any cesarean section
- It is done under S/A
- Abdominal incision is low transverse slightly larger than routine abdominal TL and smaller than cesarean section
- Uterine incision may be decided on table. If some space is available it should be low transverse, otherwise it can be low vertical
- Uterovesical fold should be opened and bladder pushed down little in either case.
- Uterine incision required is hardly 3 to 4 cm. BPD of the fetus is hardly about 4 cm and head is soft, so fetus can be delivered through very small incision
- As soon as the uterine incision is deepened amniotic sac pops out, pass a finger inside the uterine cavity and sweep it around to separate the sac from uterine wall. Fetus comes out readily intact in sac.
- Placenta also follows. If it does not come out intact, it is separated by finger and removed manually or by swab holder
- Gentle curettage may be required to scrap out decidua from the uterine wall. If required cervix should be dilated from above for lochia drainage. Although, it is not must
- As the abdominal incision is small, it may not be possible to deliver uterus out in all cases like in cesarean sections for suturing. It is not must and uterine incision can be sutured keeping it inside the abdomen.
- As uterus is small and in depth a prior stay suture taken just above the uterine incision helps in giving traction for easy suturing
- Uterus is closed by Vicryl no. 1 in two layers
- For a case of low lying placenta or scar ectopic deep stitches or uterine artery ligation may be required
- Peritoneal toilet is done, hemostasis is checked, counting is done and abdomen is closed as routine without suturing the peritoneum.

Aspirotomy

It is surgical D&E type method for second trimester MTP. As wider cervical dilatation is required, insertion of laminaria tents preoperatively is must. First the cannula is inserted to rupture the fetal membranes and aspirate the amniotic fluid. Then long heavy special ovum forceps (e.g. Sopher forceps, Hern forceps) is introduced inside the uterus and fetal parts are crushed. The vacuum cannula is reinserted to aspirate the material or to pull tissue downwards where it can be grasped with the forceps. To check the completeness of the procedure finally curettage with sharp curette is done. Intraoperative USG is helpful. It was done up to 16 weeks of pregnancy. Complications include excessive bleeding, trauma, incomplete evacuation and infections.

With prostaglandins freely available it is **not done** now.

CHAPTER 7

Drugs

The drugs kept on viva tables include ampoules, bulbs, vials, tablets, kit, gel or pessary.
1. Oxytocin, carbetocin
2. Ergometrine
3. Parenteral iron preparations
4. Magnesium sulfate
5. Isoxsuprine
6. Ritodrine
7. Prostaglandins
8. Cervical relaxants
9. Rh-anti-D immunoglobulin
10. Diazepam, midazolam
11. Furosemide
12. Tetanus toxoid
13. Sodium bicarbonate
14. Pethidine, pentazocine, tramadol
15. Promethazine
16. Metoclopramide
17. Ondansetron
18. Drugs for treatment of malaria
19. Low molecular weight heparin
20. Steroids-hydrocortisone, dexona
21. Xylocaine, bupivacaine
22. Atropine, glycopyrrolate
23. Hormones in gynecology
24. Clomiphene citrate, letrozole
25. Bromocriptine, cabergoline
26. Danazol, gestrinone, dienogest
27. Antihypertensive drugs
28. Aspirin
29. Tranexamic acid
30. Drugs used in leukorrhea
31. Antiretroviral drugs, STI/RTI kits
32. HPV vaccine—Cervarix, Gardasil

1. OXYTOCIN

It is an octapeptide. Natural one is produced in hypothalamus but stored and released from posterior pituitary. Synthesized in a purified form, it is available for clinical use.

Uses

Most commonly used drug in obstetrics.
- Induction of labor—common indications include, postdated, pregnancy-induced hypertension (PIH), eclampsia, premature rupture of membranes (PROM), intrauterine fetal demise (IUFD), malformed baby, intrauterine growth restriction (IUGR), Rh-iso-immunization and abruptio placentae
- Augmentation of labor, in case of uterine inertia
- Active management of the third stage of labor (AMTSL)—as recommended by World Health Organization (WHO) injection oxytocin 10 units I/M as soon as the baby is delivered
- Postpartum hemorrhage (PPH)—for treatment of atonic PPH 10 to 20 units in

I/V fluids (RL pint) is administered and repeated as necessary
- In lower segment cesarean section (LSCS) or hysterotomy operation (after the fetus is delivered) to prevent excessive bleeding
- Acceleration of abortion & to control postabortal bleeding
- Evacuation of vesicular mole along with suction evacuation

Central Government last year banned the manufacturing and sale of oxytocin by private manufacturers & retail chemists. This was with the apprehension that it is misused to increase milk production in animals. Only public sector undertaking (PSU), Karnataka Antibiotics and Pharmaceuticals Ltd (KAPL) was allowed to manufacture and sale throughout India. Delhi High Court quashed the notification in December 2018, allowing the manufacture and sale by private manufacturers. Now Central Government has moved to Supreme Court against Delhi High Court order. Final judgment is awaited.

Routes of Administration

Intravenous –by drip made in 500 mL of ringer lactate or 5% glucose pint.

For induction and augmentation of labor 2.5 to 5 units are injected in pint. 0.5 U/min is started initially and doubled every 15 seconds till required contractions of 3 per 10 min lasting for 40 seconds are achieved. Dose > 100 U/min is not useful as all the oxytocin receptors may be saturated.

While for abortion cases, in PPH and in LSCS 10 to 20 units are injected in pint.

Its effect starts within 20–30 seconds, but half life time in pregnant woman is only 3 min.

Available in 5 unit/mL ampoule evatocin, gynotocin, syntocinon and 5 units/0.5 mL pitocin, etc.

Contraindications

- Contracted pelvis or CPD
- Malpresentation
- Grand multipara
- Threatened rupture
- Fetal distress
- Pelvic tumors

It is used with caution in: (1) previous LSCS, and (2) cardiac disease.

Complications

- Fetal distress
- Fetal death
- Hyperstimulation with precipitate labor
- Rupture uterus
- Water intoxication if it is administered in large volume (over 4 liters) of electrolyte free solution with 40 U/min dose
- Hypotension – if given directly I/V in bolus form
- Neonatal jaundice is common in babies delivered with oxytocin if total dose of oxytocin exceeds 20 units
- Postpartum hemorrhage (PPH) – if oxytocin drip was used in labor and then not continued soon after the third stage.

Carbetocin

It is long acting analogue of oxytocin (half-life 85–100 min) which is heat stable. It is given in the dose of 100 µg I/M or I/V. It will be available in near future, but it is costly. It is recommended for treatment of PPH following vaginal delivery and at cesarean section. Its effect starts in 1–2 min and lasts for minimum 1 hour. Unlike oxytocin (and like ergometrine) it should not be used in patients with high blood pressure & cardiovascular diseases.

2. ERGOMETRINE

- It is an Amine alkaloid isolated from fungus, *Claviceps purpurea* which grows on rye.
- The drawback is that it causes tetanic contraction of whole of the uterus and closes the cervix
- Its effect starts: 10–15 minutes after oral administration, 3–5 minutes after I/M

Drugs

injection and 45–90 seconds after I/V administration.

It is available as:
- Injection methylergometrine maleate—0.2 mg/mL ampoule, e.g. methergine, utergin, lerine, mergox, etc.
- Injection ergometrine maleate 0.5 mg./mL as ergometrine.

Uses

- Prevention of PPH—as uterotonic in AMTSL. It is usually given I/M or I/V after the placenta has delivered
- Treatment of PPH. It is given I/M or I/V. It may be repeated at 2-4 hourly interval. I/V injection is given slowly over 1 minute
- During cesarean section after the baby is delivered
- Control of postabortal bleeding
- Suction MTP
- In hysterotomy.

Contraindications

- Kidney diseases
- Liver diseases
- Valvular heart diseases
- Hypertension
- Before the delivery of fetus

Adverse Effects

- Nausea, vomiting
- Sudden shoot up of blood pressure
- Peripheral vasospasm
- If given before delivery of fetus, it causes tetanic contraction of uterus, fetal death and rupture of uterus.

3. PARENTERAL IRON PREPARATIONS

Indications for Parenteral Iron Therapy

- Malabsorption syndrome –failure to absorb oral iron
- Intolerance to oral iron
- Patients with chronic bleeding where daily blood loss exceeds that of absorption from GI tract and stores are already depleted
- Noncompliance
- No response to oral iron in a confirmed case of iron deficiency anemia
- Contraindications to oral iron, i.e. inflammatory bowel disease.

Iron Sucrose

- It is FDA category B drug
- It is available as 50 mg/2.5 mL or 100 mg/5 mL ampoules
- It can be given undiluted I/V slowly 1 mL/min OR diluted 100 mg in/100 mL of normal saline and given I/V over 15 to 30 min
- It cannot be diluted in 5% dextrose as it is not stable in dextrose
- It cannot be given I/M because it has an alkaline pH, which can cause muscle damage
- Dose calculation is total iron = 2.4 x wt in kg x deficit of Hb in gm
- 500 mg (10 mg/kg) should be added for replenishment of stores
- As compared to iron dextran it is more safe, effective and well tolerated
- Test dose is not necessary. However some authorities still prefer to give it
- It is claimed that there is rapid rise of Hb than oral iron, i.e., after 1 week and also rapid buildup of iron stores
- Contraindications to I/V iron sucrose include iron overload, e.g., thalassemia, known hypersensitivity to iron-sucrose, severe infection, liver disease, acute renal failure and early pregnancy (up to 10 weeks)
- Maximum 200 mg per dose is given repeated up to three times a week.

Ferric Carboxymaltose

- It is newer formulation of parenteral iron
- Contains 50 mg/mL in 10 ml vial
- 1000 mg in 250 mL normal saline can be given over 15 minutes.

- Safety during pregnancy is not established as iron released can cross the placental barrier but it can be used postpartum.
- Side effects are nausea, dizziness, headache and hypertension.

Iron Dextran (Imferon)

- It is a compound of ferric hydrochloride and dextran in 0.9% NaCl solution
- It contained 50 mg elemental iron/mL of drug
- It was given intramuscularly or intravenously (diluted in normal saline as total dose imferorn - TDI) after test dose.

Side Effects of I/M

- Pain due to local inflammatory reactions
- Discoloration
- Injection abscess and lymphadenopathy
- Sarcoma in rats

Intravenous

Formula for total dose

$$\frac{0.66 \times \% \text{ deficit of Hb} \times \text{weight in kg}}{50}$$

$$= \text{mL of Imferon}$$

- To this 50% more is added for depleted stores
- To this 500 mg (10 mL) more is added for pregnancy.

Adverse Effects of TDI

Malaise, fever, thrombophlebitis at I/V site, lymphadenopathy, arthralgia, urticaria, exacerbation of rheumatoid arthritis, premature onset of labor. Iron intoxication if wrong diagnosis (e.g., hemoglobinopathy with excess iron).

Anaphylactic reactions and deaths have been reported.

Iron Sorbitol Citric Acid (Jectocos)

It contained 50 mg elemental iron per mL. It should be given I/M only.

Oral Iron

It is indicated in all mild and moderate iron deficiency cases. It is cheap, safe and effective in most of the cases.

- Different oral preparations are ferrous sulfate, ferrous fumarate, ferrous gluconate, ferrous ascorbate, sodium feredetate and ferrous bisglycinate chelate.
- Different iron salts with their elemental iron content is mentioned table in below:

Oral iron preparations

Salt	Tablet	Elemental iron
Ferrous sulfate	200 mg	60 mg (30%)
Ferrous fumarate	200 mg	66 mg (33%)
Ferrous gluconate	320 mg	36 mg (12%)
Ferrous succinate	100 mg	35 mg (35%)
Ferric ammonium citrate	125 mg	25 mg (17% –22)
Ferrous ascorbate	–	100 mg
IPC	–	100 mg
Carbonyl iron	–	90 mg
Sodium feredetate	–	231 mg

- Government of India (Ministry of Health and Family Welfare) has recommended at least 100 mg of elemental iron + 0.5 mg FA/day for 100 days to every pregnant woman in our country
- Ferrous salts are 3 times readily absorbed than ferric salts
- Ferrous sulfate is the cheapest and well absorbed form of iron
- Ferrous gluconate is well tolerated but it has low iron content (36 mg in 320 mg tablet)
- Ferrous fumarate is the most commonly used salt in commercial preparations
- Ferrous ascorbate is a synthetic molecule of ascorbic acid, iron and as ascorbate makes stable chelate with iron there is no dissociation in GI tract, so there is no action of food inhibitors. Also ascorbic acid reduces ferric iron to ferrous iron which is readily absorbable. Tablets

containing 100 mg elemental iron is available for use.
- *Carbonyl iron:* Newer market preparation contain this. Carbonyl refers to manufacturing process where iron is obtained by thermal decomposition of iron pentacarbonyl which when heated to above its boiling point decomposes to give iron and carbon monoxide. Iron thus obtained has high purity (> 98%), very fine spherical size (<5 U) and uniform particle size

  It is easily absorbed and less toxic than ionized forms of iron such as iron sulfate. It has a high safety range.
- *Sodium feredetate:* It contains ferric sodium EDTA. It contains iron in an unionized form. It is not astringent and does not discolors teeth. Its absorption is less affected by food inhibitors like phytates. It is also available as chewable tablet.
- *Ferrous bisglycinate chelate*: It is a chelated form of iron, where two molecules of amino acid glycine are bound to a molecule of iron. It does not cause gastric irritation and constipation. Absorption of bisglycinate is not affected by phytates in food.
- *IPC complex:* It is ferric hydroxide polymaltose complex. It is nonionic and it does not stain the teeth. There is no metallic taste and no interaction with food or other drugs. It is taken with food. Initially claimed high therapeutic results were not found in clinical practice.

4. MAGNESIUM SULFATE

It is usually available as 2 mL ampoules of 50% strength (1 gm/ampoule).

Uses

- As an anticonvulsant in eclampsia
- In severe pre-eclampsia to prevent eclampsia when labor is induced or cesarean section is planned
- As a tocolytic to arrest preterm labor
- Impending eclampsia
- For neuroprotection in very premature baby (<32 wks) it is given 1 gm/hour I/V for 24 hours just prior to delivery.

Mechanism of Action

- It exerts a rather specific anti-convulsant action on the cerebral cortex without producing generalized CNS depression
- Central action is more important than peripheral curariform action at the myoneural junction (i.e. decreases acetyl choline release in response to motor nerve impulses, reduces motor end-plate sensitivity to acetyl choline and decreases the motor end-plate potential)
- It is believed to decrease intracranial edema and enhance diuresis
- It has got direct depressant action on the uterine muscle (tocolytic effect)
- The exact mechanism of action of magnesium as a neuroprotective agent is unknown. A number of biologically actions are suggested. Magnesium sulfate may reverse the harmful effects of hypoxic/ischemic brain injury by blocking NMDA receptors, acting as a calcium antagonist.

Protection against free radical activity, vasodilatation, vascular stability and antiapoptotic activity are other suggested mechanisms.

Dose: It is given both by I/V & I/M routes.

Pritchard Regimen

- 4 gm as 20% solution I/V slowly at the rate of 1 gm/min.
- Immediately followed by 10 gm as 50% solution deep I/M one half (10 mL) in each upper quadrant of both buttocks with 1 mL 2% lignocaine. If convulsions persist after 15 min give 2 gm more as 20% solution I/V slowly.

  If convulsions still persist, give I/V pentothal.
- Repeat 5 gm $MgSO_4, 7H_2O$ every 4 hourly intramuscularly after checking urine output, knee jerk and respiration.

Zuspan Regimen

4 gm I/V initially as 20% solution slowly, over 10 min followed by 1 gm/hour I/V in drip form after checking urine output, knee jerk and respiration. Continuous slow I/V administration gives better control of fits. For proper administration infusion pump must be used.

In Sibai modification the initial dose is 6 gm in 20 min followed by 2 gm/hour I/V.

Monitoring

Before repeating or continuing the dose see that:
- Deep reflexes are present
- Respiration is not depressed, rate should be above 14/min
- Urine output must exceed 100 mL in 4 hours.

Toxicity

- Ideal plasma level 6–8 m Eq/L
- Respiratory paralysis 12–15 m Eq/L
- Cardiac conduction affected >15 m Eq/L.

It can cross the placenta but does not harm the fetus. Newborn infant may be depressed only if severe hypermagnesemia exists at delivery.

Antidote

Calcium gluconate or calcium chloride 1 gm (10 mL 10% I/V).
- $MgSO_4$ should be given up to 24 hours after delivery or after last convulsion whichever is later
- Occasionally transient fall in BP may occur within first hour of administration but otherwise an antihypertensive agent must be used along with it for control of BP.
- Use for tocolysis: 4–6 gm loading dose initially as 20% solution over 20 minutes, then continued in I/V drip 1–2 gm/hr. It is continued for at least 12 hours after cessation of contractions.

- For eclampsia various low dose regimes and single dose regimes are suggested for Asian Women with lower BMI & found effective. These are VIMS regimen, Dhaka regimen, Sardesai S, et al., and others.

5. ISOXSUPRINE

- Nonselective beta-adrenergic stimulant drugs.
- It works by binding to beta-2 adrenergic receptors on uterine smooth muscles which results in relaxation of uterine myometrium.

It is available as Duvadilan, Tidilan, Suprox, etc.

Use

It is used in the treatment of premature labor to arrest uterine contractions as tocolytic agent.

Dose

100 mg (10 ampoules) are injected in 500 cc of 5 % glucose or glucose saline and I/V drip is started at the dose of 0.2 mg/min (16 drops/min) increasing slowly up to 0.8 mg/min (64 drops/min) I/V drip is continued for at least 4 hrs after the contractions cease.

In practice lower initial dose, i.e. 40 mg (4 ampoules) instead of 100 mg I/V is used. Then 10 mg I/M is given 6 hourly for 24–48 hours. Then orally 10 mg is given 6–8 hrly up to 37 completed weeks.

Long-term tocolytics although commonly practiced is not supported by evidence based medicine.

Contraindications

- Tachycardia of more than 120 beats per min
- Positive fluid balance
- Chronic cardiac disease
- Chorioamnionitis
- Dead or severely malformed fetus

- Along with MAO inhibitors
- Concomitant use of steroids.

Side Effects

- Maternal tachycardia, hypotension, palpitation are common side effects, there may be transient dizziness, weakness, nausea, sweating and headache. Acute pulmonary edema can occur after prolonged administration. Hyperglycemia and due to it, hypokalemia are also found.
- In neonate it may cause transient hypoglycemia (due to hyperinsulinemia), hypokalemia and hypotension.

Other tocolytic drugs include:
- Ritodrine
- Salbutamol
- Terbutaline
- Orciprenaline
- $MgSO_4$
- Atosiban
- Calcium channel blockers
- Prostaglandin inhibitors

6. RITODRINE

It is a sympathomimetic drug which is preferentially active on beta-2 receptors, so it is a good tocolytic drug, with minimum β1 activity as compared to other tocolytics.

It was available as injection Yutopar or utodine 5 mL ampoule containing 10 mg per mL and tablet Yutopar, Utodine, Ritord containing 10 mg ritodrine hydrochloride.

Uses

1. As a tocolytic to arrest preterm labor.
2. Prevention of preterm labor after surgical operations.
3. Acute fetal distress in labor.

Dose

Intravenous Injection

Initially 50 µg (0.05 mg) per minute is started, then increased by 0.05 mg every 10–15 min. until contractions have ceased or maternal heart rate reaches 130 or other side effects appear. Do not exceed 0.35 mg/minute dose.

Continue treatment for 12–48 hours after contractions stop. The diluent fluid should be 5% glucose (except in diabetes).

Oral Therapy

1 tablet every 2 hourly for first 24 hours, starting 20 min before I/V infusion is stopped. Then after 1–2 tablet every 4–6 hours. Maximum daily dose is 120 mg/day.

Mechanism of Action

It binds to beta-2 receptors on uterine smooth muscle activating the enzyme adenyl cyclase which leads to increase in CAMP. This inhibits myosin light chain kinase activity through direct phosphorylation and by lowering of the concentration of intracellular calcium.

Contraindications

- Cardiac disease
- Hyperthyroidism
- Antepartum hemorrhage
- Severe PIH, eclampsia
- Chorioamnionitis
- Severe IUGR
- Fetal death or lethal malformation
- Known hypersensitivity to any component of the product.

Side Effects

They are tachycardia, palpitation, nausea, vomiting, headache, tremor. Occasionally postural hypotension nervousness, restlessness, anxiety, hyperglycemia, hypokalemia, fluid retention. Rarely chest pain, tightness, ECG abnormalities, cardiac arrhythmias, pulmonary edema and death. Because of reports of deaths its clinical use in US has been discontinued.

Precautions

- Beta-blockers inhibit the action of ritodrine
- Anesthetics used in surgery may potentiate the hypotensive effect of ritodrine

- Corticosteroids used concomitantly may increase the risk of ritodrine (fluid retention - pulmonary edema, hyperglycemia).

7. PROSTAGLANDINS

Uses of prostaglandins for MTP are already discussed in Chapter 6. Other uses of PGs are as follows:

Pre-induction Cervical Ripening

Natural prostaglandin PGE-2 is used for cervical ripening. It can be used as endocervical gel or vaginal gel, vaginal pessaries or tablets to be inserted in the posterior fornix. Vaginal route due to higher dose leads to side effects like nausea, vomiting and fever. Endocervical route (gel) is currently favored.

Dinoprostone Gel (PGE-2)

Cerviprime gel or dinoripe gel are commercially available and contain 0.5 mg Dinoprostone (PGE-2). It is available in a prefilled syringe with a catheter. Under aseptic precautions the entire contents of the syringe is administered into the cervical canal just below the level of internal os. The patient is asked to remain supine for 30 minutes.

It is used for preinduction cervical ripening and dilatation in patients at or near term with unfavorable cervix (poor Bishop score). Complete effect occurs in 12 hours. If there is inadequate response after 8 hours, a repeat application may be done.

There are no absolute **contraindications** to the use of dinoprostone gel. However, it is not recommended in patients who are hypersensitive to PG and in whom, oxytocics are generally contraindicated. It should be used cautiously in patients of glaucoma and history of asthma.

The drug should be stored in a refrigerator between 2–8° C.

Its side effects include hyperstimulation of uterus with or without fetal distress and occasional nausea, vomiting and diarrhea. Its failure rate is less than 10%. Though dinoprostone gel is developed and used for cervical ripening, in practice it also induces labor > 50% of cases apart from ripening the cervix.

Induction of Labor

Induction of labor have increased many folds in recent times. Indications are:
- Post-term and post- date pregnancy
- Intrauterine fetal death
- PIH
- IUGR
- Congenital malformations
- Suspected placental insufficiency and oligohydramnios
- PROM
- Chronic hypertension, chronic renal disease
- Elective induction.

Dinoprostone Tablet

Primiprost tablet or PG tablet is an oral PGE-2 containing Dinoprostone 0.5 mg per tablet and used for induction or augmentation of labor.

It was started at a dose of one tablet every hour. After 3 to 4 hours the dose should be increased to two tablets every hour till uterine activity is established. Then, it may be reduced to one tablet per hour. If after 10 tablets labor has not been established the drug is discontinued.

Contraindications, precautions, storage and side effects of primiprost tablets are same as for dinoprostone gel.

Due to higher failure rate and better options available it is not much used now.

Pessary: Recently dinoprostone is available as controlled release vaginal pessary (propess). It is kept high in posterior fornix. It contain 10 mg or Dinaprostone and releases 0.3 mg/hour.

Recently tablet misoprostol is officially permitted for induction of labor. 25 µg vaginally every 4 hourly is the safe dose. It can be used orally as well as sublingually. Althouth

50 µg is more successful, it leads to fetal distress. Meconium stained liquor and traumatic PPH due to hyperstimulation and should be used with caution.

Post-partum Hemorrhage

PGs are successfully used in recent years for prevention and treatment of atonic PPH. They are effective irrespective of the cause of atonic PPH and when oxytocin, ergometrine or routine uterine massage have failed.

Carboprost (15(s)-15 methyl PGF-2α) tromethamine is available now as injection Prostodin 1 mL ampoule containing either 125 µg or 250 µg of the drug/mL inj. Deviprost, Endoprost and Cystos 250 µg/mL.

Prophylaxis of PPH

125 µg (0.5 mL) is given intramuscularly, at the birth of anterior shoulder. It can be used for routine third stage management as it is better than ergometrine and causes less elevation of blood pressure.

Treatment of PPH

250 µg is given intramuscularly stat and repeated every 20–90 minutes as necessary. Maximum 8 injections are recommended. However in practice after 3 doses surgical treatment is initiated rather than waiting for too long.

It is successful in 80–95% cases. Causes of failure include chorioamnionitis, undiagnosed laceration of genital tract (traumatic cause) and retained placental tissues.

Direct intramyometrial route is of special value only in patients (1) in shock, (2) at cesarean section, and (3) after internal iliac ligation, if atony and bleeding persists.

8. CERVICAL RELAXANTS

Valethamate

It is a quaternary ammonium compound with peripheral action same as atropine, i.e., anticholinergic.

It is given as 8 mg deep I/M or I/V injection. It can be repeated after 20–30 minutes if required. Maximum 3 injections can be given.

Side effects are anticholinergic, i.e. tachycardia, dry mouth, blurring of vision, urinary retention, etc.

It is **contraindicated** in patients with cardiac insufficiency, severe hypertension, thyrotoxicosis and glaucoma.

It is available as Epidosin, Valosin and Osdil 1 mL injections containing 8 mg of valethamate bromide/mL.

Drotaverine

It is an isoquinoline antispasmodic. It relieves smooth muscle spasm by correcting cyclic AMP and calcium imbalance at the spastic site. It is given as 40 mg (2 mL) I/M injection. It is available as Drotin. Like other drugs it is given after 3 cm dilatation and can be repeated after 3 hours if necessary. Rapid I/V injection can cause fall in BP, nausea and vertigo.

It can also be used as antispasmodic in dysmenorrhea and other colics.

Hyoscine Butyl Bromide

It is anticholinergic. It is given as 20 mg I/M injection and repeated once after 20 min if necessary. It is available as Buscopan 1 mL containing 20 mg. It has selective spasmolytic effect on the parasympathetic innervation of the cervical os. So there are no undesirable side effects like dryness of mouth, visual disturbances or change in BP.

Camylofin Hydrochloride (Anafortan)

Camylofin is a smooth muscle relaxant. It has both anticholinergic action as well as direct smooth muscle action. Single dose 2 mL (50 mg) is given I/M after 3 cm dilatation. It is potent antispasmodic and shortens labor by facilitating cervical dilatation.

Side effects (anticholinergic) are mild like dryness of mouth, dilatation of pupils, paralysis of accommodation and palpitations

9. RH-ANTI-D IMMUNOGLOBULIN (IgG)

- It is prepared from serum of immunized male volunteers or naturally immunized women with high titer of anti-D antibodies.
- It is available as **RhoGAM, Rhiggal, Partobulin** and monoclonal, **Rhoclone** 300 µg/vial injection.

Indications

It is given 300 µg I/M to Rh -negative mother in following cases to prevent sensitization:
- Delivery of Rh -positive fetus
- Abortion of more than 6 wks pregnancy (50 µg)
- Amniocentesis
- Cesarean section
- Ectopic pregnancy (50 µg)
- APH
- Manual removal of placenta.
    - It is **not given** to (1) Rh positive women, (2) already sensitized Rh- negative women, (3) when infant is Rh- negative, and (4) to the neonate
    - It should be given within 72 hours of the delivery preferably, but if 72 hours have passed, it should still be given as it may still be protective
    - 20–25 µg of drug protects against 1 mL of fetal blood
    - Actual amount of feto-maternal hemorrhage may be calculated and dose should be given accordingly.

Kleihauer – Betke test to calculate FMH:
A thin smear of maternal blood is subjected to acid and then stained. The fetal cells contain Hb that is resistant to acid and will remain dark. Maternal Hb is diluted by the acid and therefore cells will appear as ghosts. Under the microscope no. of cells are counted. Then volume of fetal hemorrhage is calculated as:

$$FMH = \frac{\text{No. of fetal cells} \times \text{maternal blood volume}}{\text{No. of maternal cells}}$$

Grossly 5 fetal cells in 5 low power fields indicate FMH of about 4 mL
- Instead of 300 µg lower doses may be given (i.e. 100 µg) after delivery, if exact FMH is calculated
- Drug is given deep I/M. Adverse reactions are uncommon and include local reaction at the site of injection and occasionally fever. Rarely anaphylaxis can occur.
- To overcome failures, prophylactic antenatal administration of 300 µg anti-D at 28 wks is suggested.
- Antibodies given to the mother act by neutralizing the fetal Rh-positive cells which enter the maternal circulation. They get fixed to the binding sites on RBCs which then cannot elicit immune response in mother and are rapidly removed by RE system.

10. DIAZEPAM

- It is available as Calmpose, Valium, Anxol.
- It is Benzodiazepine derivative
- It is effective after oral, I/M, or I/V use. It is metabolized in liver and it has long half life time of 18–90 hours
- It causes sedation, hypnosis, decreases anxiety and muscle relaxation. It also has anticonvulsant effect
- If affects activity at all levels of neuraxis, but anticonvulsant effects appears to be a direct depressant effect on the thalamus and hypothalamus
- Injection is available as 2 mL ampoules containing 5 mg drug per mL.

Uses

- In the treatment of eclampsia: It was previously used. On admission 20–40 mg injection Diazepam is given I/V slowly not exceeding 2.5 mg/min. Then slow I/V drip is started containing 40 mg Diazepam in 500 cc of 5% Glucose. Every 4–6 hourly injection Diazepam is repeated 20–40 mg direct I/V as necessary and drip is continued for 24 hours after delivery.

- To prevent eclampsia in case of severe preeclampsia any time, i.e. antepartum, intrapartum or immediately postpartum period. Magnesium sulfate is preferred.
- To relieve anxiety, e.g., in cardiac patient, in cases of APH, etc.
- As hypnotic to do minor surgical procedures which are done without anesthesia or done under local anesthesia only, e.g., D&E, MTP, etc.
- As preanesthetic medication.

Now **midazolam** is commonly used as sedative instead of diazepam.

Adverse Effects

- *Maternal:*
  - It has no major side effects. It causes drowsiness, lethargy and ataxia in the patient. Long-term use causes drug dependence.
  - It may cause paradoxical increase in irritability and anxiety.
- *Fetal and neonatal*
  - If more than 30 mg is given during labor it may produce neonatal hypotonia, hypothermia, apneic spells, low apgar scores and reluctance to feed known as "floppy baby syndrome" as it readily crosses the placenta and it has doubtful teratogenic (cleft lip) effect.
  - It causes loss of beat to beat variability in the fetal heart. This variability is an important parameter of fetal well-being.
  - Its sodium benzoate and benzoic acid buffer, both compounds are potent uncouplers of bilirubin - albumin complex so free circulating bilirubin is increased and may lead to kernicterus in newborn.
  - It is secreted in milk. Regular use of high dose by the mother may cause drowsiness, lethargy and failure to thrive in the newborn.

Midazolam

- It is benzodiazepine derivative used for same purpose as diazepam
- It is faster, shorter acting and 3 times more potent than diazepam
- I/M dose is 5 mg and I/V dose is 2.5 mg
- It is water soluble and less irritant to the veins than diazepam

11. FUROSEMIDE/FRUSEMIDE (LASIX)

- It is a very potent diuretic.
- It acts along the entire nephron except distal convoluted tubules. As the chief site of action is the loop of Henle, it is also called loop diuretic.
- It can be given by oral, I/M or I/V route.
- It has rapid onset and short duration of action. After I/V administration effect starts in 2 minutes but lasts for only 2–3 hours.
- It is excreted largely unchanged from the kidney in 4 hours.
- Inj. Lasix is available in 2–4 mL ampoules containing 10 mg/mL.

Uses

It is used in obstetrics in following conditions:
- Along with blood or packed cells transfusion in cases of severe anemia
- Pulmonary edema, e.g., in eclamptic patient
- Cardiac failure in cardiac disease or severe anemia
- Massive edema not relieved by conservative measures. A short course of diuretics may be given
- Impending acute renal failure in obstetrics.

Adverse Effects

- Because of potassium depletion (hypokalemia) it causes weakness, fatigue, dizziness and cramps
- It can cause orthostatic hypotension, it produces hyperuricemia and impaired glucose tolerance.
- Sudden deaths have been reported after its direct I/V use.
- With large doses it sometimes causes temporary or permanent deafness.

- In cases of PIH as it causes further reduction in already decreased maternal plasma volume, it leads to decrease in placental perfusion, which is hazardous to the already compromised fetus.
- It can cause thrombocytopenia and hyponatremia in the fetus.
- Fetal electrolyte imbalance by direct action as well as indirectly through mother.
- **Torasemide** (Dytor) and **Bumetanide** (Bumet) are the other diuretics of the same group now available. While Furosemide and Bumetanide are FDA category 'C' drug, Torasemide is category 'B' drug.

As compared to furosemide torasemide has more prolonged diuretic effect, less potassium loss and not found ototoxic. Bumetanide has more bioavailability than furosemide and it is more potent.

12. TETANUS TOXOID

It is prepared from tetanus toxin produced by *Clostridium tetani*. Refined toxin has been rendered nontoxic by treatment with formaldehyde (Formal toxoid) and is made more effective by adsorption on to an aluminum hydroxide or aluminum phosphate carrier (adsorbed toxoid).

Given to mother during pregnancy it produces active immunity in mother and passive immunity by placental transfer of antibodies in the fetus. Thus, it prevents both maternal and neonatal tetanus.

For primary immunization 0.5 mL adsorbed toxoid is given I/M in dose with the interval of 6 weeks between 1st and 2nd while 3rd dose is given 6-12 months after 2nd dose.

Schedule during pregnancy: As per WHO. In nonimmunized pregnant mother 0.5 mL TT I/M is given as follows:
- First dose—first visit (as early as possible)
- Second dose—4 weeks after first dose

If mother is adequately immunized in past (i.e. 3 doses in infancy and one booster dose in childhood) only one dose is required in the third trimester of pregnancy, preferably 4 weeks before the expected date of delivery. Because TT vaccination status may be unknown or incomplete, we routinely give 2 doses.

Adverse Reactions

They are uncommon, incidence is 1-2%

Local: Excessive pain, redness and swelling around the site of injection persisting for 3 to 4 days.

General: Urticaria with or without angioneurotic edema, frank serum sickness and peripheral neuropathy have been rarely reported. Severe allergic reactions occur in less than one in 1,00,000 individuals.

Tetanus Antitoxin and Immunoglobulin

Tetanus antitoxin is an anti-serum (ATS) obtained from horses actively immunized against tetanus antigen. As it is heterologous in origin there are chances of hypersensitivity as well as serum sickness type of reactions. It is given in the does of 1500–3000 IU I/M prophylactic and 50,000 to 1,00,000 therapeutic.

Tetanus immunoglobulin are prepared from human male volunteers or placenta of healthy mothers especially immunized against tetanus. It is available as 250, 500 or 1000 IU/vial.

Dose: 250–500 IU I/M for prophylaxis

Therapeutic-500–10000 IU I/M in tetanus neonatorum or in adults, 250 IU intrathecal

As compared to antitoxin it is more potent with longer duration of action and can be repeated as necessary.

It is indicated in obstetrics in unimmunized mothers and in tetanus neonatorum. Simultaneously, tetanus toxoid should be given for active immunization.

The Health Ministry has recently ordered to replace all tetanus toxoid by Td vaccines in pregnancy.

Indian Association of Pediatrics (IAP) suggests immunization of pregnant women with a single dose of Tdap (contain Tetanus, Diphtheria and pertussis) during the third trimester (preferred during 27 through 36 weeks gestation) regardless of number of years from prior Td or Tdap vaccination. Tdap has to be repeated in every pregnancy irrespective of the status of previous immunization.

13. SODIUM BICARBONATE

It is available as 8.4% or 7.5% sterile solution in 10 or 25 mL ampoules for intravenous injections. 1 mL of 8.4% solution contains 1.0 mEq of HCO_3, while that of 7.5% solution contains 0.9 mEq of HCO_3.

It is used in cases if electrolyte imbalance particularly to treat acidosis as it neutralizes H+ ion as follows:

$NaHCO_3 = Na^+ + HCO_3$
$HCO_3 + H^+ = H_2O + CO_2$

CO_2 formed in above reaction is eliminated from the body through respiration.

Uses

- Metabolic acidosis, e.g. in prolonged labor, obstructed labor, hyperemesis gravidarum, septicemia, diabetic coma, etc.
- The dose is calculated as follows:
- Amount of $NaHCO_3$ (mEq) required = 0.5 × body weight (kg) × (15 − serum bicarbonate level), e.g. 50 kg weighing patient with serum bicarbonate level of 7 mEq/L requires total 200 mEq of sodium bicarbonate.
- Renal failure in obstetrics in acidotic patient 100-150 mEq is usually added in slow I/V dextrose drip
- Asphyxia neonatorum 5 mL 8.4% solution diluted in equal amount of 5% glucose is injected slowly through umbilical vein to combat acidosis, only after respiration is established.
- Respiratory distress syndrome to correct acidosis the drug injected by diluting it in equal amount of 5% dextrose in the dose calculated as mEq of sodium bicarbonate required = 0.3 x base deficit x body weight (kg). 5-10 mL is usually required. It is repeated at 4-6 hourly intervals as necessary.

14. PETHIDINE (MEPERIDINE)

- It is synthetic narcotic analgesic 1/10th as potent as morphine as an analgesic on weight basis.
- It is available as 2 mL ampoules containing 50 mg of the drug per mL. It can be given direct I/M or I/V or in drip form.
- As it can cause drug addiction, it is not available freely. It is in the list of controlled substances under the NDPS Act. Special license is required for the doctor or hospitals for its use.

Uses

- *Obstetrics analgesia:* It was used in the past for labor analgesia. Apart from pain relief it causes rapid dilatation of the cervix. It can cause significant neonatal depression.
- Acute LVF, acute pulmonary edema.
- *Eclampsia:* Lytic cocktail therapy, i.e., Krishna Mennon's regimen (Not used now): On admission 100 mg pethidine and 25 mg chlorpromazine (largactil) in 20 mL of 5% glucose are given intravenously and 50 mg chlorpromazine + 25 mg promethazine (phenergan) are also given intramuscularly.

  An intravenous drip of 10% glucose containing 100 mg pethidine in 500 mL pint is started slowly at the rate of 20-30 drops per minute.

  Subsequently injection phenergan 25 mg I/M and injection largactil 50 mg I/M are given alternatively every 4 hourly up to 48 hours. If causes heavy sedation and does not control convulsions adequately, so it is not used since many years.

Magnesium sulfate is the drug of choice for eclampsia.
- It was used in past for preanesthetic medications, postoperative analgesia and as a sedative in obstetric patients with hemorrhage.

Side Effects
- Nausea, vomiting, tachycardia, sweating, euphoria, dizziness
- Respiratory depression
- Significant depression of respiration in the newborn if administered to mothers within 2 hours before child birth
- Drug addiction.

Contraindications
- Liver disease
- Kidney disease
- Diminished respiratory reserve
- Patients receiving MAO inhibitors or tricyclic antidepressants.
- *Antidote:* **Naloxone** (Narcan) in the dose of 0.01 mg/kg is injected into the umbilical vein of the depressed newborn.

Pentazocin (Fortwin)
- Pentazocine, is a benzomorphan derivative
- As analgesic it is about half as effective as morphine and also it has shorter duration of action
- It crosses the placental barrier rapidly, but to a lesser extent than pethidine.

As it is psychotropic substance, it is now not freely available on prescription. Only hospital with narcotic license can obtain from medical distributors and its usage is to be recorded in a register.

Uses
- Postoperative analgesia.
- As an analgesic for minor operations: Along with phenergan or diazepam it is used in many operations like D & C, D & E, MTP, Lap TL, abdominal TL done under local anesthesia.
- It is not used for pain relief in labor as it can cause hypertension and it decreases renal plasma flow.
- Preanesthetic medication.

Side Effects
- Respiratory depression
- Nausea, sweating, headache
- Sedation
- Tolerance, physical dependence.

Tramadol
- It is a centrally acting synthetic analogue of codeine
- It is one-tenth as potent as morphine in terms of analgesia.
- It has a lower affinity for opioid receptors and as it selectively acts on the µ receptors it causes less respiratory depression than other opioid analgesics
- It has very low abuse or dependence potential
- It is available as tramadol HCl 50 mg/100 mg per mL inj. e.g., tramazac, supridol.
- It is also available as 50 and 100 mg tab
- Maximum daily dose is 400 mg.

Uses
- In Ob-Gy it is used for postoperative pain after major surgery
- For labor analgesia 100 mg I/M is given in first- stage of labor.

Side Effects
It can cause sweating, dizziness, nausea, vomiting, dry mouth, fatigue, confusion, constipation.

15. PROMETHAZINE (PHENERGAN)
- Promethazine hydrochloride is a phenothiazine group antihistaminic agent

- It has antiemetic and sedative properties
- It increases respiratory rate so along with narcotic analgesic it can be helpful in controlling respiratory depression and vomiting
- It is available as 25 and 50 mg/mL solution 2 mL ampoules.
- It can be given I/M or I/V.

Uses

- Obstetrics analgesia—as an adjunct to narcotic analgesic because of its antiemetic and sedative properties.
- To control postoperative nausea and vomiting
- Preanesthetic medication
- Prevention of postoperative adhesions after pelvic surgery for infertility, e.g., tuboplasty
- Allergic reactions
- In lytic cocktail therapy for eclampsia it was used in past.

Side Effects

- Hypotension with large doses
- Sedation (when used for other indications).

16. METOCLOPRAMIDE (PERINORM)

- It is a potent antiemetic agent acting both centrally as well as locally
- By increasing lower esophageal sphincter pressure it prevents reflux esophagitis and heart burn
- It normalizes and coordinates the peristaltic movements in the stomach, duodenum and ileum
- Inhibiting prolactin inhibiting factor it increases the prolactin secretion
- It is available as 5 mg/mL 2 mL ampoules for I/M or I/V use.

Uses

- Hyperemesis gravidarum
- Control of postoperative nausea, vomiting and distension
- In emergency surgery when anesthesia is given on full stomach not only it prevents vomiting but, it also promotes gastric emptying.

Side Effects

It is relatively safe drug. It may cause drowsiness, dystonic reactions, methemoglobinemia and galactorrhea.

17. ONDANSETRON

- It is specific 5-HT_3 receptor antagonist
- It acts on 5-HT_3 receptors present peripherally on vagal nerve terminals and centrally in the chemoreceptor trigger zone
- It is a potent antiemetic
- It is available as 4 mg, 8 mg tablets and 2 mg/mL, 2 mL and 4 mL injections, e.g., Emeset, Osetron, Vomiz.

Uses

- It was developed to control vomiting induced by cancer chemotherapy and radiotherapy
- It is highly effective in postoperative nausea and vomiting. It is used preoperatively as well
- Vomiting during pregnancy. It is successfully used for excessive vomiting associated with early pregnancy as a second line of drug. Its safety in pregnancy is proved by studies (category 'B' drug).

Side Effects

It is generally well tolerated. It can cause headache, constipation, flushing and rarely allergic reactions. It does not cause sedation.

Use of ondansetron is associated with prolongation of QT interval, which can produce potentially fetal heart rhythm.

18. DRUGS FOR TREATMENT OF MALARIA

As per recent national guide lines drugs treatment for malaria is as follows:
- Presumptive treatment with chloroquine is no more recommended.
- Treatment is based on parasitological diagnosis. In nonavailability of timely microscopy or rapid diagnostic test, suspected malaria cases will be treated with full course of chloroquine, till the results of microscopy are received.

Acute Attack

- **Treatment of uncomplicated P. vivax cases:** Chloroquine (25 mg/kg wt) 4 tablets on day 1, 4 tablets on day 2 and 2 tablets on day 3 (Primaquine is given for 14 days to prevent relapse in nonpregnant patients).
- **Treatment of uncomplicated P. falciparum cases:** Artemisinin based combination therapy (ACT).
    - 1st trimester—Quinine 10 mg/kg 3 times/day for 7 days
    - 2nd trimester and 3rd trimester—Artesunate 4 mg/kg daily for 3 days and sulphadoxine 25 mg/kg, pyrimethamine 1.25 mg/kg on 1st day (Primaquine 0.75 mg/kg body weight is given on day 2 in nonpregnant patients).
- **Treatment of severe malaria cases:**
  Antesunate—2.4 mg/kg I/V or I/M at 0, 12 and 24 hours and then once a day; OR
  Artemether—3.2 mg kg I/M on admission then 1.6 mg/kg per day;OR
  Arteether—150 mg I/M daily for 3 day; OR
  Quinine—20 mg/kg on admission I/V (5 mg kg/hour) followed by maintenance dose 10 mg/kg 8 hourly.
  After parenteral artemisinin Rx patient should receive full course of oral ACT for 3 days.
  In Quinine 10 mg/kg oral tablets three times a day for 7 days.

Resistant malaria is suspected if within 72 hours patient does not respond clinically or parasitologically and there is no history of diarrhea or vomiting.

19. LOW MOLECULAR WEIGHT HEPARIN (LMWH)

LMWH are heparin salts having an average molecular weight of less than 8000 Da. They are obtained by various methods of fractionation or depolymerization of Heparin.

Uses

- Recurrent pregnancy loss due to anti phospholipid antibody syndrome (APS). It is started as soon as the pregnancy test is positive
- History of thromboembolic events
- Known case of hereditary thrombophilia.

Dose

Enoxaparin (Lonopin) 40 mg subcutaneously daily. **Dalteparin** 5000 U SC daily. Therapeutic dose is twice a day.

Side Effects

- Bleeding, Monitoring of LMWH is done by mensuring antifactor Xa level. 0.5 of 1.2 IU/mL is adequate for therapeutic purpose
- Protamine sulfate does not fully reverse the effects of LMWH. It requires blood components to treat the overdose.
- It is contraindicated in patients who are allergic to the drug, who have active major bleeding and in patients with kidney disease.
- It does not cross placenta like heparin and it is administered from confirmation of pregnancy (intrauterine) till term. After 36 weeks it can be changed to heparin, which is stopped as soon a labor starts.
- As compared to UF heparin
    - It has long half- life
    - Increased bioavailability
    - Less risk of bleeding

- Less risk of osteoporosis
- Less risk of thrombocytopenia
- No need of monitoring (prophylactic dose).

20. STEROIDS – HYDROCORTISONE, DEXAMETHASONE

- These are glucocorticoids. Hydrocortisone is a natural one, while dexamethasone is synthetic preparation
- Both these have number of pharmacological actions on different systems of the body. Important actions for Ob-Gy purpose are strong anti-inflammatory, anti-allergic and anti-immunological actions.

Comparison of hydrocortisone (HCS) and dexamethasone (DMS):

	HCS	DMS (Dexona)
Therapeutic efficacy	1	16
Mineralocorticoid activity	Present	Absent
Plasma half-life (minutes)	80	300
Half-time of glucocorticoid	8–12	36–72

- Hydrocortisone is available as hydrocortisone hemisuccinate injection (Efcorlin) for I/M and I/V use. 133 mg of salt contains 100 mg of hydrocortisone
- Dexamethasone is available as dexamethasone sodium phosphate injection containing 4 mg of the salt per mL. It is also given by I/M or I/V route. It is available in 2 mL ampoules or bulbs.

Uses

Hydrocortisone

- *Anaphylactic shock:* 100–200 mg hydrocortisone is given I/V stat and repeated after 6 hours if necessary
- *Septic shock:* Large doses of hydrocortisone, i.e., 50–75 mg/kg/day is given I/V
- *Acute stressful conditions*: 100–200 mg I/V
- *Mendelson's syndrome*: 200–400 mg I/V

- *During microsurgery:* In a point of ringer lactate 100 mg hydrocortisone with 5000 units heparin are added and constant irrigation is done to keep the tissues moist and prevent postoperative adhesions
- *Hydrotubation:* Postoperatively after tuboplasty. It has very few advocates at present.

Dexamethasone

- **To enhance lung maturity:** In preterm pregnancies between 26 to 34 weeks, injection dexona is given 6 mg I/M 6 hourly 4 doses. Effect starts after 24 hours of initiation of treatments and reaches peak at 48 hours. Instead, inj. **Betamethasone (Betnesol)** is given in doses 12 mg/IM twice, 24 hours apart. In past repeat courses were given every 7 days, but this is not done now as it leads to fetal IUGR and brain damage
- *Rescue dose:* Second course may be given just before delivery or CS, if more than 2 weeks have passed after first dose. Recently, it has been advocated to give till 36 weeks of pregnancy or even after that in elective cesarean section.
- *Cerebral edema:* Inj. dexona 8–12 mg is given I/V and repeated 6 hourly as necessary
- **Postoperatively in microsurgery:** To prevent adhesions, injection dexona is given 8 mg 8 hourly for 24 hours along with injection phenergan and the dose is tapered in next 2 days.

Side Effects

Toxic effects are related to individual susceptibility, dosage and duration of therapy. Single large doses of short-term therapies as required for Ob-Gy purpose are harmless. Its adverse reactions on long-term use include, acute gastritis with hemorrhage, peptic ulceration, hypertension, precipitation of diabetes, spread or aggravation of infection, osteoporosis and fractures, proximal myopathy, acute psychotic reactions.

Precautions

Except Cushing syndrome there is no absolute contraindications, relative contraindications include TB, other infections, peptic ulcer, diabetes, hypertension.

21. LIGNOCAINE (LIDOCAINE)

- It is the most commonly used local anesthetic agent
- It can be stored at room temperature and can be autoclaved repeatedly
- It has a rapid onset of action and as local anesthetic its effect lasts for 30 to 60 minutes. Its duration of action can be doubled by adding very dilute adrenaline (vasoconstrictor) to it
- Maximum safe dose is 200 mg, i.e., 20 mL of 1% solution.

Uses

- It is used for local infiltration as 0.5 to 1% solution for lap TL, abdominal TL, episiotomy, and resuturing of wound gap
- *Paracervical block:* For D & C, MTP, D & E, hysteroscopy and for pain relief in labor
- *Pudendal block:* For low forceps, vacuum extraction and assisted breech delivery
- The drug without preservative is used as antiarrhythmic for ventricular arrhythmia. It is available as Xylocaine, Lidocaine 1% or 2% 20 mL vial and 5% (heavy) 2 mL ampoule.

Side Effects

- It is safe drug. Allergic reactions rarely occur.
- Systemic absorption leads to CNS stimulation and cardiovascular effects. Convulsions after direct I/V injection and sudden death are also reported.

Bupivacaine

- It is amine, amide group local anesthetic marketed as Marcaine, Sensorcaine
- As compared to lignocaine it has slower onset of action but anesthetic effects lasts for longer time. Its half-life in adults is 2.7 hours.

Uses

- It is used for local regional anesthesia. It is now commonly used for obstetrics and gynecology major surgeries performed under spinal anesthesia as 0.5% solution of bupivacaine hydrochloride
- 0.125 to 0.250% dilution is used along with fentanyl for obstetric analgesia (painless labor) by lumbar epidural catheter.

Side Effects

- Adverse drug reactions are rare when it is correctly administered
- Systemic exposure results in CNS and cardiovascular effects
- It is more cardiotoxic than other local anesthetics.

22. ATROPINE

- It is a Belladonna alkaloids which blocks the muscarinic effects of both endogenous as well as externally administered acetylcholine, so it is parasympatholytic in nature
- It is available as 0.6 mg/mL atropine sulfate 1 mL ampoule. It can be given I/M or I/V.

Uses

- As preanesthetic medication before minor or major surgery, e.g., hysterectomy, D & C, TL, MTP, etc.

  It is given 0.6 mg I/M 1/2 hour before operation. Due to its parasympatholytic action it prevents reflex bradycardia and hypotension induced by vagal stimulation.

It also reduces salivary and respiratory secretions.
- Severe bradycardia.

Contraindications

- Congestive heart failure
- Chronic lung diseases.

Glycopyrrolate is synthetic anticholinergic agent. It is used before surgery to reduce salivary, tracheobronchial, and pharyngeal secretions, as well as decreasing the acidity of gastric secretion. It blocks cardiac vagal inhibitory reflexes during induction of anesthesia and intubation. It is also used in conjunction with neostigmine, a neuromuscular blocking reversal agent, to prevent neostigmine's muscarinic effects such as bradycardia..

Glycopyrronium blocks muscarinic receptors, thus inhibiting cholinergic transmission. Glycopyrrolate, being about twice as potent as atropine in the clinical situation and it is associated with a more stable cardiovascular system, fewer arrhythmias and better control of oropharyngeal secretions at the time of reversal. Glycopyrrolate inj 1 mL contains 0.2 mg. It is given intramuscular (I/M) or intravenous (IV).

Side Effects

Hyperthermia, dry mouth, headache, difficulty in micturition, diarrhea and constipation.

23. HORMONES IN GYNECOLOGY

Estrogens

They are naturally occurring steroidal sex hormones with 18 carbon atoms. They are produced in the body by the ovary, adrenal gland and by the placenta during pregnancy. Estradiol is the most active estrogen produced in the body. It is metabolized to form estrone and estriol mainly in the liver. Estradiol is 10 times more potent than estrone and 25 times than estriol. Natural estrogens given orally are rapidly metabolized in the liver and so they are ineffective. Synthetic compounds can be used orally and have replaced the natural products.

Preparations for Clinical Use

- *Conjugated estrogen:* Premarin tablet 0.625 mg, 1.25 mg 20 mg/5 mL injection.
- *Ehinyl estradiol:*
  - Lynoral 0.01 mg, 0.05 mg tablet
  - In oral pills: 0.02 to 0.05 mg with different progestogen
- *Estriol:* Evalon 1.0 and 2.0 mg tablet
- *Estradiol valerate:* 10 mg/1 mL Progynon Depot I/M inj.
- *Estradiol benzoate:* 1.0 mg along with estradiol phenyl propionate and testosterone in inj. Mixogen
- *Dienesterol:* 0.01% topical cream for vaginal application
- *Estradiol pellets:* Subcutaneous implants 25, 50, 100 mg.

Uses

- *Contraception:* 20 or 35 µg ethinyl estradiol is commonly used in currently available low dose and phasic pills.
- *Menopause:*
  - Menopausal symptoms: To control hot flushes, sweating, depression, insomnia, etc. Lynoral 0.01 mg, Premarin 0.625 mg or Evalon 2 mg daily for 3 wks with one week rest is advocated
  - Postmenopausal osteoporosis: Estrogen is useful in prevention and treatment of osteoporosis. Premarin 0.625 mg tablet is given daily
  - Senile vaginitis, Dyspareunia: **Dienestrol** cream is used

  In recent times SERMs and Tibolone are more used in menopausal patients.
- *AUB:* High doses are required for the acute episode, while cyclical therapy by OC pills is given for at least 3 months
- *Menstrual problems:* Estrogens in OC pills are commonly used for (1) primary

dysmenorrhea, (2) regularization of cycles, and (3) postponement or advancement of cycles
- *Amenorrhea:* In primary and secondary amenorrhea estrogen—progesterone challenge test for investigating the cause and for cyclical therapy to have cyclical bleeding if necessary
- *Endometriosis:* OC pills as pseudo-pregnancy treatment
- *Hypogonadism* to stimulate secondary sexual characters
- *Vulvovaginitis* in young children
- *Acne* vulgaris and **hirsutism**
- *Asherman syndrome* after breaking the adhesions to stimulate the endometrial growth
- Low dose estrogen is used along with clomiphene in infertility cases to counter the antiestrogenic effects on cervical mucous and endometrium however there is no strong scientific evidence.

Side Effects

Nausea, vomiting, painful breast, water retention, weight gain, impaired glucose tolerance, growth of fibroid, breast carcinoma, endometrial carcinoma, gallbladder disease, thromboembolic disease, coronary disease and cerebrovascular disease.

Progestogens

Progestogens are a class of steroids that bind to or activate progesterone receptors. Progesterone is a natural steroid with 21 carbon atoms. It is mainly produced by corpus luteum from the ovary and during pregnancy from placenta. Adrenal contributes to very little amount. It is metabolized in liver. Natural micronized and synthetic progestogens are useful orally for clinical use.

Progestogens are divided in following groups:
1. Natural progesterone
2. Derivatives of progesterone

i. *Derivatives of progesterone (C-21) Pregnane progestogens:*
   - 17 alpha hydroxyl progesterone caproate
   - Medroxypogesterone acetate
   - Chlormadinone acetate
   - Stereoisomer of progesterone—Dydrogesterone

ii. *Derivatives of 19 testosterone (C-18):*
   a. Estrane steroids:
      - Norethisterone
      - Norethisterone acetate
      - Norethynodrel
      - Allylestrenol
   b. Gonane steroids:
      - Norgestrel (dl-norgestrel)
      - Levonorgestrel

      Newer Gonanes:
      - Desogestrel
      - Gestodene
      - Norgestimate

Preparations for Clinical Use

- *Progesterone:* Natural micronized progesterone as 100, 200, 300 and 400 mg soft capsule or 50 and 100 mg I/M injection, e.g. Susten, Hernmp, Naturogest.
- *17 α HPC:* Proluton depot 250–500 mg I/m injection
- *Medroxyprogesterone acetate:* Modus, Meprate, Deviry tablets 5–10 mg, DMPA injection 150 mg/mL (Depot provera)
- *Dydrogesterone:* Duphastone tablet 5 mg.
- *Norethisterone:* Primolut-N, Sysron tablet 5 mg
- *Norethisterone acetate:* Regestrone tablet 5 mg
- *Lynestrenol:* Orgametril tablet 5 mg.
- *Norgestrel (dl-norgestrel) Levonorgestrel:* In oral pills 0.5 mg
- *Allylestrenol:* Gestanin, Fetugard, Gravidin 5 mg tablets.

Uses

- *Contraception:* Along with estrogen in oral pills different progestogens are used.

Only progestogens are used in minipill, injectable contraceptives and implants.
- *AUB:* Primolute-N, Regestrone, Orgametril, Meprate are used 10–20 mg oral for 5–10 days in acute episode and then after, in last 10–14 days of each cycle 5–10 mg per day is given for 6 months.
- *Infertility due to luteal phase defect*: Natural micronized progesterone is used—it is used through oral or vaginal route and I/M injections. Vaginal route is preferred unless there is bleeding. Due to direct vaginal absorption and hepatic bypass it gives better blood levels and better results. It is used in the dose of 200 to 300 mg/day from 16th day of cycle for 10 days
- *Threatened abortion:* Habitual abortion—as mentioned above. As compared to synthetic progesterone natural micronized progesterone has better bioavailability and minimal side effects
- *Dysmenorrhea:* Duphaston 5 mg twice or thrice a day from 5th to 25th day of cycle. Instead of cyclical oral pills this may be given for 6 months
- *Premenstrual tension:* Duphaston, Primolut-N, orgametril, etc., 10 mg bid from 15th to 26th day of cycle; OR cyclical oral pills
- *Endometriosis:* 1. With oral pills as pseudopregnancy treatment, 2. tablet Meprate 30 mg per day for 6 months (c) Newer progestogen Gestrinone (R-2323) 2.5 mg orally twice weekly or Dienogest 2 mg daily
  - Endometrial hyperplasia: Adenomatous hyperplasia – Oral pills for 6 months. Atypical hyperplasia –Injection Depot provera 100 mg/wk; OR Injection proluton 500 mg/wk.
- *Endometrial carcinoma:* For treatment of endometrial carcinoma large doses of progesterone are used
- *Primary or secondary amenorrhea:* Progesterone challenge test- any of the synthetic oral tablet is used 10 mg for 5 days; OR Natural injection progesterone 50 mg I/m for 2 days
- *Postponement of menses:* Any oral tablet is given 5–10 mg daily at least 4–6 days before expected date. Menses can be safely postponed for maximum of 15 days. Period starts 2–3 days after stopping the drug
- *Uterine hypoplasia:* Proluton depot I/M is given after pretreatment with progynon, weekly I/M for 8 wks
- *Fibrocystic disease of breasts:* Provera, Dubogen 10–20 mg is used
- *Precocious puberty:* MPA is found useful in the treatment of precocious puberty in children.

Side Effects

Nausea, vomiting, diarrhea, water retention, weight gain, break through bleeding, amenorrhea, hypertension, masculinization of female fetus, deep vein thrombosis and pulmonary embolism.

Gonadotropins

There are 2 gonadotropic hormones secreted from the anterior pituitary, i.e., follicle stimulating hormone (FSH) and luteinizing hormone (LH). Gonadotropins available for human therapy are:
1. *Human menopausal gonadotropin (HMG, Menotropin)*: It is prepared from urine of postmenopausal women
2. *Human chorionic gonadotropin (hCG)*: It is prepared from urine of pregnant women.

Preparations for Clinical Use

- *Menotropins (HMG)*: It is a combination of FSH and LH in equal amount, i.e., 75 IU each per mL of ampoule. Preparations available are *Menogon, Gonotrop-M*,etc.
- *Chorionic gonadotropin:* It has a predominantly luteinizing action. Preparation available are *Corion* (1000, 2000, 5000, 10000, IU), *Pregnyl* (1500, 5000 IU), *Hucog, Ovutrig. Fertigyn,* etc. Highly

purified (HP) hCG injections are now available
- *Urofollitropin:* It provides pure FSH 75.0 IU/mL of drug (amount of LH is negligible < 1.0%)

Metrodin HP is highly purified FSH preparation.

Now, recombinant FSH preparation are available, e.g., Gonal F which are highly purified which can be administered subcutaneously (75–150 IU). It is purified by using monoclonal antibodies to FSH.

Human Menopausal Gonadotropins (HMGs)

Uses
- For induction of ovulation in than ovulatory infertile patient and who fail to respond to clomiphene citrate or letrozole therapy
- Luteal phase defect in cases with defective follicle ripening and consequent corpus luteum insufficiency if other treatments have failed
- Controlled hyperstimulation to produce multiple ovulation for assisted reproductive techniques (ART) like IVF-ET, ICSI
- Unexplained infertility
- For stimulation of spermatogenesis in men who have primary or secondary hypogonadotropic hypogonadism.

For induction of ovulation 75–150 IU are started daily from day 2 of spontaneous cycle and day 5 of induced cycles for 3–4 days. Monitoring is done by noting the growth of the follicles and no. of follicles growing on USG and measuring serum levels of estradiol (E2) daily. The dose may be increased to stimulate the growth of the follicle. Non-responding patients may require high dose of 4–6 ampoules per day. 5000–10000 IU hCG is administered when the follicle has reached 18–19 mm size and serum E2 concentration is 300 pg/mL.

In male HMG is administered 1 ampoule (75 IU) three times a week for 4 months, only after pretreatment with hCG.

Contraindications
- Pituitary tumor
- Primary ovarian failure
- Thyroid or adrenal dysfunction
- Infertility due to other factor
- Ovarian enlargement other than PCOD
- Pregnancy
- Abnormal uterine bleeding of unknown origin
- In males it is contraindicated in testicular tumor and elevated gonadotropins suggesting primary testicular failure.

Human Chorionic Gonadotropin (hCG)

Uses
- Anovulatory infertility– 5000–10000 IU is given one day after the last dose of menotropin when follicle size on USG and serum E2 levels are optimum
- Corpus luteum insufficiency up to 3 repeat injections of 5000 IU are given within 9 days following the 1st injection
- Recurrent pregnancy loss (RPL) – 5000 to 10000 IU are used twice or thrice a week for up to 14 weeks
- Along with HMG for controlled hyperstimulation for assisted reproductive techniques and in cases of unexplained infertility
- In male patient with (1) hypogonadotropic hypogonadism– hCG 2000 IU/wk, and (2) cryptorchidism– hCG 1000 IU/wk for 8 wks.

Contraindications
- Precocious puberty
- Prostatic carcinoma (male) or other androgen dependent tumor
- Prior allergic reactions to hCG.

Adverse reactions to HMG/hCG therapy
- Ovarian hyperstimulation syndrome (OHSS)
  - *Grade I (Mild hyperstimulation):* Includes patients with variable ovarian enlargement and sometimes small cysts.
  - *Grade II (Moderate hyperstimulation):* Includes patients with ovarian

enlargement along with symptoms like abdominal distension, nausea, vomiting, diarrhoea and weight gain. Hospitalization is advisable.
- *Grade III (Severe hyperstimulation):* Includes patients with large ovarian cysts, ascites and sometimes hydrothorax.

Although mild hyperstimulation is common, severe variety rarely occurs, i.e. 4%. With proper monitoring OHSS can be prevented in most of the patients. If the follicle growth is more, number of follicles are more and estrogen level rises more than double for more than 2 consecutive days or reaches 2000 pg/mL HMG should be stopped and hCG should not be given. With newer **assisted reproductive technology** (ART) and better monitoring OHSS is less now.

- Rupture of ovarian cyst with hemoperitoneum
- Multiple births – 15 to 40% of cases
- Torsion of ovary can also occur
- Skin rashes, headache, restlessness and fatigue may rarely occur.

Gonadotropin Releasing Hormone (GnRH)

Gonadotropin releasing hormone (GnRH) is a decapeptide synthesized by neurones within the median basal and preoptic area of the hypothalamus. It is secreted in a pulsatile fashion and it has a plasma half-life of few minutes only. It stimulates the gonadotropic cells of anterior pituitary to produce luteinizing hormone and follicle stimulating hormone.

GnRH analogues are of 2 type: (1) Agonists, and (2) antagonists.

Agonists

They are synthesized by amino acid substitution at position 6, 9 or 10 of GnRH molecule. This increases the potency and duration of action. Plasma half-life of different agonists varies from 35 min to 5 hours. Different agonists in clinical use include: (1) leuprolide, (2) buserelin, (3) nafarelin, (4) goserelin, (5) triptorelin, (6) histrelin.

GnRH agonists cause initial flare-up effect resulting in increased FSH and LH levels. After 1-3 weeks of administration it results in down regulation and desensitization of pituitary leading to hypogonadotropic hypogonadal state.

Downregulation means chronic exposure to agonist induces a loss of pituitary GnRH receptors.

Desensitization means the inability of the pituitary to respond to any residual natural GnRH.

Preparations available:
- Triptorelin 3.75 mg (Decapeptyl) depot and 0.1 mg I/M daily
- Leuprolide depot (Lupride, Leuprodex) 3.75 mg I/M and 11.25 mg I/M
- Goserelin (Zoladex) 3.6 mg SC.

Clinical uses: Due to complete inactivation in gut parenteral routes (i.e., intramuscular, subcutaneous and intranasal) are used for administration.
- *Assisted reproduction:* It is used for pituitary downregulation prior to ovulation induction. This not only increases the pregnancy rates but also decreases the incidence of OHSS
- Endometriosis—monthly for 3-6 months as sole therapy or as an adjunct to surgery
- Fibroids (prior to surgical treatment)—monthly for 3-4 months
- Central precocious puberty
- Menorrhagia as a therapeutic treatment or endometrial thinning prior to ablation.

Side effects: Hypoestrogenic side effects like vasomotor symptoms, vaginal dryness, mood changes and most important osteoporosis. Due to this, long-term use for > 6 months is never indicated. To prevent this add back therapy by estrogen progesterone combined preparation or tibolon (synthetic steroid) is indicated.

Antagonists

They can produce immediate therapeutic effects by producing a decline in gonadotropin levels. Cetrorelix is now available as cetrotide 0.25 mg and 3 mg SC injection. Its advantage over agonist is that there is no initial flare-up.

24. CLOMIPHENE CITRATE

It is a nonsteroidal triphenylethylene compound with potent antiestrogenic and weekly estrogenic action. It is rapidly absorbed orally and metabolized in liver.

Mechanism of Action

It interferes with hypothalamic or pituitary cytosol estrogen receptor binding, blocking estrogen feedback and leading to increasing levels of serum gonadotropins. The increased FSH and LH acts on ovary and brings about follicular growth and ovulation. It's is direct effect on ovarian steroidogenesis is also suggested.

Uses

- In female patients with anovulatory infertility to bring about ovulation who have potentially functional **hypothalamic-pituitary-ovarian** axis and who have adequate endogenous estrogen
- Ovulation induction in cases of PCOD
- In male patients with oligozoospermia.

Method of Administration

- It is started from 2nd or 3rd day of period and is given in 50 mg daily dose for 5 days.
- Response is checked by detecting ovulation either clinically or by hormonal assay or commonly by serial USG examination.
- If ovulation does not occur the dose may be increased to 100 mg for 5 days in the subsequent cycle. Dosage may be increased to 150 mg/day maximum. Also in resistant cases 50 mg for 10 days can be tried. If ovulation is occurring, but there is no pregnancy for 6 months, therapy should be discontinued.
- To improve the ovulation rate clomiphene may be combined with injection hCG (5000 IU I/M when the follicle is 18–20 mm on USG) or with dexamethasone tablet (for suppression of androgens) or bromocriptine (in cases of hyperprolactinemia)
- In male patients 25 mg is given daily for 24 days with 6 days rest in every month for 3–6 months to stimulate spermatogenesis.

Preparations available: Clomiphene citrate is available as 50 and 100 mg tablets, e.g., Fertyl, Fertomid, Ovofar, Siphene, Mature ova and 25 mg tablets for use in male patients, e.g., Fertyl-m, Siphene-M, Clofert.

Contraindications

- Liver diseases
- Abnormal uterine bleeding of unknown origin
- Pregnancy
- Neoplastic diseases of genital tract
- Ovarian cyst other than PCOD

Success rate: Ovulation 70–80%, pregnancy rate 40–50%

Adverse Reactions

- *Hyperstimulation:* It occurs infrequently with clomiphene as compared to gonadotropins and mainly it is found in cases of PCOD.
- Multiple pregnancy
- Increased incidence of abortion
- Hot flushes
- Abdominal discomfort
- Blurring of vision
- Luteal phase defect
- *Miscellaneous:* Breast tenderness, vertigo, allergy.

Enclomiphene: It is trans- stereoisomer of clomiphene. As compared to clomiphene it is short acting, improves cervical mucous and endometrial thickening (No antiestrogenic effect). It is given in the same way as clomiphene and side effects are also same.

Tamoxifen: 20 mg for 4 days from day 2–5. Increase the dose to 40 mg and maximum 80 mg/day can be given. Side effects include fluid retention, hot flushes, pruritus, vaginal bleeding and ↑↑ tendency to thromboembolic effects.

Letrozole: It is 3rd generation aromatase inhibitor compound. It inhibits cytochrome P 450 enzyme. It affects final conversion of androgen to estrogen.
- If was banned in October 2011 as research has shown that babies born to mothers who has consumed letrozole have suffered from bone malformations, cardiac stenosis and cancers.
- The most common side effects are sweating, hot flashes, arthralgia (joint pain), and fatigue
- In 2017 after ICMR recommendation from systemic review and meta-analysis the Government revoked the ban and allowed it for insuction of ovulation in anovulatory infertility
- It is used in the dose of 2.5 mg/day from 2nd to 6th day.
- As compared to clomiphene it has no negative effect on endometrium and cervical mucous
- It is the drug for treatment of postmenopausal women with metastatic breast cancer.

25. BROMOCRIPTINE

It is a semisynthetic ergot alkaloid. It has potent dopamine receptor agonistic action. It inhibits the secretion of the anterior pituitary hormone prolactin without affecting other hormones. It is available as 2.5 mg tablet of bromocriptine as mesylate, e.g., Parlodel, Sicriptin, Proctinal, B-crip, etc. Also available as 1.25 mg tablet, e.g. Proctinal 1.25.

Uses

- Suppression of puerperal lactation
- Pathological hyperprolactinemia causing galactorrhea with or without amenorrhea
- Prolactin induced female infertility – anovulation, luteal phase defects
- Hyperprolactinemia in male causing oligospermia, decreased libido and impotence.
- Prolactinoma – micro and macroadenoma
- Other uses in female include polycystic ovarian syndrome, premenstrual syndrome and benign breast diseases.

Contraindications

- Hypersensitivity to any ergot alkaloid.
- Pregnancy.

Dosage

- *Suppression of lactation:* One tablet (2.5 mg) bid for 14–21 days
- *Female infertility:* Starting dose is 1.25 mg/day for one week increasing gradually to maximum dose of 2.5 mg tid. The treatment is continued for 3–4 cycles. The drug is immediately stopped when pregnancy is confirmed
- *Male infertility:* 1.25–2.5 mg 3 times daily for 3 months.

Side Effects

Nausea, vomiting, orthostatic hypotension, nasal congestion, fatigue, rarely drowsiness, psychomotor excitation or hallucinations may occur. Because of side effects it has been largely replaced by cabergoline.

Cabergoline

- A long acting dopamine receptor agonist with a high affinity for D2- receptors
- It exerts a direct inhibitory effect on the secretion of prolactin by pituitary lactotrophs.

Uses

- Hyperprolactinemia
- Inhibition of lactation

- Treatment of uterine fibroids
- Prolactinoma
- Parkinsonism

Dose

For hyperprolactinemia it is given 0.5 mg orally weekly and increasing by 0.5 mg every month till response in achieved (usually by 2 mg/wk). For inhibition of lactation 1 mg single dose in the first postpartum day and for suppression of established lactation 0.25 mg 12 hrly for 4 doses.

Side Effects

Nausea, vomiting, constipation, abdominal pain, headache, dyspepsia, dizziness. It causes less nausea and vomiting as compared to bromocriptine so patient compliance is better and relapse is also less.

It is contraindicated in cases of uncontrolled hypertension and patient with history of puerperal psychosis. Available as Caberlin, Cabergoline 0.5 mg tablets.

26. DANAZOL

Danazol is isoxazole derivative of a synthetic steroid 17 ethinyl testosterone. It has antiestrogenic, mixed progestogenic and androgenic properties. It is available as tablets of 100 of 200 mg, e.g., Ladogal, Danocrine, Danogen.

Mechanism of action of Danazol is complex. It includes interference with pulsatile GnRH secretion, inhibiting mid-cycle gonadotropin surge, direct inhibition of ovarian steroidogenesis, blockage of endometrial receptors and suppression of sex hormone binding globulin SHBG from liver, binding directly to androgenic receptors in implants inhibiting its growth and also immunosuppressive effect.

Uses

Danazol was used in endometriosis. It is used as medical treatment either alone or in combination with surgery either before or after. It is used in the dose of 200–800 mg per day in divided doses for 3–9 months. As it produces hypoestrogenic environment and amenorrhea, it is called pseudomenopausal treatment.

Contraindications: Apart from pregnancy and breastfeeding contraindications are liver disease, renal disease and cardiac disease.

Side Effects

- *Anabolic and androgenic*: Weight gain, acne, oily skin, voice changes and hirsutism.
- *Hypoestrogenic:* Breast atrophy, hot flushes, night sweats, insomnia, irritability, depression, atrophic vaginitis.
- *General:* Muscle cramps, skin rash, nausea, headache, dizziness and edema.

Drawbacks

- In 20–40% cases there is recurrence in 2 years.
- It causes virilization of female fetus if pregnancy occurs.
- It is not much effective in chocolate cysts of ovary, scar endometriosis and adenomyosis.

Other Uses

- Benign cystic mastopathy
- DUB
- Fibroid
- Precocious puberty
- In autoimmune disorders like systemic lupus erythematosus and idiopathic thrombocytopenic purpura.

Gestrinone

Is a synthetic trienic 19 nor-steroid compound. It is anti-estrogenic, antiprogestogenic and mild androgenic. It is used in the treatment of endometriosis since last 10 years in western world but not available in India. The proprietary name is Dimitrios It is given in the dose of 2.5 mg twice a week orally for 3–6 months. It has been found very useful with good compliance and fewer side effects.

Dienogest

It is semisynthetic progesterone. It is new drug now available for endometriosis. It has antiandrogenic activity. 2 mg is given orally as monotherapy for 3-6 months.

Along with ethinyl estradiol it is available for use as an oral contraceptive in western countries. Apart from contraception it is used for control of menorrhagia and treatment of menopausal symptoms. Adverse effects include menstrual irregularities, headache weight gain, breast tenderness, nausea and increased blood pressure.

27. ANTIHYPERTENSIVE DRUGS

Commonly used drugs for hypertension in pregnancy are discussed.

Alpha Methyldopa

It is the oldest drug commonly used and more completely studied than any other drug during pregnancy.

Mechanism of action: It induces the synthesis of a methylnorepinephrine that stimulates alpha-2 adrenergic receptors and decreases the sympathetic outflow from the central nervous system. The effect of methyldopa is mainly on peripheral vascular resistance with little effect on cardiac output.

After oral administration effect reaches peak in 4-6 hrs. The drug is completely excreted in urine in 12 hrs. It crosses the placenta and is excreted in low concentration in human breast milk but no neonatal adverse effect are found.

It improves the pregnancy outcome by controlling BP and it reduces the occurrence of severe hypertension late in pregnancy or during labor.

Preparation

250 mg/500 mg oral tablets as Am dopa, Alphadopa.

Dosage

250 mg 2 to 3 times a day is started. The dose is gradually increased to total 2 gm per day. If > 2 gm is required to control the BP combination of other drug is advisable.

Contraindications

Acute hepatic disease, depression, pheochromocytoma, postpartum period.

Adverse Reactions

Sedation, depression, headache, nightmares, drowsiness, fatigue, nasal congestion, salt and water retention, postural hypotension, liver and hemolytic anemia.

Nifedipine

It is a calcium channel blocker. It is an excellent peripheral vasodilator. It lowers the BP by blocking the calcium entry into the vascular smooth muscle cell, thus decreasing the availability of intracellular calcium required for contraction which in turn results in vasodilatation. It is used for both routine control of BP as well as hypertensive emergencies. It is effective after oral administration and effect reaches peak in 30 minutes after ingestion. The plasma half-life is approximately 2 hours. Sublingual use is not favored as it can cause sudden severe lowering of blood pressure.

It may improve uteroplacental perfusion by preventing platelet activation and aggregation.

Preparation

Nifedipine tablet 5 mg, 10 mg; OR Depin, Calcigard, Nifedipine, Myogard; OR 10 to 20 mg as sustained release tablets, e.g., Calcigard retard, Depin retard, Nifedipine SR.

Dosage

It is started 5-20 mg orally three times daily and increased to 20 mg tds. Dose more than 120 mg/day is rarely necessary. It is also useful as tocolytics agent. Initial dose is 20 mg orally, followed by 20 mg after 30 minutes. Maintenance dose is 20 mg 3–6 hourly for 48 hours. As per Cochrane review 2009, Nifedipine is preferred to other tocolytics when tocolysis is indicated in preterm labor.

Side Effects

Headache, dizziness, exaggerated hypotension, flushing, nausea, vomiting, sedation, chest pain and congestive heart failure may be precipitated with beta-blockers.

Beta-blockers

Beta-adrenergic receptors are of 2 types beta-1 or beta-2. Beta-1 receptors produce cardiac stimulation, while beta-2 receptors produce **bronchodilatation** and vasodilatation.
- Cardioselective beta- blockers (β-1): Atenolol, Metoprolol, Practolol
- Non-selective beta-blockers (both β-1 and β-2): Oxprenolol, Propranolol, Alprenolol, etc.
- Beta-blockers (β-1, β-2) with alpha blocking property: Labetolol.

Commonly used drugs are:

Labetalol

It is used orally in the dose of 100 mg twice daily gradually increased to 400 mg twice daily. It can also be given I/V slowly or by slow infusion. Its ratio of alpha to beta blockade is 1: 3 for oral form. It lowers blood pressure without causing bradycardia.

Preparation: Labebet, Gravidol, Lobet 100 mg tablet and Gravidol 2 mL ampoule having 5 mg/mL Labetalol hydrochloride.

In severe hypertension it is given 20 mg I/V over a period of 2 minutes. Then 40–80 mg I/V every 10 min till desired supine BP is achieved or maximum 300 mg/day has been injected.

Contraindications: Bronchospasm, allergic disorders, CCF, pulmonary hypertension, severe bradycardia.

Side effects: Postural hypotension, headache, angina, dreams, jaundice, dryness of mouth, fluid retention.

Atenolol

Its effects starts within 1 hour of oral administration and maximum reaches at 2–4 hours. Its plasma half-life is 6–8 hours, but the effect on the blood pressure is relatively long so it is given in a single daily dose.

Dose: 50 to 100 mg tablet daily.

Preparation: Tab Altol, Atecor, Betacard, etc., 50 mg, 100 mg.

Contraindications: Sinus bradycardia, heart block, cardiac failure.

Side effects: Headache, dizziness, fatigue constipation, hypotension, angina, bradycardia.

As compared to emdopa it is well tolerated. It is excreted in breast milk but quantity is clinically insignificant. Because of its β-1 selectivity it does not cause bronchospasm like propranolol and may be given in asthma.

Hydralazine

Hydralazine is vasodilator drug and it acts directly on arteriolar smooth muscle to reduce peripheral vascular resistance. There is compensatory tachycardia and increased cardiac contractility. It is effective orally and also by I/V and I/M routes.

Its action peaks in 3–4 hours after oral administration and lasts for 6–12 hours. It is metabolized by acetylation in liver. It tends to improve renal, uterine and cerebral blood flow, so it is useful even in the presence of renal damage.

Tachyphylaxis occurs with prolonged use. Hypotensive effect is largely offset by compensatory increase in heart rate and renin release so it should be given in association with beta-blockers.

Presentation: Dihydralazine sulfate 25 mg tablet *(Nepresol)* Hydralazine hydrochloride 25–50 mg tablets Hydralaze and 20 mg/mL injection.

Dosage:
Oral: 25–50 mg bd to total 200 mg/day
I/M: 5–20 mg
I/V: 5–40 mg by slow I/V injection

Contraindication: Tachycardia.

Side effects: Headache, tachycardia, palpitation, nausea, vomiting, skin rashes, flushing, tremors, dizziness, tolerance, fever, polyneuritis and rheumatic symptoms or SLE syndrome on prolonged heavy use.

28. ASPIRIN

Aspirin a non-steroidal anti-inflammatory drug is found useful for prevention of severe pre-eclampsia and IUGR due to its antiplatelet effect.

If produces irreversible inhibition of the enzyme cyclo-oxygenase which is necessary for thromboxane and prostacyclin generation. In low doses aspirin selectively reduces only thromboxane production, so vasodilator prostacyclin is spared. It also has an inhibitory effect on platelet aggregation.

There are many studies of low dose aspirin for prophylaxis of PIH in last 20 years, but recent multicenter study has shown that it is useful in preventing PIH in only high-risk patients. It is suggested that even, if it does not prevent PIH it at least decreases its severity.

Other Uses

Apart from preventing PIH and IUGR it is also used in:
- Women with recurrent abortion in whom anticardiolipin antibody and lupus anticoagulant antibody is raised, i.e., primary APS (antiphospholipid antibody syndrome)
- Pregnant women with autoimmune disease like systemic lupus erythematosus (SLE).

Dose

It is used in 60 to 100 mg/day starting from 12 weeks onwards. In confirmed case of APS it is started even prior to conception.

Contraindications

Hepatic disease, kidney disease and severe acid-peptic disease.

Side Effects

No harmful effects on fetus are found till today. In mothers also it is safe, but slight increase in accidental hemorrhage (not statistically significant) is reported.

29. TRANEXAMIC ACID

- It is antifibrinolytics agent
- It is an analogue of amino acid lysine. It combines with lysine binding sites on plasminogen. Activation of plasminogen to plasmin is inhibited and so lysis of fibrin is inhibited which results in stabilization of clot.
- It is 7–10 times more potent than EACA.
- It is available as 500 mg tab and 500 mg/ampoule injection.

Uses

- It is used in menorrhagia in the dose of 1 to 1.5 gm 3 to 4 times/day.
- Postoperatively 10 to 25 mg/kg body weight is given 3 to 4 times per day by slow I/V or oral route.
- For treatment of all cases of PPH it is recommended 1 gm in 10 mL I/V at 1 mL per minute with a second dose of 1gm IV if bleeding continues after 30 min.

Side Effects

Nausea, diarrhea, headache, giddiness, fatigue and potential risk of thrombosis.

30. DRUGS USED FOR LEUKORRHEA

Common vaginal infections which give rise to leukorrhea are as follows:

Trichomoniasis

Treatment of male partner is important.

Oral

- *Metronidazole:* 400 mg bd for 7 days; OR 2 gm single dose
  - Available as Flagyl, Metrogyl, Unimezol, etc.
  - Common side effects include metallic test, gastric upset and dark yellow staining of urine
  - During first trimester of pregnancy vaginal pessary is preferred.
- *Tinidazole:* 300 mg bd X 7 days or 2 gm single dose—available as Tiniba, Tinibid, etc.
- *Secnidazole:* 2 gm single dose available as Secnil, Tagera.

Vaginal

Clotrimazole vaginal pessary 100 mg for 6 days or 200 mg x 3 days is effective. Metrogyl gel or combination of Clotrimazole + Tinidazole, e.g., Tinicide-V are also used.

Candidiasis

Treatment of predisposing factor is important.

Oral

- *Fluconazole:* 150 mg single dose available as Syscan, Forcan, Flucon, etc. The dose is repeated in chronic or recurrent case.
- *Itraconazole:* 200 mg bd for 7 days available as Sporanox, Canditral, Ketoconazole is less used due to hepatotoxicity.

Vaginal

Pessary or cream form is used.
- *Imidazole (Azole) group*: Clotrimazole, Econazole, Miconazole, Terconazole, Ticonazole, Fenticonazole.
  - Clotrimazole: Imidil, Canesten, Cansoft, etc. 100 mg for 6 nights or 200 mg for 3 nights or 500 mg single dose
  - Econazole: Ecanol vaginal 150 mg for 3 nights
  - Miconazole: Zole ovules 200 mg for 6 nights
  - Terconazole: 80 mg for 3 nights
  - Ticonazole: Vaginal gel zilsa 5 gm of the drug as single application
  - Fenticonazole: 600 mg single capsule is used. It is available as Fentin, Fenza (Fenticonazole nitrate).
- *Polyene derivative:* Nystatin available as Mycostatin 1,00,000 units per pessary. One pessary intravaginally for 10 days.

	Trichomoniasis	Candidiasis	Bacterial vaginosis
Discharge	Copious, frothy, yellow green	White, curdy, adherent	Thin, homogenous grey, moderate
pH	5–6.5	< 4	> 4.5
Odour	Unpleasant	Odourless	Malodorus discharge
Pruritus	May be present	Intense	Absent
Burning	Minimal	Moderate	Absent
Erythema	Mild	Severe	Absent
Petechiae	Present	Absent	Absent
Microscopy	Motile organisms, plenty WBCs	Budding hyphae, spores	Clue cells few WBCs

Bacterial Vaginosis

Oral

- Metronidazole 2 gm single dose or 400 mg bd for 7 days
- Secnidazole 2 gm single dose
- Clindamycin 300 mg bd for 7 days.

Vaginal

- Metrogyl gel 5 gm vaginally for 5-7 days
- Clindamycin 2% cream 5 gm for 7 days
  - During first trimester of pregnancy vaginal clindamycin or ampicillin 500 mg 4 times orally for 7 days is used
  - Combined vaginal pessary is available containing Clotrimazole 200 mg + Clindamycin 100 mg, e.g., Cansoft CL for mixed vaginal infections.

31. ANTI-RETROVIRAL (HIV) DRUGS

They are of six groups:
1. *Nucleoside reverse transcriptase inhibitors (NRTIs):* Zidovudine, Stavudine, Lamivudine, Didanosine, Zalcitabine, Abacavir.
2. *Non-nucleoside reverse transcriptase inhibitors (NNRTIs)*: Nevirapine, Efavirenz and Delavirdine
3. *Protease inhibitors (PI):* Indinavir, Nelfinavir, Saquinavir.
4. *Fusion inhibitors:* Enfuvirtide
5. *Chemokine co-receptor antagonist*: Maraviroc.
6. *Integrase inhibitors:* Raltegravir.

Post-exposure Prophylaxis (PEP)

Basic Regimen

Zidovudine (AZ) 300 mg bid + Lamivudine (3TC) 150 mg bid;
OR
Stavudine (d4T) 30 mg bid + Lamivudine (3TC) 150 mg bid.

Expanded Regimen

Basic regimen + Lopinavir 400 mg twice daily or 800 mg 1 daily. (First choice);
OR
Basic regimen + Nelfinavir 1250 mg twice daily or 750 mg thrice daily with empty stomach (Second choice);
OR
Basic regimen + Indinavir 800 mg 8 hourly (Third choice).

Prophylaxis must start in 72 hours ideally 2 hours of exposure. The drugs are to be taken for 4 weeks, i.e., 28 days. Which regimen is to be recommended depends upon Exposure code (EC) and HIV source code (HIVSC).

NACO Guidelines

As per new guidelines by WHO (June 2013) NACO has decided to provide life long ART (Triple drug regimen) for all pregnant and breastfeeding women living with HIV from January, 2014 in which all pregnant women living with HIV receive a triple drug ART regimen regardless of CD4 count or WHO clinical stage both for their own health and to prevent vertical transmission to child. This strategy will reduce the transmission to < 5% in breastfeeding population.

First line regimen recommended is Tenofovir (TDF, 300 mg) + Lamivudine (3 TC, 300 mg) + Efavirenz (EFV, 600 mg).

Alternate regimens are AZT 3 TC + EFV, AZT + 3TC + NVP and TDF + 3TC + NVP. Recent evidence has shown that Efavirenz can be safely used in all trimesters of pregnancy.

For Newborn 15 mg (1.5 mL) of NVP is given daily till 6 wks whether exclusively breastfed or exclusively replacement fed, if wt is > 2.5 kg between 2-2.5 kg NVP dose is 10 mg (1 mL) and for < 2 kg wt NVP is given 0.2 mL/kg.

In pregnant women presenting directly in labor TDF (300 mg) + TC (300 mg) + EFV (600 mg) is started intrapartum and continued postpartum Nevirapine prophylaxis for breastfeeding infants should be for 12 weeks, as mother did not receive any ART during antenatal period.

STI/STI Kits

NACO has adopted syndromic approach as a primary strategy to control and prevent STIs/

RTIs. Syndromic approach is a scientifically proven approach which ensures complete treatment for common organisms responsible for a particular syndrome.

There are total 7 different color coded drug kits for different syndromes.
Commonly used kits in gynec are:

Kit 1: It is for cervicitis and urethral discharge.
It is gray colored.
It contains tab Azithromycin 1 gm and tab Cefixime 400 mg, both are given statement.

Kit 2: It is for vaginitis
It is green colored
It contains tab Secnidazole 2 gm and tab Fluconazole 150 mg to be given statement

Kit 6: It is for lower abdominal pain (PID).
It is yellow colored.
It contains tab Cefixime 400 mg which is given stat + tab Metronidazole 400 mg bid for 14 days + tab Doxycycline 100 mg bid for 14 days.

32. HPV VACCINES FOR CERVICAL CANCER

- Currently 2 vaccines are available: Cervarix and Gardasil.
- Both vaccines protect against the two HPV types (HPV-16 and HPV-18) that cause 70% of cervical cancers, 80% of anal cancers, 60% of vaginal cancers and 40% of vulvar cancers
- HPV 16 and 18 are responsible for only 70% of all cervical cancer cases. So cervical cancer screening should be continued even after vaccination
- The World Health Organization (WHO) recommends HPV vaccines as part of routine vaccinations in all countries, along with other prevention measures. Vaccinating girls around the ages of nine to thirteen is typically recommended. In India routine vaccination is yet not started. HPV vaccines are very safe. Pain at the site of injection occurs in about 80% of people. Redness and swelling at the site and fever may also occur.
- Women who have already been exposed to HPV 16 or 18 will not be protected by the vaccine.
- HPV 6 and 11 are responsible for 90% of genital warts
- Side effects to the vaccines are usually minor reactions to intramuscular injections sites
- The vaccine is contraindicated in females with a history of immediate hypersensitivity to yeast or to any vaccine component.

Cervarix	Gardasil
Bivalent vaccine	Quadrivalent
Effective against HPV virus 16 and 18	Effective against HPV virus 16, 18, 6 and 11
0, 1 and 6 months	0, 2 and 6 months
Uses L1 protein	Made from L1 protein of the viral capsid (virus like particles)
Not to be used in pregnant women	Not to be used in pregnant women
Age 10 to 25 yrs	Age 9 to 26 yrs

- In 2014 FDA approved a nine-valent Gardasil based vaccine Gardasil 9, to protect against five other HPV strains responsible for 20% of cervical cancers (HPV – 31, 33, 45, 52 and 58).

CHAPTER 8

Obstetric Operations

Forceps delivery, vacuum extraction and surgical methods of MTP are already discussed in chapters 6. Remaining obstetric operations minor or major, are discussed here.

EPISIOTOMY (PERINEOTOMY)

Definition

It is a deliberate incision made on the perineum during the second stage of labor for its various benefits.

Benefits

- It cuts short the duration of second stage of labor
- It is a surgical incision, so it is easy to repair and healing is better than that of irregular tears which may occur if episiotomy is not given
- Soft tissues are not unduly stretched, which otherwise may be damaged leading to prolapse of vaginal wall or deficient perineum in future life.
- It widens out the birth passage so: (a) any instrumentation or maneuver, if required can be done comfortably, and (b) fetal head is saved from sudden compression and decompression during its birth.

Indications

- *Primigravida patients:* Evidence based medicine suggests restrictive episiotomy however due to rigid perineum, it is routinely given in all primigravida
- *Fetal indications:* Prematurity, postmaturity, twins, fetal distress
- Threatened laceration of perineum–large size of fetus, deflexed head, rigid perineum in some parous patients
- Instrumental delivery – forceps, vacuum
- Abnormal presentation–breech, face-mento-anterior, persistent occipito-posterior-face to pubis delivery.
- History of previous plastic surgery, e.g., third degree perineal tears repair.

Types of Episiotomy

- *Mediolateral:* 60° from midline on any side, i.e., starting from fourchette and directed towards right or left side. After delivery it automatically becomes 45°.
- *Median:* Strictly in midline starting from fourchette directed backward

towards anus. It is practiced in Western countries.

J shaped and lateral episiotomies are not practiced.

Lateral (90°) episiotomy is also not practiced due to excessive bleeding and risk of injury to Bartholin's duct or gland.

Mediolateral episiotomy: It is commonly performed.

Advantages

- No danger of extension into anal sphincter causing third degree perineal tear,
- No danger of injury to Bartholin's duct or gland, and
- Less bleeding as compared to lateral episiotomy.

Disadvantages

As compared to median episiotomy there is more bleeding, less better apposition and healing.

Contraindications

Apart from patient's absolute refusal to consent contraindications are very few. They include:
- Lymphogranuloma venereum
- Severe painful scarring or malformation of perineum, and
- Coagulation disorders.

The structures cut in episiotomy from outside inwards are skin, perineal fascia with fat, superficial perineal muscles (bulbospongiosus, superficial transverse perineal), deep transverse perineal muscles and posterior vaginal wall. In deep episiotomy lower fibers of levator ani may be cut.

Suturing of Episiotomy

- *Posterior vaginal wall*: It is sutured with "o" number chromic catgut continuous locking sutures on curved round body needle.
- *Perineal muscles:* They are sutured with "1" number chromic catgut interrupted sutures in two layers on curved round body needle.

Skin: It is sutured by vertical mattress sutures with silk or with absorbable chromic catgut, or subcuticular stitches may be taken.

Removal of stitches: Nonabsorbable stitches are removed after 7 days.
- Vicryl rapide is used for suturing all layers of episiotomy
- Recent evidence from the western world suggests that episiotomy should not be given to all primigravidas. It does more harm than benefits. It should only be given to indicated primigravidas. However, it is difficult to practice in our patients.

Complications

Immediate: Excessive bleeding, third degree perineal tears, episiotomy hematoma.

Late: Wound gap (non-union), infection, painful scar, dyspareunia. Rarely rectovaginal fistula and necrotizing fasciitis and scar endometriosis.

Most common complications are incomplete healing, wound gap and infection.

DILATATION AND EVACUATION (D&E)

Dilatation and Curettage, (D&C) usually implies gynec procedure, while complete obstetric procedure is dilatation, evacuation and curettage.

Indications

- Inevitable abortion– suction evacuation is better and faster
- Incomplete abortion
- Missed abortion
- Septic abortion (under antibiotic cover)
- Vesicular mole evacuation
- Following second trimester MTP by medical methods: In some cases to remove remaining placental tissues.

In conditions where cervix is already dilated, straight away evacuation is performed, while in other cases cervical dilatation may be carried out either by rapid method (metal dilators) or by slow method (prostaglandins).

Preoperative Measures

Except in emergency, full routine preoperative preparations are done, i.e., local shaving, antiseptic cleaning, minor preoperative profile, evacuation of bowel, nil by mouth for minimum 6 hours and sedatives. Written consent is taken.

Anesthesia

General anesthesia or local anesthesia, i.e., paracervical block with premedications. When cervix is already dilated evacuation can be easily done without anesthesia under the effect of I/V sedation.

Procedure

- Steps are same as those described under suction evacuation method up to dilatation of cervix. But here dilatation required is more
- When uterus is more than 10 wks size, prior separation of products by index finger passed inside the uterine cavity may be done
- Ovum forceps is introduced and products are completely removed one by one
- Check curettage with blunt or sharp curette is done to remove the left out products
- Injection methyl ergometrine is given I/V
- Completion of evacuation is indicated by:
  - No active bleeding
  - Grating sensation with curette
  - No products with ovum forceps, and
  - No irregularity felt inside the cavity.
- Bimanual examination is done to check that the uterus is well contracted and decreased in size
- All the products removed should be preserved for examination to check that it is complete

- Type of curette – blunt curette is less traumatic, but grating sensation and removal of adherent products are better with sharp curette. Use of sharp curette when uterine ecbolic are given is safe.

Post-operative Care

- Prophylactic antibiotics are given
- Patient is discharged after 2-6 hours depending upon her general condition and type of anesthesia used
- Avoidance of sexual relations for 5 days.

Complications

They are same as those described under suction evacuation in chapter 6.

MCDONALD'S OPERATION

It is known by different names like os tightening, cervical suture, cervical cerclage, nylon wiring.

Indications

- Incompetent cervical os.
- Prophylactically in cases with history of repeated second trimester abortions or history of premature labor without obvious cause
- Twin pregnancy to prevent preterm labour. However, role of prophylactic cervical cerclage is not scientifically proved
- Uterine malformation, e.g., unicornuate and bicornuate uterus may be beneficial.

Time of Operation

During pregnancy around 12-14 wks is ideal time. It can be done as early as 10 wks and in indicated cases up to as late as 32 wks. Reasons for doing operation at 14 wks:

- After 14 wks risk of abortion increases in proved case of cervical incompetence
- Before 14 wks, i.e., in first trimester the abortion is commonly due to defect in the fertilized ovum or defect in the placenta.

- Even in proved cases there is very little risk of abortion before 14 wks because only at the end of 12 wks uterine cavity is completely filled up by the growing fetus, so as to exert strain on the cervix at internal os.

Anesthesia: It is performed under short GA (I/V pentothal / propofol). It can be performed in local anesthesia + sedation. Preanesthetic medication in the form of inj. atropine 0.6 mg 1/2 hour before operation is given.

Steps of Operation

- Emptying of bladder, lithotomy position, painting and draping
- Anesthesia is given per vaginal examination is done
- Per speculum examination is done to see that there is no bleeding or leaking or herniation of membranes
- Cervix is swabbed with dry sterile swabs
- Anterior and posterior lips are held with swab holders. Instead, 4 Allis forceps are commonly used as they give better grip
- Double strands of No. 2 braided silk or No. 1 nylon or prolene on round body half-circle curved needle is used for suture. Purse string suture is taken as high as possible on the cervix without incising the epithelium. Suture is started anteriorly and minimum 4 bites are taken, i.e., at 1–2, 10–11, 7–8 and 4–5 o'clock position anticlockwise. Bites should be deep in the cervical substance, but avoiding endocervix.
- The knot is tied anteriorly tight enough to grip the tip of the assistant's finger kept in the cervical canal. Ligatures are cut long for ease of identification and removal at term. Usually about 2 mm diameter of cervical canal remains at the end of the operation
- *Postoperative treatment:* Patient is kept in the hospital for 1–2 days. Antibiotics, uterine relaxants and sedatives are given. P/S examination is done before discharge
- Patient is advised for weekly antenatal check-up and should report immediately if she develops pains, bleeding P/V or leaking.

Removal of stitch: Suture is removed after 38 weeks. But, if the patient is not sure of her LMP it may be removed immediately after the onset of labor.

Long ends of the ligature are caught with an artery forceps and ligature is cut with the scissors beyond the knot close to the cervix and then pulled out.

Contraindications

Local infection, bleeding p/v, rupture of membranes, irritable uterus, cervical dilatation more than 3 cm, intrauterine fetal death, fetal abnormalities, suspected intrauterine infection.

Complications

Bleeding, accidental injury to membranes leading to rupture or ascending infection (amnionitis) or abortion. During labor cervical dystocia (due to fibrosis) can occur. If stitch is not removed immediately after labor pains have started cervical tears can occur.

History-indicated Cerclage

- Insertion of a cerclage as a result of factors in a woman's obstetric or gynecological history which increase the risk of spontaneous second-trimester loss or preterm delivery
- A history-indicated suture is performed as a prophylactic measure in asymptomatic women and normally inserted electively at 12–14 weeks of gestation.

Ultrasound-indicated Cerclage

Insertion of a cerclage as a therapeutic measure in cases of cervical length shortening seen on transvaginal ultrasound.

Ultrasound-indicated cerclage is performed on asymptomatic women who do not have exposed fetal membranes in the vagina. Sonographic assessment of the cervix is usually performed between 14 and 24 weeks of gestation.

Rescue (Emergency) Cerclage

Insertion of cerclage as a salvage measure in the case of premature cervical dilatation with exposed fetal membranes in the vagina.

This may be discovered by ultrasound examination of the cervix or as a result of a speculum examination performed for symptoms such as vaginal discharge, bleeding or 'sensation of pressure'.

Steps

- Regional anesthesia or general anesthesia
- Steep Trendelenburg position
- Perioperative antibiotics is must
- Fill the bladder with 600 mL saline
- Vagina is washed with dilute Betadine solution
- McDonald purse string suture with prolene 1-0 or nylon 1-0 is usually taken
- Insert small caliber Foley's catheter in the cervix, inflate the balloon 30 mL to push the membranes back. Membranes can be pushed back by moistened sponge on sponge holder also, but Foley's catheter is better. Deflate the balloon of the catheter removing it gradually while tying the suture
- Tocolytics should be given for 24 hours.

Cervical Incompetence

Etiology

- Mechanical injury to cervix, e.g., Dilatation of cervix, D&C, suction MTP, breech extraction, difficult forceps delivery, deep lateral cervical tear, deep conization, high amputation, precipitate labor
- Developmental, i.e., congenital
- *Dysfunctional:* Functional abnormality which causes premature triggering of the factors normally responsible for effacement of cervix at term.

Diagnosis

- *Specific history:* Repeated midtrimester abortions with painless dilatation of cervix, herniation of membranes, rupture of membranes, short painless labor with delivery of live fetus
- Pervaginal examinations during pregnancy, repeated frequently if necessary.
- *Vaginal ultrasonography (TVS) during pregnancy*: Y or V shape of cervical canal are suggestive. Normal cervical canal is T shape. U shape suggests obvious dilatation. Cervical length of < 25 mm is suggestive.
- *Other tests:* They are not done now, they were done in nonpregnant state:
  - Passage of No. 8 size Hegar dilator without resistance
  - HSG– funnelling at internal os with isthmic width of 8 mm or more.

Conservative Treatment

- Complete bed rest with foot end of the bed raised
- Tocolysis— its value is doubtful because uterine contractions are not at fault
  - Surgical treatment other than McDonald's operation include Shirodkar's operation, Lash and Lash operation, Benson and Duffy operation. Electrocauterization, i.e., internal scarification of cervix, etc.
  - Material used for suturing other than silk include Mersilene tape, nylon, teflon.
  - The first true cervical encerclage operation was reported by Shirodkar in 1955. The material he used originally was fascia lata.
  - In **Shirodkar operation** as against McDonald's operation the suture (now mersilene tape is used) is tied at the level of internal os. For that purpose both anterior and posterior vaginal walls are incised and anteriorly bladder is dissected away up to internal os. The knot is tied posteriorly and kept out

of the vaginal wall while closing the posterior incision for easy removal of tape at the time of delivery.
- **Benson and Duffy operation:** It is an abdominal cerclage operation where mersilene tap is tied at the level of uterine isthmus. It is indicated where there is very short and badly damaged cervix and in cases of repeated failures of vaginal procedures.

CESAREAN SECTION

Definition

It is abdominal delivery of fetus by putting an incision over the abdominal wall and the uterine wall after 20 weeks of pregnancy (Laparotomy + Hysterotomy).

Types

- Lower segment — more than 98% of today's operations are of this type (LSCS)
- Classical or upper segment, very rarely performed
- Extraperitoneal—not performed in modern obstetrics
- Cesarean hysterectomy— performed for specific indications.

Incidence

In last two decades incidence has increased tremendously.

It varies from 10% to 40% in different institutes. It is more in tertiary care centres and private clinics. WHO had issued a consensus statement (1985) that there were no additional health benefits associated with cesarean section above 10–15%.

However in 2015 WHO said that every effort should be made to provide cesarean section to woman in need rather than striving to achieve specific rate. WHO proposed to implement Robson 10 group classification for accessing, monitoring and comparing cesarean section rates as a global standard.

Current cesarean section rate in India on an average is 25–30%.

Indications

Maternal

- *Contracted pelvis:* In major degree contraction LSCS is required in every case, while in minor degree contracted pelvis if there is any associated complicating factor LSCS is carried out otherwise trial of labor is given (As such in any case cephalo-pelvic disproportion, i.e., CPD is more important than pelvis alone
- Previous 2 or more LSCS scars (vaginal delivery is still possible if indications are nonrecurrent)
- Previous one LSCS with some adverse obstetric factor this time
- Failure of progress of labor due to cervical dystocia, abnormal uterine action or any other cause
- Major degree placenta previa, i.e., second degree posterior or more. Even in minor degree if there is excessive bleeding
- Severe hypertension in pregnancy, i.e. preeclampsia, eclampsia.
- Failed induction of labor
- Accidental hemorrhage — in early cases when fetus is still alive or in late cases of concealed type to save mother, even if the fetus is dead and rapid vaginal delivery is not possible
- Failed trial of labor. Unsuccessful trial forceps
- Selected cases of diabetes.

Fetal and Placental

- Fetal distress during first stage of labor
- Breech presentation — primigravida, BOH, IUGR, large baby, hyperextended head, footling presentation, prematurity.
- IUGR, oligohydramnios.
- Malpresentations like shoulder, brow and face mentoposterior
- Arrested occipito-posterior position

- Bad obstetric history— recurrent pregnancy wastage, repeated unexplained intrauterine deaths or intrapartum deaths
- Some cases of twin pregnancy— first nonvertex, fetal distress in first baby, conjoined twins, locked twins
- Cord prolapse before full cervical dilatation (if fetus is alive)
- Selected cases of Rh- incompatibility.
- HIV positive mother to decrease the vertical transmission to the baby.

(There are some absolute indications but they are rare. They include previous classical cesarean scar or rupture uterus scar, undilatable and indivisible strictures of cervix or vagina, soft tissue pelvic tumors of pelvic bones, previously repaired vesicovaginal fistula and fetal monsters).

Common indications of cesarean section in present times include fetal distress (FHR abnormality, thick meconium stained liquor), nonprogress of labor, previous cesarean section, failed induction of labor, oligohydramnios and breech presentation.

Contraindication

In modern obstetrics there is no absolute contraindication to CS. Only disseminated intravascular coagulation remain the important contraindication, but here also the operation can be done after correction of the coagulation defect.

In case of dead fetus, grossly premature fetus or severely malformed fetus CS is preferably avoided but may be required when mother is at risk.

LOWER SEGMENT CESAREAN SECTION

Anesthesia

SA: Bupivacaine (Sensorcaine) 0.5% 2 to 2.5 cc is used. Xylocaine 5% 0.8 to 1.4 cc was previously used. Spinal anesthesia is the most commonly used method.

GA: Induction is by 250 mg I/V pentothal and 75 mg scoline. Patient is maintained on oxygen and nitrous oxide till baby is delivered then ether or trilene is added.

Epidural analgesia: Single shot technique or continuous by epidural catheter – Bupivacaine is used.

Steps

In emergency cases full preoperative preparation may not be possible but following measures are done:
- Injection glycopyrrolate 0.2 mg half an hour before operation
- Intravenous line with wide bore intracath is set up
- At least 500 mL of RL should be pushed before starting CS
- Prophylactic antibiotics are given
- Blood is sent for grouping and cross - matching
- Local preparation, i.e., abdomen and back
- Evacuation of bladder – usually Foley's catheter No. 16 is kept during operation
- 5–15° Trendelenburg with slight left lateral tilting is ideal position
- Painting and draping
- Under anesthesia abdomen is opened in layers, commonly by Pfannenstiel incision (low transverse curved)
- Parietal peritoneum is opened in upper part of the incision to avoid bladder
- With the scissors the peritoneal incision is extended above and down
- Doyen's retractor is introduced in the lower end of the incision and the uterus is exposed
- Uterus is examined for dextrorotation in the right side by inspecting or palpating the round ligaments
- Dextrorotation is corrected manually (Abdominal pack may be inserted one on either side, first on the left side to prevent recurrence of dextrorotation. Packs are

- preserved by artery forceps attached to it). Most of the doctors do not insert packs in present times
- Loose visceral peritoneum of the lower uterine segment is identified, lifted with toothless forceps and small transverse cut is put by scissors
- Visceral peritoneum is dissected on either side by passing scissors between it and lower uterine segment and then the incision is extended on both sides
- The lower peritoneal flap is lifted up with forceps and by finger pressure or swab on holder, it is pushed down for about 3–5 cm along with the bladder
- Doyen's retractor is adjusted to retract the bladder
- Site of the incision of lower uterine segment is at least 2 cm above the bladder reflection
- Small transverse incision is put in the lower segment in the midline by knife till the membranes are reached
- Incision can be extended on either side by stretching it with index fingers or cutting it with the curved scissors
- Adequacy of incision for easy delivery of head is checked
- Hand is passed in the uterus below the head, Doyen's retractor is removed, head is flexed, lifted up to the incision and delivered by lateral flexion in combination with fundal pressure
- Injection ergometrine is given I/V stat and injection oxytocin 10–20 units are injected in the drip
- Mouth and nose of the fetus are sucked out
- Rest of the fetus is delivered simply by gentle traction on the head aided by fundal pressure
- Umbilical cord is clamped and cut. Baby is handed over to the nurse or neonatologist on a tray covered by sterile towel
- Angles and edges of the lower uterine segment incision are caught with Allis forceps or swab holders (or green armytage hemostatic forceps).
- Placenta is delivered by gentle cord traction and fundal pressure. Only if it does not separate readily it can be removed manually. Care must be taken to remove the membranes completely
- Uterine cavity is explored as a routine before closure by swab holder or manually
- Uterus is closed in one or two layers. First layer is by No. 1 polyglactin 910, i.e., Vicryl on curved round body needle, taking continuous locking suture with good tension. Suture must extend beyond the angles on both sides. Care is taken to exclude decidua in stitch if possible so that the scar does not become weak.
  Second layer by No. 1 Vicryl on curved round body needle, taking continuous or interrupted stitches burying the first layer, i.e., lambert suture
- Uterine closure is now done in single layer by more and more obstetricians. Although evidence is still not clear on the status of uterine closure single layer closure decreases the operative time and additional hemostatic stitches are required less often.
- Visceral peritoneum if sutured it is done by 1-0 chromic catgut or Vicryl taking simple continuous stitches
- Before the abdomen is closed following measures are taken:
  - Suture line and broad ligament are examined for bleeding and hematoma
  - Peritoneal toilet is done
  - Uterus is felt to check that it is firmly contracted
  - Ovaries are examined
  - Counting of mops and instruments should be done to confirm that nothing is left behind inside the peritoneal cavity.
- Abdomen is closed in layers
- Recent studies have shown that not suturing both the peritoneum (visceral and parietal) results in less postoperative adhesions. It saves the operative time and there are no disadvantages

- While the patient is still under anesthesia uterine fundus is firmly pressed downwards to expel the blood clots from the uterus and vagina
- Dressing is applied over the wound and vagina is cleaned with Savlon.

Difficulty in delivering the head: Following measures are tried —
- Assistant may be asked to put the hand in vagina and push the head above
- If the incision is higher up at the level of fetal shoulder delivery by Patwardhan method (shoulders first) is better alternative
- Catching the lower limb by passing the hand towards fundus and delivering as breech is successful and easy (modified Patwardhan) in arrested occipito-posterior position
- Outlet forceps may be used instead of hand when head is deeply impacted or high floating
- Small vertical midline incision may be put in the upper edge of the incision (i.e. inverted T) to get more space but only in desperate situations.

Induction delivery interval if operation is done in general anesthesia should be between 4 to 8 minutes. Uterine incision delivery interval under any anesthesia is quite safe up to 3 minutes. If it exceeds 3 minutes it may cause neonatal asphyxia.

Complications of Lower Segment Cesarean Section

Maternal
- *Profuse bleeding (Postpartum hemorrhage):* From the edges of the incision, from placental site (atony of uterus), or from injury to uterine vessels
- Hematoma-over the angles or edges of incision or in board ligament
- Extension of the incision with irregular tearing of lower uterine segment
- *Sepsis:*
  - Wound sepsis
  - Pelvic— pelvic thrombophlebitis, pelvic peritonitis, pelvic cellulitis
  - Septicemia.
- Shock
- *Bladder complications:*
  - Injuries during dissection of visceral peritoneum, due to extension of lower segment incision downwards or during suturing of uterus
  - Postoperative retention of urine
  - Hematuria
- *Bowel complications*— paralytic ileus, distension of abdomen, peritonitis and rarely injury to cecum or sigmoid colon during suturing of uterus
- *Anesthetic complications*
  - Pulmonary embolism-amniotic fluid embolism
  - Disseminated intravascular coagulation
  - Death-maternal mortality from CS is around 0.1 to 0.3% (includes emergency cases).
- *Late complications:*
  - Scar on the uterus can lead to simple dehiscence or rupture during next pregnancy or labor
  - If by chance placenta is implanted on the scar, the risk of rupture is increased and placenta may be morbidly adherent (accreta)
  - Abdominal scar can lead to incisional hernia or keloid formation. There may be intraperitoneal adhesions.
- *Perinatal complications:*
  - Respiratory distress syndrome (RDS)
  - Injury to fetal presenting part by knife
  - Asphyxia due to anesthetic agent or delay in delivery
  - Fetal blood loss if placenta is cut through or torn during delivery, e.g., in placenta previa
  - Intracranial hemorrhage by difficult delivery through small uterine incision or secondary to asphyxia.

Misgav Ladach Technique

Misgav Ladach technique of cesarean section was suggested by Dr Michael Stark from Misgav Ladach Hospital, Israel. It is minimalist surgical approach. There is less disruptive opening of the abdominal wall, minimal instrumentation and minimizing the procedures for abdominal closing:

- Joel Cohen's incision— a straight transverse incision about 3 cm below a line joining the anterior-superior iliac spines
- Minimal use of instruments— using the fingers, abdominal wall layers are stretched in a caudal cranial direction thereby enabling separation of layers. Parietal peritoneum is also opened in the same way transversely to avoid damage to the bladder
- Manual lateral stretching of the uterine incision
- Exteriorization of the uterus
- Single layer uterine closure
- Nonclosure of the visceral and parietal peritoneal layers
- Closure of the abdomen in two layers: (1) skin, and (2) fascia.

Advantages

- Reduces operation time
- Less postoperative morbidity
- Faster—less delivery time
- Less anesthesia required
- Less dose of postoperative analgesia
- Less blood loss
- Less suture material
- Quicker return of bowel activity
- Early ambulation.

Classical Cesarean Section

Because of its various disadvantages and complications it is very rarely performed. Here the incision on the uterus is put in the midline vertically in the upper uterine segment. Its indications in modern obstetrics are as follows:

- Severe adhesions in the lower segment due to previous surgery or infection
- Fibroids in lower uterine segment
- Severe kyphosis where distance between symphysis pubis and sternum is so reduced that lower segment is not accessible
- Carcinoma of cervix
- Conjoint twins
- When hysterectomy is contemplated at the same time
- Postmortem cesarean section
- Anterior placenta previa and transverse lie with dorsoinferior are relative indications of classical CS.

Advantages of LSCS Over Classical Cesarean Section

- Less vascular so less bleeding
- Scar is strong because:
  - Lower segment is the quiescent part of the uterus in postoperative period (Rest is important for good healing)
  - Due to thinness of wall it can be sutured better.
- Minimal intraperitoneal adhesions
- Seals off infection. No extension to general peritoneal cavity if infection occurs
- Postoperative convalescence is better- pain, abdominal distension and paralytic ileus are less common
- Muscle fibers are transverse so it is anatomical
- There is minimum handling of uterus and abdominal contents
- Less chances of placenta to be implanted over the scar in future pregnancy
- Overall mortality is less.
- *Scar rupture:*
  - Previous classical CS: 2–9%
  - Previous LSCS: 0.2–1.5%

Disadvantages of LSCS Over Classical Cesarean Section

- Injury to bladder or ureter more
- Lateral extension of incision may cause profuse hemorrhage or broad ligament hematoma due to involvement of large vessels

- In case of large fetus, because of limited space delivery may be difficult
- Technically more difficult and more time consuming. With LSCS now being exclusively done this is not true.

Extraperitoneal CS

Here the peritoneal clarity is not opened so these is no contamination of peritoneal cavity and loess infectious morbidity.

With good antibiotics available, it is not done in modern obstetrics. It has following disadvantages:
- Technically more difficult
- More time consuming
- Chances of injury to bladder more
- Buttoholing of peritoneum offsets the main purpose of operation
- Troublesome oozing, from venous plexuses during operation
- Incidence of pelvic cellulitis and thrombophlebitis greater.

Cesarean Hysterectomy

Here after delivery of the fetus during cesarean section, hysterectomy is performed. Ideally total hysterectomy should be done, but if the patient's general condition is low subtotal hysterectomy is the best for her as it is less dangerous and less time consuming. In well dilated cervix may be difficult to find out where cervix ends and where vagina begins.

Indications

- Uncontrollable hemorrhage at the time of CS – atonic or traumatic
- Placenta accreta, increta
- Significant myomas
- Intrauterine severe infection
- Operable malignant diseases of cervix.
    1. *Rupture uterus:* Here no incision may be put on the uterus to deliver the baby so even if hysterectomy is done, it is an obstetric hysterectomy and not truly a cesarean hysterectomy.
    2. In atonic PPH after vaginal delivery hysterectomy may be required as a last resort to save the patient's life, which is also obstetric hysterectomy.

In *obstetric hysterectomy* deviation from normal abdominal hysterectomy steps are as follows:
- Clamp, cut and drop technique (Plauche) is recommended. Here you require more clamps
- All pedicles should be ligated as close to the uterus and cervix as possible
- Keep small tissues in pedicle and keep adequate size of the stump
- Round ligament should be separately ligated
- Cornual pedicles are doubly ligated
- Clamps on vascular pedicles should be manipulated as little as possible
- Subtotal hysterectomy is recommended. It is simple, safe, quick, with less blood loss and avoids injury to bladder and ureter. But, it is not useful in placenta previa-accreta, tear extending in LUS and in cervical tear
- Before closing the abdomen copious irrigation is done, all the pedicles are inspected several times, hemostasis is checked and drain is kept.

Vaginal Birth after Cesarean Section (VBAC)

- In case of previous one CS if the indication is recurrent, i.e., contracted pelvis, next time also CS is performed. But, if indication was non-recurrent, i.e., fetal distress, breech, etc., vaginal delivery in the hospital is permitted. This is also called trial of labor after cesarean section (TOLAC). Once successfully completed it is called vaginal birth after cesarean section (VBAC). The success rate of VBAC is from 60% to 80%
- Criteria for selection of VBAC are:
    - One previous lower segment cesarean section
    - Clinically adequate pelvis

- Vertex presentation
- Facilities to carry out immediate cesarean section
- Patient's consent, i.e., willingness to take trial after proper understanding of risks and benefits.
- Recent studies have shown that in cases of non-recurrent indications vaginal delivery is possible without any adverse outcome even in cases of two previous LSCS. However, this is rarely practiced.
- If there are no high-risk factors for scar rupture patient may be admitted in the hospital only after labor pains start
- The patient is watched for signs and symptoms of threatened scar rupture. Signs are unexplained tachycardia and scar tenderness. Symptoms include persistent suprapubic pain and vaginal bleeding. If any of these develop CS is to be done. Second stage of labor is cut short by episiotomy, and outlet forceps or vacuum
- To given oxytocin drip in scarred uterus was contraindicated in past. But, guarded pitocin drip just enough to bring about normal uterine contractions can be given without danger in case of uterine inertia
- After vaginal delivery lower segment is not routinely explored. It is only explored when there is excessive bleeding after delivery.

High-risk factors for scar rupture in next pregnancy or labor:
- Type of previous CS—classical CS – more chances because scar is weak as compared to lower segment scar (rare now)
- Post-operative infection leads to weak scar
- Surgical technique at previous CS, i.e., excessive foreign body reaction due to thick suture material, tissue ischemia by continuous locking suture, improper hemostasis and inclusion of decidua in stitches - all these lead to weak scar.
- Implantation of placenta at the site of incision of previous CS leads to weak scar due to unsatisfactory suturing
- Risk is increased if there is no vaginal delivery before, i.e., CS in primigravida.
- Over distension of uterus (large fetus, hydramnios or multiple pregnancy) in this pregnancy
- Interdelivery interval of <24 months (i.e., 15 months between last cesarean and this pregnancy). There is 2–3 times increase in scar rupture
- *Induction of labor*: There is more risk than spontaneous labor. Use of prostaglandins led to more incidence of scar rupture, so it is banned in some countries
- Repeated vaginal deliveries after CS— with each delivery scar gets weakened, so risk of rupture increases
- If USG with full bladder show scar thickness <2.5 mm, it points against TOLAC. Ultrasonic windows are more important than thinned out lower segment.

DESTRUCTIVE OPERATIONS

These operations were done to reduce the bulk of the fetus so as to have easy delivery through the birth canal. They are **rarely performed** in modern obstetrics. With exception of major congenital malformations they are performed only when the fetus is dead.

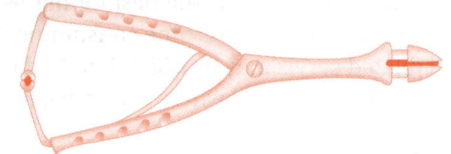

Fig. 8.1: Simpson's perforator.

Operation	Instrument
Craniotomy	Craniotome (perforator)
Cranioclasm	Cranioclast
Cephalotripsy	Cephalotribe
Decapitation	Decapitation hook, knife or saw, Gigli saw wire
Evisceration, cleidotomy, spondylotomy	Embryotomy scissors

Complications

Injuries to uterus, cervix, vagina and rarely to bladder, rectum or sacral promontory, PPH, shock and sepsis.

Craniotomy

This is the only operation which is rarely carried out in modern obstetrics as cesarean section in cases of deeply impacted head has increased risk.

If means perforation of the fetal head, to evacuate the cranial contents, before its extraction. Simpson's perforator is the best instrument for the purpose. In absence of it embryotomy scissors is used.

Simpson's Perforator

It is a heavy stainless steel instrument. Blades have triangular tips with outer cutting edges (jaws). The jaws are limited by shoulders. A malleable narrow metal plate, running obliquely between the two handles acts as a spring. There is locking system at the proximal end of the handles. Handles can be compressed only when the lock is pressed inwards. When the handles are pressed, blades open and when the handles are wide apart the blades are closed.

Indications of Craniotomy

- Cephalopelvic disproportion in vertex presentation with dead fetus.
- Malpresentations with dead fetus, i.e., impacted brow, face mentoposterior, aftercoming head of breech
- Malformation of fetal head, i.e., hydrocephalus, fetal monster. Here, it can be performed even in living fetus.

Contraindications

Major degree pelvic contraction and threatened rupture of uterus.

Prerequisites: Same as those for forceps + the fetus must be dead.

Procedure: It is done in operation theater:
- Lithotomy position, aseptic precautions
- G/A or S/A
- Empty the bladder by catheter. Examination under anesthesia
- Under guidance of 2 fingers of left hand in vagina, the instrument held in right hand is passed. The two fingers of left hand kept anteriorly protects the bladder
- Assistant fixes the head from above. Blades are kept closed and the tip is held perpendicular to the part to be perforated
- A bold perpendicular thrust is made, in the dependent and accessible part of the head. Scalp tissue at the site of perforation may be cut by scissors, before the introduction of perforator
- Push the instrument inside up to the shoulder, open the blades by pressing the handles to make a linear tear. Then close the blades, rotate the instrument through 90° and again press the handles to make a cruciate incision on the skull
- The instrument is then passed further in the cranial cavity with closed blades and then by closing and opening the blades brain matter is destroyed in all directions up to the base of skull
- Contents of cranial cavity come out spontaneously as they are under pressure or removed by a sponge holder or suction cannula.
- Perforated head can be extracted by Vulsellum traction or forceps
- After delivery uterine cavity must be explored to exclude the rupture.

Sites of perforation:

Vertex:	Parietal bone near anterior fontanelle
Brow:	Frontal bone

Face: Orbit or hard palate
Aftercoming head of breech: Through occipital bone or hard palate through floor of the mouth

Better not to perforate through the joint or fontanelle.

Complications

Injuries to uterus, cervix, vagina and rarely to bladder, rectum or sacral promontory, PPH, shock and sepsis.

Other destructive operations are not described as they are very rarely performed.

CHAPTER 9

Gynecological Procedures and Operations

CERVICAL CAUTERIZATION

Introduction

This is performed by electric cautery or diathermy cautery. In electrocautery there is simple burning of diseased tissue while with diathermy cautery there is electrocoagulation (i.e., both incision and coagulation) of diseased tissue. Electrocoagulation (with high frequency monopolar electrode) is better than electrocautery, because the penetration of heat and destruction of diseased gland tissue are uniform and controllable.

Indications

- Cervical erosion (ectropion) not responding to conservative management
- Chronic cervicitis
- Nabothian follicles on cervix.

Contraindications

- Acute cervicitis, vaginitis
- Pregnancy
- Acute pelvic inflammatory disease
- Suspected early invasive carcinoma of cervix under evaluation.

Procedure

- Pap smear examination is must and if necessary cervical biopsy should be taken to rule out invasive carcinoma of the cervix
- It should be done within 7 days after cessation of menstrual period
- Superficial cauterization can be done on OPD base, as no cervical dilatation and no anesthesia is required. For deep cauterization in case of extensive erosion short general anesthesia or local anesthesia with sedation is must.

Steps

- Emptying of bladder
- Lithotomy position
- Aseptic and antiseptic precautions
- Pervaginal examination
- Cervix is exposed, cleaned and caught with tinaculum
- Cervix is dilated up to 8 No. Hegar's dilator in case of deep cauterization
- Point of the cautery is inserted into the cervical canal. Usual method is making linear strokes from just below internal os to erosion bearing area at external os. These are made in radial fashion. No intervening area should be left. The entire affected area of the cervix should be cauterized. Any Nabothian follicles present are punctured by the cautery tip and their contents are boiled out
- Small dilator or uterine sound is passed at the end of the procedure to ensure against cervical stenosis.

After-treatment

- Inform the patient that there may be excessive vaginal discharge for 3–4 weeks
- Abstinence from sexual intercourse for four weeks
- Vaginal pessary or antiseptic cream is usually not necessary. Only, if the discharge becomes infective they are indicated
- Follow-up after six weeks:
  - If erosion has not healed completely repeat cauterization once, is indicated
  - Pass a uterine sound to check that cervix is not stenosed.

Complications

- Cervical stenosis
- Secondary hemorrhage
- Accidental burns of vulva and vagina
- Sepsis.

CRYOSURGERY

Introduction

This is cold cauterization of tissue by freezing it with the use of refrigerants. Refrigerants used are nitrous oxide (– 80°), liquid nitrogen (– 90°), carbon dioxide (– 60°) and freon (–60°), equipment consists of cryoprobe attached to cryogun with rubber tubing. The other end of tube is attached to refrigerant tank. Cooling effect of gas circulated through cryoprobe brings about freezing. Different varieties of tapered ended probes are available to fit into different cervical shapes.

Indications: Cervical Lesions

- Cervical erosion
- Chronic cervicitis
- Nabothian follicles
- Condyloma acuminate
- Cervical intraepithelial neoplasia

Contraindications

Same as electrocautery.

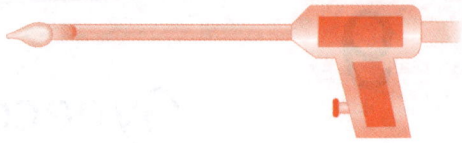

Fig. 9.1: Cryoprobe.

Procedure

- Pap smear examination is must. It may take three months before cytological findings come to normal after cryosurgery
- Like cauterization it is also done immediate postmenstrually. It is an OPD procedure. As it is a painless procedure anesthesia is not required (freezing itself produces some anesthesia).

Steps

- Emptying of bladder, lithotomy position, aseptic and antiseptic precautions.
- Cervix is exposed with Cusco's speculum and cleaned
- Properly selected cryoprobe is applied at external os. By pressing the trigger of cryogun the gas circulates through the cryoprobe and freezing starts. Application of lubricating jelly to the probe facilitates the freezing process. Within 15 seconds probe firmly adheres to the cervix (That is why tenaculum or vulsellum may not be required to catch the cervix during the procedure)
- For benign cervical lesion, the ice ball should extend at least 3 mm onto the normal epithelium, but for cervical intraepithelial neoplasia entire affected area (detected by colposcope) plus 5 mm of normal surrounding an epithelium is also freezed
- Freeze-thaw-freeze technique is used taking 2 minutes for each step
- The probe carrying rewarming system gets detached within 15 seconds, otherwise it gets detached on its own due to natural heat within 30 seconds.

Gynecological Procedures and Operations

After Treatment
Same as for electrocautery.

Advantages Over Electrocautery
- Less discomfort and pain to the patient
- Ease of administration
- Anesthesia not required
- Postoperative stenosis less
- Postoperative hemorrhage is also less.

Disadvantages Over Electrocautery
- Costlier than electrocautery and requires constant supply of gas
- Profuse watery discharge for 3 weeks.

Other Uses of Cryosurgery
- Condyloma acuminate of vulva or vagina
- Ca in situ vulva
- Vaginal adenosis.
- Vaginal intraepithelial neoplasia and
- Granulation at the vault following hysterectomy.

RUBIN'S TEST (RT)

It is tubal insufflation test which was introduced by Rubin in 1920. It is not done now because other better diagnostic facilities are available.

Time: From 6th to 10th day of menstrual cycle (i.e. soon after the period is over).

Procedure
It is an OPD procedure. No anesthesia is required. Injection atropin is given. After emptying of bladder patient is taken and lithotomy position is given after proper aseptic measures cervix is exposed and anterior lip is caught by tenaculum. Rubin's cannula is fitted to kymographic apparatus (CO_2 gas) or simple air insufflator. The cannula is gently introduced through the cervical canal. The acorn (rubber collar) of cannula is firmly pressed against external os and cervix is pulled by tenaculum for air tight fitting. Rate of CO_2 flow is 10–30 cc/min. Total 100 cc gas is usually sufficient for single test.

Contraindications
- Local or pelvic infection
- Suspected pregnancy
- Uterine bleeding
- Recent curettage
- Heart or lung disease.

Complications
- Spreading or activating pelvic infection
- Collapse and vomiting
- Embolism
- Rupture of uterus or tubes.

Criteria for positive RT (Patent tubes):
- Hissing, gurgling or bubbling sound heard on auscultation of the lower abdomen
- Typical kymographic tracing.

Rubin's Test Negative—Blocked Tubes
False negative, i.e., failure to pass gas in the peritoneal cavity even when the tubes are patent. 33% reasons include tubal spasm, block in the instrument, functional closure at uterine end due to edema and hypertrophy of endometrium.
- Besides its diagnostic value it had therapeutic effect in 20% of cases, due to temporary clearance of secretions from the tubes
- A positive test does not exclude the presence of significant tubal damage and peritubal adhesions. In case of negative test it does not given the site of block.

Other Tubal Patency Tests
- Hysterosalpingography (Described in the chapter of X-rays)
- *Endoscopic technique*: Diagnostic laparoscopy with chromopertubation. Dilute methylene blue is injected through vaginal route and seen at fimbrial ends by laparoscope. This is the best method

as it gives complete inner view of the pelvis. Video laparoscopy by attaching video camera to the laparoscope gives, continuous display on video monitor, which can also be recorded on a CD or DVD.
- *Sonosalpingogram*: Saline is injected from below through pediatric Foley's catheter under USG monitoring. If it is seen collected in pouch of Douglas it confirms patency of one or both tubes.
- *HyCoSy (Hysterosalpingo contrast sonography):* It uses of sonography contrast media like Echovist or Levovist. It avoids radiation, but it is costly and results are inferior
- *Starch test:* Starch granules are injected in the posterior cul-de-sac followed in 48 hours by iodine staining of the cervical mucous. Positive iodine test indicates tubal patency. It is not done.

COLPOSCOPY

The colposcope is a stereoscopic binocular microscope of low magnification usually from 4x to 40x. With the help of colposcope the illuminated cervix and lower genital tract are examined for detecting or eliminating precancerous and early cancerous (microinvasive) lesions. Colposcope was invented by Professor Hinselmann of Germany in 1925.

Indications

- Evaluation of abnormal Pap smear. ASCUS or persistent LSIL (CIN 1)
- Evaluation of clinically suspicious cervix regardless of cytology
- To direct the biopsy of most suspicious site
- To define size and extent of the lesion and also to detect endocervical or vaginal invasion of multicentric lesion on the cervix
- CIN 2 or CIN 3 (HGSIL) on cytology
- Acetopositivity detected by VIA or VILI.

Method

- It is an OPD procedure. However, patient should not have douche, vaginal tampon, medication or sex in last 24 hours.
- No specific preparation is required. The patient is placed in lithotomy position and bivalve speculum is inserted
- The colposcope is then focused on cervix
- The cervix is cleaned by a swab soaked in normal saline. This clears the mucous and if the epithelium is dry, it moistens it
- Usually the examination is done in 16x magnification
- 3–5% acetic acid is applied on the cervix and examination is continued. Acetic acid produces dehydration of cells and transient coagulation of nuclear proteins, so it reduces the transparency and epithelium of larger nuclear size (e.g., CIN) becomes temporarily white—acetowhite epithelium
- As the effect of acetic acid is transient it may be repeated as necessary
- A green filter can be employed to absorb the red light so optimal contrast of the vessels is achieved. Normal blood vessels branch like a tree
- The basic features studied at colposcopy are sharply delineated acetowhite epithelium and abnormal vascular pattern.

Colposcopic findings are described under following headings:
- *Normal colposcopic findings*: Original squamous epithelium, columnar epithelium, normal transformation zone
- *Abnormal colposcopic findings*: These include cellular changes and vascular changes. Cellular changes are leukoplakia and acetowhite epithelium. Vascular changes include punctations (fine or coarse), mosaicism (fine or coarse) and atypical vessels. Punctation is due to influx of capillary loops, mosaicism is due to arborization and coalescence of intraepithelial vessels and atypical vessels is due to nonuniform growth.

- *Colposcopy suspicious invasive carcinoma*—Lesion is not visible on clinical examination but evident on colposcopy as a raised lesion with irregular nodular surface contour or ulceration and bizarre abnormal blood vessels.
- *Unsatisfactory colposcopy findings:* When the squamocolumnar junction is not visible
- *Miscellaneous findings*: These include inflammatory changes, atrophy, ulcer, condyloma or papilloma.

Swede scores devised by Strander, et al., (2005) is useful. Score of 8 or more has 100% specificity and can be used for performing direct excisional procedures as see and treat method.

DILATATION AND CURETTAGE

Definition

Dilatation and curettage (D&C) means dilatation of cervical canal and curetting (scrapping out) of the cavity of uterus.

Indications

Diagnostic

- Abnormal uterine bleeding (AUB): To rule out the organic cause of bleeding and to know the exact type of AUB from endometrial histology (i.e., hormonal pattern).
- Post-menopausal bleeding
- *Infertility*: To find out any pathology and hormonal pattern of endometrium. Secretory endometrium suggests ovulation. This is not done now as ovulation can be easily detected by transvaginal sonography
- Suspected endometrial cancer (fractional curettage)
- Suspected pelvic tuberculosis
- Along with Manchester and like operations for prolapse by vaginal route, where uterus is retained.

Therapeutic

- *AUB*: It may act as hemostatic measure when hormonal treatment has failed
- Infertility: D & C also has some therapeutic value in cases of infertility
- Along with polypectomy
- Removal of embedded IUCD
- *Ectopic pregnancy*: Required along with other definitive treatment of ectopic, to remove thick decidua to stop uterine bleeding. In suspected ectopic, it was done in past to see the presence of chorionic villi in curetted material, which rules out ectopic.

Now with transvaginal sonography with color Doppler and serial serum β-hCG ectopic can be accurately diagnosed.

Prognostic

- Follow-up cases of vesicular mole when need arises
- Follow-up cases after medical treatment of endometrial carcinoma or endometrial tuberculosis.

Contraindications

- Suspected pregnancy
- *Infections*: Local or pelvic. If indicated it is done under adequate antibiotic cover.

Instruments

Arranged in chronological order of use:
- Swab holder
- Sims' speculum
- Anterior vaginal wall retractor
- Uterine sound
- Cervical dilators
- Curette
- Uterine dressing forceps

Procedure

- Pre-medication: Injection glycopyrrolate 0.2 mg I/M
- Anesthesia: Short G/A is preferred.
  In patients with medical risks and in parous patients operation can be done under L/A (paracervical block) with sedation.

Steps of Operation

- Emptying of bladder
- Lithotomy position
- Painting and draping
- G/A is given. Examination under anesthesia
- Expose the cervix by speculum and anterior vaginal wall retractor
- Swab out the cervix. Catch the anterior lip by Vulsellum
- Sounding of uterus is done to determine the length and direction of the utero-cervical canal
- Dilatation by well lubricated cervical dilators is done in increasing number gradually
- Dilatation up to 8-9 No. Hegar's dilator is sufficient for easy introduction of curette
- Sterile gauze piece is kept over the speculum below the cervix for collection of curettage material
- Curette is introduced, passed up to the fundus and cavity is curetted in longitudinal direction from the fundus to the internal os
- A useful routine is to start at 12 o'clock and work round the cavity in clockwise or anticlockwise direction
- Top of the cavity is explored by side to side movement and both Cornu are explored separately
- Curetting is done till grating sensation is felt
- If prior USG (TVS) has shown polyp, polypectomy should be carried out by polyp forceps
- Material is collected for histopathology in a container having 10% formalin solution.
- Uterine cavity is cleaned by gauze soaked in antiseptic solution (Savlon) with uterine dressing forceps
- Instruments are removed. See that there is no bleeding from the uterus or Vulsellum bite of cervix
- Vagina is cleaned and sterile pad is applied.

Complications

- Failure to dilate the internal os
- Injury—laceration or tear of cervix, perforation of uterus
- Introduction of infection or flare-up of pre-existing infections
- Hemorrhage—from the injuries of cervix or uterus, or from the endometrial cavity.

Late

- Vigorous curettage leading to secondary amenorrhea—Asherman's syndrome
- Deep scar of curettage on the uterine wall may lead to adherent placenta or rupture uterus in future pregnancy or labor.

Medical Curettage

To convert the hyperplastic endometrium of metropathia into secretory phase by giving progesterone and to precipitate withdrawal bleeding has been called "Medical curettage".

Fractional Curettage

It is done in case of suspected endometrial carcinoma. First the endocervical curettage is done. Then cervix is dilated and thorough curettage is done. Previously, it was done by obtaining different specimens from different parts of uterus, i.e., isthmus, anterior wall, right lateral wall, posterior wall, left lateral wall and lastly fundus. This is not done now as management of endometrial cancer does not depend upon the site of cancer but the stage of cancer.

FEMALE STERILIZATION

Female sterilization refers to all operations performed on a woman which permanently prevent conception. Though most commonly it involves Fallopian tube, it can involve ovary or uterus:

Tube: Infundibulum—amputated, buried, plugged or capped
Isthmic and ampullary portion—removed, cut, tied, occluded, buried, frozen or burnt
Uterotubal junction—closed, plugged or scarred.

Ovary: Removed, irradiated, buried or covered with silicone rubber.
Uterus: Removed.

Tubal procedures may be classified as follows:
- *Traditional surgical methods*:
    - Abdominal approach   – Laparotomy
    -                       – Minilap
    - Vaginal approach   – Colpotomy
- *Endoscopic methods*:
    - Abdominal approach   – Laparoscopy
    - Vaginal approach   – Hysteroscopy

Only laparotomy and laparoscopy tubal operations (Lap TL) are commonly done at present.

In laparotomy procedures modified Pomeroy method is commonly performed at present.

Abdominal Tubal Ligation (Abdo TL)

Modified Pomeroy Technique

- *Time*:
    - Interval sterilization (gynec TL).
    - Post-abortal.
    - Post-partum.
    - During cesarean section.
- *Anesthesia*: It can be done under any anesthesia. L/A, S/A or G/A.

Steps

- After premedication, written consent and emptying of the bladder patient is taken on the operation table
- Supine position with foot end of the table slightly raised
- Painting and draping.
- Under anesthesia, abdomen is opened by transverse incision 3–5 cm long
- Site of incision in interval sterilization is 1 inch above the symphysis pubis, while in postpartum patient it is put just below the fundus of uterus
- Rectus sheath is cut opened, rectus muscles are separated, peritoneum is identified and cut opened taking care not to injure bladder or bowel
- C-retractor or Morris's retractor is introduced inside the incision and retraction is done as required
- In obstetric cases tubes can be caught under direct vision by babcock or toothless forceps, otherwise one or two fingers are slipped laterally to catch the tube which is then delivered through the incision
- Tube is confirmed by its tubular structure, soft consistency, pink-red color, fimbrial end and its attachment to the uterus medially
- A loop is made by holding the tube with babcock forceps, usually at the junction of medial one-third and lateral two-third. TL at isthmic region is better than ampullary part as it has (1) less failure rate, and (2) subsequent tuboplasty if required in future will have better results
- Strong artery forceps is applied at the base of the loop to crush it. Below the crushed part, through an avascular area of mesosalpinx needle is passed and tube is ligated doubly by No. 1 chromic catgut
- Loop of the tube above the artery forceps is cut-off. Minimal adequate portion should be removed so that tuboplasty, if required in the future, can have adequate length of the tube available
- Additional second ligation of the cut ends of tubes may be done separately
- After checking that there is no bleeding from cut ends of the tube or mesosalpinx, ligated tube is released back in the abdomen
- Opposite tube is ligated in the same way through the same incision
- Abdomen is closed in layers and sterile dressing is applied over the wound. From a medicolegal point a portion of the tube removed should be sent for histological examination for confirmation.

Postoperative Care

- Prophylactic antibiotics for 5–7 days
- If there is no complication, postoperative I/V fluid is not required

- Patient can start liquid diet orally within 4–6 hours of operation depending upon which anesthesia is given
- Stitches are usually removed on 7th postoperative day.

Complications

- Tearing of tubes
- Hemorrhage, if vessels of mesosalpinx are injured and it may cause hematoma also
- Infection
- Wound gap
- Rarely injury to bowel or bladder
- Complications of anesthesia.

Late complications

- Failure, i.e., pregnancy 3/1000 operations, (Modified Pomeroy).
- Ectopic pregnancy
- Menorrhagia— interference of blood supply to ovary leading to congestion may be the cause.
- Wound complications—incisional hernia, scar endometriosis and adhesions
- Torsion of unsupported outer end of the tube (rare).

Other Methods

- *Classic Pomeroy:* No crushing of the loop. Tie with plain catgut No. 0 and cut-off the loop
- *Mendlener*: Make loop of midportion of the tube, crush the base for 1 minute. Apply silk. No cutting of the loop. Failure rate is high.
- *Uchida:* Inject saline in mesosalpinx. Strip-off the peritoneum from the tubal musculature. Cut-off 5 cm of the tube. Medial end is tied and buried inside the mesosalpinx. Lateral end is tied outside the mesosalpinx. In between peritoneum is sutured in purse string fashion. 100% effective.
- *Irving*: Tie with catgut No. 0 chromic doubly. Cut the tube between 2 ligatures. Medial end is buried in the myometrium posteriorly (in tunnel), the lateral end is buried in mesosalpinx (It was designed for TL following CS). 100% effective.
- *Modified Irving*: Same except no burial of lateral end
- *Kroener's fimbriectomy*: Distal portion of ampulla doubly ligated with silk and fimbria is excised. Irreversible.
- *Parkland procedure*: Introduce hemostate in the avascular area of mesosalpinx. By opening the jaws make 2.5 cm space. Tube is ligated proximally and distally by 2-0 chromic suture and intervening segment of about 2.5 cm is excised:
  - Oxford method: Tube is cut. Medial end is tied with catgut and brought to the back of the round ligament. Lateral end is sutured with linen thread and brought anterior to the round ligament. Plication of the round ligament
  - Shirodkar method: Tube is cut in the middle part. Cut ends are ligated half inch away from their ends. Then they are folded on themselves and tied again with silk
  - Crossen's operation: Cornual end of the tube with wedge of the uterine muscle are removed. Distal cut end is ligated and buried between the two layers of broad ligament.
    - Disadvantages—hemorrhage, recanalization is difficult.
  - Aldridge method: Burying fimbrial end of the fallopian tube extraperitonealy by means of mattress suture in the broad ligament through a hole made in the anterior leaf, posterior to the round ligament
- *Ovariotexy*: Mechanical obstruction by silastic pouch.
- *Fibriotexy*: Applying silastic cap over fimbria-reversible.
- *Salpingectomy*: Total bilateral, with or without excision of cornual area.

Gynecological Procedures and Operations

MINILAP TECHNIQUE

Originally described by Uchida in 1971 as a postpartum procedure. But, now it can be done at any time, postpartum, postabortal or interval sterilization. It is safe, effective and convenient method of sterilization. Usually done under local anesthesia, but G/A may be used. Small (2.5 cm) transverse incision is put at the level of fundus or an inch above the symphysis pubis in interval cases. Uterus is manipulated by uterine elevator from vaginal route to bring the tube at the site of abdominal incision.

VAGINAL TL

In vaginal TL tubes can be approached from either anterior fornix or posterior fornix (preferred) after opening the uterovesical pouch or pouch of Douglas respectively. Methods commonly done are Pomeroy's, fimbriectomy or salpingectomy. Certain prerequisites are essential for vaginal TL:
- Uterus should not be enlarged,
- Uterus should be reasonably mobile,
- No local infection,
- No pelvic pathology,
- There should be adequate space in the vagina. Prolapse of uterus is not necessary for vaginal TL. It is rarely practiced in present times.
    - As it avoids laparotomy advantages over abdominal TL are obvious
    - Disadvantages are increased risk of infection, technically more difficult, limited space, and can be done in interval cases only.

LAPAROSCOPY

It is an endoscopic visualization of the peritoneal cavity through the anterior abdominal wall.

Laparoscope

Actual telescope consists of an objective, an eyepiece near the proximal end and light conducting image relay system connecting the two. In operative laparoscope there is separate channel for operative instrument. Now for video-laparoscopy 0° or 30°, 10 mm laparoscopes are used.

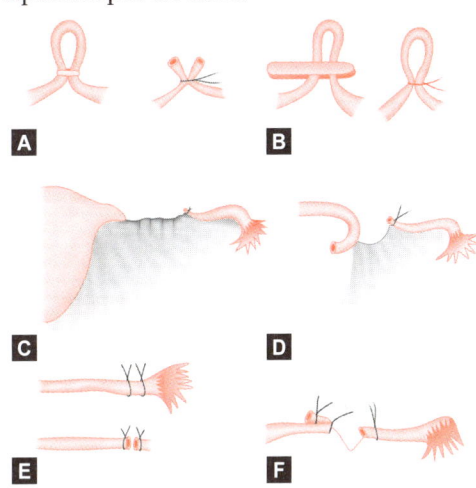

Figs. 9.2A to F: (A) Modified pomeroy; (B) Mendlener; (C) Uchida; (D) Irving; (E) Kroener's; (F) Shirodkar.

Veress Needle

It is double cannula metal needle, outer one is sharp and pointed, while inner-cannula is blunt pointed and projecting beyond the sharp point of outer cannula, with a spring action which prevents injury to abdominal viscera during insertion. Internal diameter is 16 gauge. It is available in 3 different lengths.

Trocar and Trocar Sleeve

Made of metal or nonconducting substance. Trocar has a sharp endpyramidal or conical in shape. Usually they are 5–10 mm sizes. Trocar sleeve (cannula) has got a valve to prevent gas leakage when trocar or scope is introduced inside or removed out from it.

There are two types of valve:
1. Trumpet or piston type,
2. Flapper or clip type valve.
- *Light Source:* Fiber optic system. It is cold light system located outside and light is transmitted through glass fibers, in the

light cable. Halogen, Xenon and LED light sources are used in endoscopy.
- *Gas Insufflator*: Special instrument supplying CO_2 gas with different indicators on it, indicating:
  – How much gas is going,
  – Pressure of the site where it is going (i.e., intraperitoneal pressure), and
  – How much gas is used and whether the cylinder is empty or not.

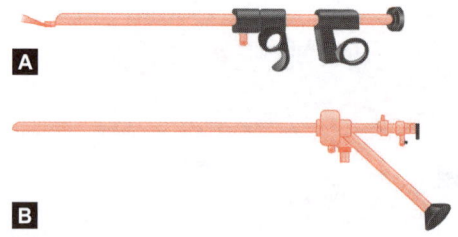

Figs. 9.3A and B: Laparoscopes: (A) Laprocator-KLI; (B) Storz.

Sterilization: Cidex solution or ethylene oxide gas or formalin vapor sterilization. No autoclaving.

Laparoscopic TL

Different methods are as under:
- *Falope ring:* It is made up of silicone rubber with 5% barium sulfate impregnated. Its outer diameter is 3.6 mm, inner diameter is 1.0 mm and it is 2.2 mm thick. It exerts 0.3–0.4 pounds per inch pressure. It is available in sterilized form presterilized by gamma rays. It destroys 2–3 cm segment of the tube. Lap TL is most commonly done with falope rings.
- *Hulka–Clemens clip:* It is made up of plexin. It has teeth and a hinge and is closed and locked in place by a goldplated stainless steel spring. The clip is 3 mm wide and 15 mm long. Clips are better for postabortal and puerperal cases.
- *Filshie clip:* It is made up of titanium lined on its inner surface by silicone rubber. It destroys only 4 mm wide segment of the tube, so recanalization success (like Hulka's clip) is better than that of falope ring, but failure rate is slightly higher.
- *Diathermy coagulation:* Unipolar or Bipolar cautery.

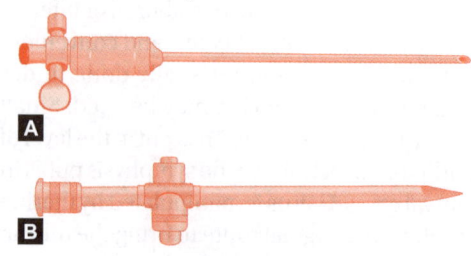

Figs. 9.4A and B: (A) Veress needle; (B) Trocar with trocar sleeve.

Indications of Laparoscopy

Diagnostic
- *Infertility:* Primary or secondary
- Examination for tubal patency, as well as evaluation of uterine, ovarian and pelvic factor for infertility
- *Endometriosis*—for diagnosis, staging, treatment and in follow-up
- Suspected ectopic pregnancy
- Primary amenorrhea—to check the development of uterus and ovaries
- To differentiate between septate uterus and bicornuate uterus (along with hysteroscopy).
- *Pelvic malignancy:*
  – Staging
  – Second look to assess therapy or to detect early recurrence
- Uterine perforation evaluation
- Undiagnosed pelvic pain
- Undiagnosed pelvic mass
- Intersexuality—to take gonadal biopsy.

Therapeutic
- Sterilization—laparoscopic TL
- *Infertility:*
  – Lysis of adhesions
  – Dilatation of phimotic fimbrial end
  – Salpingostomy
  – End to end anastomosis—tuboplasty

- Laparoscopic hysterectomy (TLH), laparoscopy assisted vaginal hysterectomy (LAVH)
- Removal of ovarian cyst, ovarian drilling for PCOD
- *Endometriosis:*
  - Fulguration of small implants
  - Treatment of chocolate cysts
  - Adhesiolysis
- Ectopic pregnancy—salpingostomy, segmental resection, salpingectomy or injection of drugs like PGs, KCI, Methotrexate in the sac
- Laparoscopic myomectomy
- Removal of displaced IUCD
- Laparoscopic sling operation, vault suspension
- Laparoscopic radical surgery for malignancy, i.e. Wertheim's
- Laparoscopic vaginoplasty
- Transaction of uterosacral ligaments for pelvic pain—LUNA.
  Almost every gynec surgery can now be done by operative laparoscopy.

Advantages of laparoscopic surgery over laparotomy include minimal total size of skin incisions—cosmetic, less blood loss, reduced postoperative pain and discomfort, more rapid Convalescence, shorter hospital stay—less cost, lower risk of postoperative adhesions and less infectious morbidity.

Video-laparoscopic surgery is now routinely done. Attaching a video camera to the endoscope (0 or 30° 10 mm telescope), surgery is performed by looking at the picture in TV monitor with laproscopic hand instruments introduced through two or three second puncture hole ports.

Contraindications

- Acute inflammation of:
  - General peritoneal cavity
  - Pelvis
- Intestinal obstruction
- Severe cardiorespiratory diseases
- Abdominal or diaphragmatic hernia
- Paralytic ileus
- Extensive abdominal scarring
- Massive hemoperitoneum
- Extreme obesity
- Advanced pregnancy
- Large intra-abdominal masses—widespread carcinomatosis

Laparoscopic TL

Anesthesia: It is done under general anesthesia or local anesthesia with sedation.

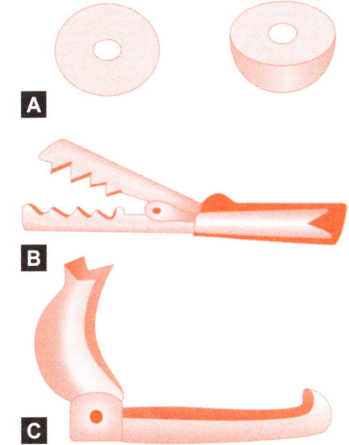

Figs. 9.5A to C: (A) Falope ring; (B) Hulca's clip; (C) Filshie clip.

Procedure

- After preanesthetic medications (Glycopyrrolate + Fortwin + Phenergan), written consent and emptying of bladder patient is taken on the operation table.
- There must be full surgical preparation of abdomen (it should be the principle that for any laparoscopy, diagnostic or therapeutic, patient should be prepared fully for laparotomy)
  Position: Lithotomy initially, head low is done after trocar is inserted and then increased as required
- Painting and draping.
- 2-3 cc 1% xylocaine is injected subcutaneously just below the umbilicus

- Small nick is put with the knife
- Anterior abdominal wall is raised from either side of the umbilicus by hands or clips
- Veress needle is passed through the nick obliquely with 45° angle to horizontal and directed towards the pelvis till it reaches the peritoneal cavity
- Gas tube from the insufflator is attached to the needle. CO_2 gas is commonly used. Flow rate should be 0.5 to 1 L/min with pressure indicator reading between 10–15 mm Hg. If pressure meter shows indicator moving to more than 15 mm Hg. It indicates that either the needle is not in the peritoneal cavity or bowel or omentum is obstructing it
- Between 1.5–2.5 L gas is usually required depending upon laxity of the abdominal muscles and obesity of the patient
- With the knife skin incision is extended in semilunar fashion with concavity towards umbilicus. Incision should be of optimum size so that there is no difficulty in the insertion of trocar and at the same time gas will not leak out
- Trocar with trocar sleeve are then introduced. After raising the abdominal wall as in needle insertion, trocar with sleeve are passed at 45° angle in the middle towards the sacrum
- As soon as the peritoneal cavity is entered there is loss of resistance and hissing sound may appear due to leakage of gas. Trocar is withdrawn and trocar sleeve is advanced to further short distance to ensure that it remains into the peritoneal cavity
- Now laparoscope loaded with falope rings is introduced, light cord is attached. Light is put on and pelvic cavity is visualized. Uterus is manipulated as required, by the assistant from vaginal route, by uterine manipulator, Rubin's cannula, uterine sound or dilator
- Tube is identified and inner tongs are extruded. Tube is grasped usually 2.5–3 cm from cornual end (i.e., isthmic part). Care must be taken to include only the tube but the entire thickness of it
- By means of slide mechanism the tongs are brought within the central sleeve bringing with them a loop of tube. Slide mechanism is pulled tightly so central sleeve is also withdrawn inside the outer sleeve. So the ring is extruded past the end of the applicator over the knuckle of the tube
- Tongs are now extruded again, so loop is released. Loop of the tube with the strangulating falope ring at its base can be visualized
- The procedure is repeated on the opposite side
- Finally examination of pelvic contents is done—it is also checked that there is no active bleeding or hematoma in mesosalpinx
- After completion of the procedure laparoscope is removed. Valve of trocar sleeve is opened by simple toothless forceps or trocar or by pushing the piston in to exhaust the pneumoperitoneum.
- Before removing the trocar sleeve, trocar is inserted into it, then it is changed to more horizontal position and then removed to prevent extrusion of omentum through the incision
- Skin incision is closed by taking subcuticular or simple stitches and dressing is done. Patient can be discharged after 3–4 hours.

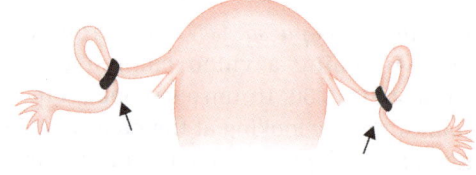

Fig. 9.6: Falope rings in situ.

Important Points

- *Site of pneumoperitoneum*: Subumbilical area is the best site because:
  - Abdominal wall is thinnest here
  - Cosmetic reason—scar merges in umbilicus.

Other sites are:
- 4 cm below the midpoint of left costal margin
- Left McBurney's point.
- Confirmation for right insertion of Veress needle, i.e., inside the peritoneal cavity.
  - Free side to side movement of needle
  - Hissing sound on introduction of Veress needle, it is due to atmospheric air being sucked in rapidly
  - A drop of normal saline placed on the needle is immediately sucked in by elevation of abdominal wall
  - Indicator on insufflator remains between 10 and 15 mm Hg, i.e., normal intraperitoneal pressure
- CO_2 is commonly used gas because:
  - More tissue solubility so rapidly absorbed through peritoneal surfaces
  - It does not support combustion and it is nonexplosive
  - It is easily cleared from the blood stream and excreted easily.
  N_2O and air are also used but N_2O is
  - Less soluble then CO_2, and
  - When used with electrocautery it can support combustion. With air, rare danger of air embolism is there, but it is very economical. So in camp set-up in absence of CO_2 insufflator, air is commonly used.

Difficulties and Minor Complications

- Fogging of lens
- Falling of ring into the peritoneal cavity
- Poor mobility of tube, which may lead to tubal transaction or tear
- Leaking of gas
- Perforation of uterus by manipulator
- Abrasion on the fundus
- Small hematoma in mesosalpinx

Failure

Failure rate of the Lap TL: 2–4/1000 operations. Common causes of failure are:
- Misapplication of rings on round ligament, broad ligament fold or ovarian ligament
- Small loop
- Poor quality of ring (breaking or slipping)
- Development of tuboperitoneal fistula
- Natural recanalization

Advantages of Lap TL Over Surgical TL

- Operative time is less.
- Very little blood loss
- Hardly visible scar
- Less postoperative pain
- Low incidence of complications
- Postoperative rest required is also less
- Outpatient procedure so less hospital load, less cost to the patient

Disadvantages

- Require of costly equipment
- Require of special training
- Not suitable for immediate postpartum cases
- Although complications are few and rare, some of them are life threatening
- It may not be done, if there are adhesions covering the tubes or tubes are badly thickened due to chronic infection

Complications of Laparoscopy

During Creation of Pneumoperitoneun

To avoid some of these complications some gynecologists are now doing direct trocar insertion without creating prior pneumoperitoneum by Veress needle.
- Subcutaneous emphysema
- Gas insufflation of abdominal wall layers, i.e. between rectus sheath and peritoneum
- CO_2 embolism — rare but dangerous
- Insufflation of retroperitoneal space, bowel or omentum
- Rarely diaphragm may be torn at one of the weak points leading to mediastinal emphysema
- Injury to the vessels of abdominal wall-may cause hematoma
- Puncture of major vessels like inferior vena cava

- Perforation of bowel, if it is adherent to the abdominal wall
- Cardiorespiratory embrassment.

Complications of Rest of the Procedure

- *Infections*: New infection, flare-up of silent tuberculosis lesion, wound sepsis
- Hemorrhage, if vessels are not properly cauterized and tissues are cut
- Bowel injury by hand instruments. Electric burns of bowel and mesentery if cautery is used
- Injury to bladder and ureter in operative laparoscopy
- Perforation of the uterus
- Injury to large abdominal vessels by Veress needle or trocar
- Omental hernia
- Peritoneal fistula
- Complications of anesthesia
- Laser burns, if it is used in operative laparoscopy

HYSTEROSCOPY

It is an endoscopic visualization of uterine cavity, tubal openings and endocervix by means of a fiberoptic hysteroscope passed through the cervical canal.

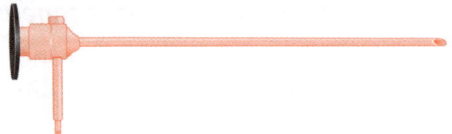

Fig. 9.7: Hysteroscope

Instruments

Routine instruments for any vaginal procedure. Hysteroscopic equipment includes actual telescope, sheath, its obturator, distension media, e.g., CO_2, Hyskon (dextran 32) 5% dextrose, Glycine, Sorbitol or normal saline, hysteroflator and a light source.

For operative hysteroscopy operative sheath, operative scissors, resectoscope, cutting loop, roller ball and bar, under water cautery and fluid delivery apparatus, etc. are required.

Indications

Diagnostic

- *Infertility:* To study the uterine factor
- Unexplained abnormal uterine bleeding
- Endometrial carcinoma to visualize the lesion and to obtain biopsy
- Recurrent pregnancy loss to find out the local cause if any
- For diagnosis of polyps and misplaced IUCDs
- For diagnosis of uterine synechiae (Asherman's syndrome).

Therapeutic

- Endometrial ablation in case of AUB-electrocoagulation or Nd-YAG:laser ablation through hysteroscope
- Endometrial resection—TCRE. Less commonly done at present
- Division or lysis of intrauterine adhesions
- Division of uterine septum
- Excision or endometrial polyps and small submucous fibroids
- Transcervical tubal cannulation and balloon tuboplasty in case of proximal tubal occlusion
- Retrieval of lost IUCDs and other foreign bodies
- *Tubal sterilization*: Different methods include diathermy, thermal coagulation, introduction of ceramic preformed tubal plugs, silastic plugs formed in situ, microcoil insertion (Essure) and use of chemical agents (sclerosants), e.g., Quinacrine (250 mg pellets), methyl cyanoacrylate.

Contraindications

- Excessive uterine bleeding
- Intrauterine pregnancy
- Infection—cervicitis, vaginitis and acute or chronic PID
- Invasive carcinoma of the cervix.

Technique

- Diagnostic hysteroscopy may be done without anesthesia as an office procedure, otherwise it is done either under G/A or L/A (paracervical block) + sedation
- Emptying of bladder
- Lithotomy position
- Strict aseptic and antiseptic precautions
- Pervaginal examination
- Sounding of the uterocervical canal
- Dilatation of the cervix up to 6 mm for diagnostic hysteroscopy. More dilatation is required for operative hysteroscopy
- If CO_2 is to be used for distension, a cervical suction cap is applied on the cervix to make it leak proof. This is not required for fluid media
- Sheath with obturator is introduced through the dilated cervix and obturator is removed
- Hysteroscope is introduced and 50–100 mL of dextran 32% is injected slowly with flow pressure of 100 mm Hg.
- Uterine cavity is now systematically examined, i.e. fundus, tubal ostia, anterior, posterior and lateral uterine walls and lastly the endocervix. Any operative procedure, if required is carried out through the hysteroscope with special instruments.

Complications

Procedure-related
- Cervical laceration
- Uterine perforation
- Infection
- Hemorrhage
- Visceral injuries: Thermal injuries in operative hysteroscopy.

Media-related
- Hyponatremia, fluid overload (rarely death can occur)
- CO_2 embolism
- Anaphylactic reactions (Dextran)
- Hemolysis (when water is used)

In fluid media electrolyte free media are required when monopolar cautery is used (in electrolyte media current gets transmitted). These when absorbed, causes hyponatremia. One should be vigilant in OT to calculate the fluid deficit continuously. Fluid deficit up to 1000 mL is a safe limit and it should never cross 1500 mL.

LASER IN GYNECOLOGY

The word laser is an acronym for light amplification by stimulated emission of radiation. Laser was first used in gynecology by Kaplan in 1973. The primary tissue effects of the surgical lasers are produced by laser heat energy. The tissue destruction occurs by:
- Vaporization of cells
- Thermal necrosis, and
- From heat conduction.

The laser unit consists of laser head which contains the lasing medium, an excitation source and an aiming beam. Unit also has a power amplifier, cooling system and delivery system (fiber or mirrors).

Commonly used lasers are CO_2, Nd : YAG (Neodymium: yttrium-aluminium garnet), Argon and KTP (Potassium titanyl phosphate) lasers.

The basic properties and characteristics of different lasers are as follows

	CO_2	Argon/KTP	Nd : YAG
Color	Infrared	Green, blue	Infrared
Delivery system	Articulated mirrors	Fiber	Fiber
Absorption	Water, glass, plastic	Heme, Melanin	Proteins
Penetration	0.1 mm	2.0 mm	4–6 mm
Maximum power	100 W	20 W	100 W
Precision cut	+++	+	+
Coagulation	+	+	+++
Wavelength (nm)	10600	515/532	1064
Lasing medium	Gas	Gas	Solid

Uses

- *Lower genital tract surgery*: In the treatment of cervical intraepithelial neoplasia (conization), vaginal intraepithelial neoplasia, vulval intraepithelial neoplasia, condyloma accuminata (HPV).
- *Gynec endoscopic surgery:*
  - Laparoscopic laser surgery: Adhesiolysis, endometriosis, PCOD drilling, ovarian cystectomy, myomectomy, ectopic pregnancy. Salpingo-oophorectomy and laparoscopic hysterectomy
  - Hysteroscopic laser surgery: Endometrial ablation, septal incision, lysis of intrauterine adhesions and myomectomy.
- *Open abdominal surgery*: Laser may be used at laparotomy for adhesiolysis, endometriosis—fulguration or excision, tubal reconstructive surgery and myomectomy.

Advantages

Laser surgery include less bleeding, less tissue handling, precise tissue destruction and less postoperative pain.

Disadvantages

High cost, not portable, special training required, risk of fire and injury to operation theater personnel.

HYSTERECTOMY

Hysterectomy: Hysterous (uterus) + ectomy (removal). It is an operation of removal of uterus. It can be done through abdominal route (abdominal hysterectomy), vaginal route (vaginal hysterectomy) or by laparoscopy.

Abdominal Hysterectomy

Types

- *Total*: Removal of uterus along with cervix.
- *Subtotal*: Removal of uterus only, leaving behind the cervix
- Total with unilateral salpingo-oophorectomy
- *Panhysterectomy*: Total with bilateral salpingo-oophorectomy (both tubes and ovaries removed)
- *Radical hysterectomy*: Pan hysterectomy + removal of parametrium, upperpart of vagina, pelvic lymph nodes, etc. for malignant diseases (Wertheim–Meigs operation for carcinoma cervix).

Indications

Gynecology

- *DUB:* Any case of excessive, prolonged and/or frequent menstruation not controlled by hormonal treatment or D & C, age more than 35 and she has completed child-bearing
- *Fibroid uterus*: Symptomatic fibroid of any size and asymptomatic fibroid >12 weeks size, when child-bearing is completed
- Adenomyosis.
- Carcinoma in situ cervix (Ca cervix stage 0), cervical intraepithelial neoplasia—CIN Gr II or III, i.e., HGSIL.
- Invasive carcinoma of cervix—Wertheim-Meigs' radical hysterectomy is performed up to stage II-a.
- Pelvic endometriosis
- Endometrial hyperplasia (complex and atypical)
- Endometrial carcinoma. Radical hysterectomy
- Ovarian tumors
- Bilateral chronic pelvic inflammatory diseases not responding to conservative treatment.

In some of the above indications of abdominal hysterectomy, vaginal hysterectomy (NDVH) or laparoscopic hysterectomy (TLH) is done now a days.

Investigations

These include ABO-Rh, hemogram, RFT, LFT, PPBS, urine-routine and microscopy, Pap

Gynecological Procedures and Operations

smear, ECG and X-ray chest. Hbs-Ag and HIV testing after patient's consent are also done.

Preoperative Preparations

- Admission at least 6–8 hours before operation
- Counseling of the patient regarding hysterectomy (i.e. procedure, risks, alternative treatment) and written consent
- NBM for minimum 6–8 hours. Low residue diet on the day before operation
- Shaving of the abdomen, back, vulva and then antiseptic applications including vaginal cleaning (Povidone iodine) in the ward
- Bowel is evacuated by enema in the morning, mild purgatives may be given on the previous night.
- Sedative (tablet Alprazolam) on the night before operation
- One unit of PCV should be kept cross-matched and ready
- One dose of antibiotics 2 hours before the operation
- Foley's catheter is introduced.

Anesthesia

Operation can be done under general anesthesia, spinal anesthesia or epidural analgesia. Preanesthetic medications I/M are given half an hour before the operation.

Technique

- After all routine preliminaries of laparotomy, abdomen is opened under anesthesia by Pfannenstiel (low transverse) incision or subumbilical vertical incision
- Abdominal retractor (Doyen's) is introduced and uterus is delivered through the incision and held by either retinaculum applied at the fundus, or 2 straight or curved clamps, one applied at each cornu
- Position of the patient is changed to head low (Trendelenburg) and intestines are packed away by roller gauze pack or mops. End of the pack or mop is preserved by an artery forceps kept outside
- Ovaries and tubes are examined and decision regarding their preservation or removal is taken
- First pair of clamps is applied to one round ligament about one inch away from the cornu, it is cut between 2 clamps, ligated by Vicryl no. 1 and preserved
- Second pair of clamps is applied on the same side on Fallopian tube, ovarian ligament and part of the broad ligament at cornu (if ovaries are to be preserved) or on infundibulopelvic ligaments (ovaries removed). It is cut and doubly ligated (first simple ligation and second transfixation) by 1 no. Vicryl
- Procedure is repeated on the opposite side
- Uterovesical fold of peritoneum is cut opened transversely from one cut round ligament to other, after dissection and at the level of isthmus
- Bladder along with its peritoneum is pushed down by blunt and sharp dissection and retractor is adjusted
- Posterior leaf of broad ligament is cut on either side obliquely up to the insertion of uterosacral ligaments on the cervix taking care not to injure ureter
- Uterine vessels are skeletonized (making it clearly visible) at the level of isthmus by sharp and blunt dissection
- A pair of curved clamps is applied at the level of isthums transversely on the uterine vessels (identification of ureter at this junction is a wise step to avoid injury to it). A third medial clamp is applied higher up to prevent retrograde bleeding. Opposite uterine vessels are ligated in the same way
- After checking that the bladder is adequately retracted next step is to apply clamps on paracervical ligaments medial to the stump of uterine vessels. On both the sides they are cut and transfixed

- Successive medial clamps are applied (depending upon the length of the cervix) till the vaginal vault is cut and transfixed in the same manner. Some gynecologists prefer to clamp and transfix uterosacral ligaments separately
- Usually the vagina gets opened at one angle while cutting the last pedicle at vault, otherwise it should be opened by a stab incision transversely on the anterior vaginal wall just below the cervix. Cut edge of the vagina is held with long Allis forceps. Cutting the vagina around the cervix, with traction on the uterus, the specimen is completely removed
- Povidone iodine may be applied to the vaginal vault and it is sutured by continuous locking or interrupted figure of 8 stitches with 1 no. Vicryl. The angle sutures must include ligaments to prevent vault prolapse in future.
- Hemostasis is secured. As mentioned under cesarean section suturing of both visceral and parietal peritoneum is not necessary. It is proved by evidence that nonsuturing lead to less adhesions and saves operative time
- Peritoneal toilet is done, all packs are removed and abdomen is closed in layers taking nonabsorbable (Prolene) or delayed absorbable material (Vicryl) for rectus sheath.

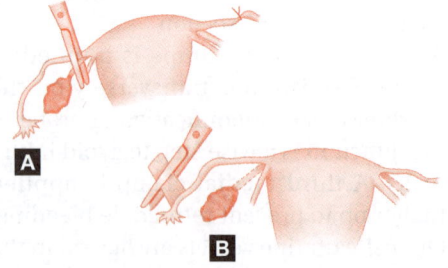

Figs. 9.8A and B: (A) Ovaries preserved and cornual structures tied together; (B) Ovaries removed.

Postoperative Management

- Nil by mouth till peristalsis appears (usually 24 hours)
- TPR half hourly and BP is recorded 2 hourly on the first day in every patient
- I/V fluids: 2.5–3 L (RL+ D5 + DNS) are given on the first day.
- Broad spectrum antibiotics (cephalosporins + amnioglycosides + metronidazole are commonly used)
- Analgesics (Diclofenac sodium or Tramadol or paracetamol) are used by I/M, slow I/V route or rectal suppository
- Urine output is measured (Foley's catheter is removed after 48 hours)
- Dressing is checked daily and changed at least once after 3rd day
- Patient is observed for any other complaint like vomiting, giddiness, distension, etc.

Complications

- *Intraoperative*: These include primary hemorrhage, injury to bowel, bladder or ureter, difficulty in dissection requiring subtotal hysterectomy and anesthetic complications
- *Postoperative*: They are as follows:
  - Infection—would sepsis, peritonitis, pelvic abscess, septicemia
  - Hemorrhage—reactionary (within 24 hours) or secondary (up to 14 days)
  - Wound complications—infection, wound gap, discharge, burst abdomen
  - Bladder—urinary tract infection, undiagnosed injury leading to fistula, retention of urine
  - Bowel—vomiting, distension, paralytic ileus, intestinal obstruction, undiagnosed injury leading to peritonitis and fecal fistula.
  - Shock–Hypovolemic, septicemic.
  Thromboembolic: Deep vein thrombosis, pulmonary embolism.
- *Remote:* Vault prolapse, cystocele, rectocele or enterocele, incisional hernia, scar endometriosis, fimbrial prolapse through vault, granulation at vault. Acute menopausal symptoms if ovaries are removed and post-hysterectomy psychosis in some patients.

Important

- *Time*: Emergency hysterectomy can be performed at any time while for planned surgery late secretory phase and menstrual phase is avoided. There may be excessive bleeding due to pelvic congestion if hysterectomy is done premenstrually. During menstruation there is risk of infection and imperfect healing
- Some gynecologists favor intrafascial approach, i.e., after uterine vessels are clamped and ligated all successive clamps are placed inside the pubovesicocervical fascia after cutting open it on the anterior surface of cervix below the isthmus. This prevents injury to bladder and ureter during operation and good support to vaginal vault is maintained so, there is less chance of vault prolapse in future.
- Subtotal hysterectomy is only done in emergency cases (i.e., mostly obstetric hysterectomies) or when further dissection is impossible without damaging the bladder, ureter or rectum because of severe adhesions.

Advantages of Total Over Subtotal Hysterectomy

- No risk of stump carcinoma. It is rare and can be prevented by regular Pap smear in follow-up
- No risk of leukorrhea due to unhealthy cervix (cervicitis, erosion) as it is removed
- Better drainage of operative site, if small hematoma or pelvic infection occurs.

Disadvantages of Total Over Subtotal Hysterectomy

- Time required is more and technically difficult
- Vault prolapse—with proper technique this is less
- Dyspareunia—only when much of the vagina is removed
- More chances of injury to bladder, ureter and rectum
- Vault granulation or fallopian tube prolapse.

VAGINAL HYSTERECTOMY

Removal of uterus through vaginal route is called vaginal hysterectomy. Vaginal hysterectomy is favored more and more in recent times due to its various advantages mentioned below. Popularly this is called **nondescent vaginal hysterectomy (NDVH)**, however in reality it is nonprolapse vaginal hysterectomy as some descent is always there if patient has delivered at least one child vaginally.

Advantages of Vaginal Over Abdominal Hysterectomy

- Less postoperative discomfort and pain
- Less overall morbidity
- Cosmetically good as there is no scar on the abdomen
- Scar related complications like incisional hernia, keloid, intraperitoneal adhesions do not occur
- Less incidence of vomiting, abdominal distension, ileus, peritonitis and intestinal obstruction
- Early ambulation leading to less pulmonary complications, deep vein thrombosis and embolism
- Vaginal wall prolapse can be corrected adequately and without changing the position of the patient
- Better drainage of operative area.

Disadvantages Vaginal Over Abdominal Hysterectomy

- Difficult and unsafe in presence of adhesions
- Less accessibility so less suitable for radical hysterectomy
- Other abdominal viscera cannot be explored
- Infectious morbidity may be slightly more because of vaginal bacterial flora
- Difficult to perform when uterus >10 weeks size
- Removal of ovaries (if required) is difficult

Indications
- All cases of prolapse when child-bearing is completed and age >35 years
- AUB not responding to medical treatment
- Small fibroids
- Adenomyosis.
- Cervical premalignant lesion—CIN II, III, Ca in situ
- Endometrial hyperplasia
- Chronic PID not responding to medical treatment and causing pelvic pain and menstrual abnormality.

Contraindications
- Severe adhesions in pelvis
- Suspicion of malignancy
- Restricted mobility of uterus
- Less lateral space in the vagina
- Uterus >14 weeks size (larger size uteri are removed by experts)
- Inexperienced surgeons.

Preoperative Preparations
As mentioned in abdominal hysterectomy.

Anesthesia
As mentioned in abdominal hysterectomy.

Steps of Operation
- Patient is given lithotomy position
- Painting and draping
- Foley's catheter is inserted
- P/V examination under anesthesia is done to reconfirm the feasibility of vaginal route
- Labial stitches are taken to widen the operative field at introitus.
- Speculum and anterior vaginal wall retractor are introduced and cervix is caught by 2 Vulsellum.
- To decrease blood loss, both vaginal walls are infiltrated with adrenaline (3-4 drops) in 100-200 mL saline (adrenaline is not used in hypertensive and cardiac patients). Some gynecologists use only saline. Only saline does not decrease blood loss but helps in dissection in correct planes created by saline injection
- Anterior vaginal wall is incised about 1-2 cm above the external os (or depending upon the limit of cystocele)
- Cut edges are held with Allis forceps
- Pubovesicocervical ligament is cut in midline and vaginal wall with bladder is pushed up by blunt or sharp dissection
- If anterior peritoneum (vesicouterine fold) is visualized (thin, smooth) at this point it is held by artery forceps and cut opened
- Landon's retractor or speculum is inserted to retract the bladder away for rest of the operation
- Holding the cervix anteriorly posterior vaginal wall is cut almost at the same level as anterior incision and vaginal wall is pushed away from cervix by blunt finger dissection
- In the midline between 2 uterosacral ligaments peritoneum of pouch of Douglas can be identified, caught between artery forceps and cut opened. Speculum is readjusted to retract the rectum
- Vaginal wall incisions on the cervix are completed laterally and the edge is caught with Allis forceps. With blunt and sharp dissection wall is separated form ligaments laterally and posteriorly
- First pedicle is thus exposed, it is clamped cut and ligated by 1 no. Vicryl and ends are held long
- Procedure is repeated on opposite side
- If cervix is elongated (as in case of prolapse) successive clamps are applied on either side medial to previous clamp upwards till isthmus is reached. 2 to 3 such clamps may be required
- At the level of isthmus the clamps occlude the uterine vessels. Uterine vessels pedicles are properly clamped, cut and securely ligated
- Next successive clamps are applied medial to uterine vessels pedicles on the broad ligament either side till cornu is reached.

- Last pedicle is cornual. If ovaries are to be preserved (young patient) clamps are applied medial to ovary and if they are to be removed clamps are applied lateral to ovary on infundibulopelvic ligaments. In latter situation as pedicle becomes broad, round ligaments may be tied separately first (as in abdominal hysterectomy) and then infundibulopelvic ligaments can be reached
- Pedicles are cut, doubly ligated with Vicryl No. 1 and held long
- All pedicles are examined for bleeding and hemostasis is secured by extra stitches, if necessary
- Anterior colporrhaphy if required (cystocele) is done at this stage
- Vault is finally closed, paracervical ligaments (first pedicle) and cornual pedicles are incorporated in the sutures or tied with vaginal vault to suspend the vault
- Different techniques of vault suspension, e.g., Heaney's, TeLinde, Mattingly, Shaw's Bonney's, Campbell's are used to prevent vault prolapse in future
- Posterior colpoperineorrhaphy is done as per the need (presence of rectocele, wide hiatus urogenitalis) after cutting labial stitches
- Vagina is packed with roller gauze soaked in Betadine.

Postoperative Management

It is same as described under abdominal hysterectomy. The difference is early ambulation and early oral intake. Vaginal pack is removed after 12–24 hours. Foley's catheter is removed after 2–3 days. Patient is advised to avoid weight lifting for 6 months to prevent vault prolapse.

Ovaries at Hysterectomy

Current evidence suggests that ovaries should be preserved while doing hysterectomy for benign disease at least up to 50 years of age (preferably 65 years of age). Premenopausal oophorectomy causes an immediate loss of all ovarian hormones. Following natural menopause, the ovary continues to produce androstenedione and testosterone in significant amounts until age 65 and these androgens are converted in fat, muscle and skin into estrone. Surgical menopause may impact negatively on future cardiovascular, psychosexual, cognitive and mental health, bone health and long-term survival of the patient.

Bilateral salpingectomy, the removal of both fallopian tubes while preserving the ovaries, is considered a safe way of potentially reducing the development of ovarian serous carcinoma, the most common type of ovarian cancer. Evidence points toward the fallopian tubes as the origin of this type of cancer. Removing the fallopian tubes does not cause the onset of menopause, as does the removal of the ovaries.

OPERATIONS FOR PROLAPSE

Complete list of operations for prolapse of different organs is as follows:

Prolapse of Uterus

As shown in the following table:

Functions to be preserved				Operations of choice
Child bearing	Menstrual	Sexual		
Yes	Yes	Yes		Abdominal sling, operations
No	Yes	Yes		• Sling + Tubal ligation • Manchester
No	No	Yes		Vaginal hysterectomy with repair
No	No	No		• Vaginal hysterectomy with repair • LeFort's operation

Prolapse of Vagina

- Cystocele, cystourethrocele → anterior colporrhaphy
- Rectocele → posterior colporrhaphy, colpoperineorrhaphy
- Enterocele → (1) Culdeplasty during vaginal hysterectomy, (2) Repair during Manchester operation or with extended posterior colporrhaphy (3) Moschcowitz operation, (4) Operations for vault prolapse.

Vault Prolapse

Discussed at the end of the chapter.

Only the main principles of different operations are described below:

Abdominal Sling Operations

These are specially devised for young nulliparous or low-parity group patients with first, second & incomplete third degree prolapse.

Contraindications to sling operations include procidentia, stress incontinence, lacerated or infected cervix and markedly elongated cervix. They are as follows:

- *Purandare's cervicopexy* : Described by Dr B N Purandare in 1956. Sling is made from strip of anterior rectus sheath cut transversely. Medial cut end is passed extraperitoneally, along the course of round ligament, between the two layers of broad ligament and fixed anterior to (or less commonly posterior to) cervix by nonabsorbable sutures. It is a dynamic sling. Round ligament plication and uterosacral approximation, are done along with it and vaginal walls repairs is also done from below if required.
- *Shirodkar's sling:* 5" long 1/2" wide sling is made from patient's fascia lata or mersilene tape. It is split longitudinally to obtain 10" long sling. Posteriorly it is fixed to anterior longitudinal ligament in front of sacral promontory and anteriorly it is tied to supravaginal cervix posteriorly by nonabsorbable stitches (It can be tied anterior to cervix after encircling it). On left side a small loop of sling is made on psoas muscle passing the original sling through this loop avoids compression of sigmoid colon. Unlike Purandare's it is a static sling
- *Khanna's operation:* Sling is made from artificial material (e.g. mersilene tape). It is tied laterally to the periosteum of anterior superior iliac spine (or lateral ends of inguinal ligament) and passing medially, between the two layers of broad ligament, the other end is fixed posteriorly on the cervix
- *Virkud's composite sling operation*: Mersilene tap is anchored from the posterior aspect of the isthmus subperitoneally to the sacral promontory on right side and on left side the tap is passed anteriorly between 2 layers of board ligament and sutured to rectus sheath. All difficulties and complications on left side in making psoas loop and passing the sling (Shirodkar's sling) are avoided. It is easy to perform and gives equally good results. Plication of left uterosacral ligament prevents dextrorotation of uterus

Currently different endoscopic sling operations are done by expert endoscopists. It has obvious advantages of minimally invasive surgery including magnification and exposure.

Fothergill–Manchester Operation

Archibald Donald from Manchester city devised it in 1888. Fothergill, his pupil, later on modified and popularized it. It is now done infrequently, in cases of elongated bad cervix with I° and II° descent and child-bearing completed. It includes: (1) D & C, (2) Amputation of cervix, (3) Shortening and tying of cardinal ligaments anterior to cervix, (4) Anterior and posterior colporrhaphy.

Shirodkar's Extended Manchester

As compared to Manchester it is useful where cervix is short, child-bearing is to be preserved and where retroversion is to be corrected. Vaginally uterosacral ligaments with their peritoneal covering are mobilized after cutting them from cervix and than tying them anterior to cervix by nonabsorbable sutures. High suturing of cut peritoneum on the back of cervix takes care of hernia of pouch of Douglas.

Le Fort's Operation

It is done in very old frail patients, who are not fit for major surgery under GA. Quadrilateral same size flaps from anterior and posterior vaginal walls are removed from 2 cm proximal to external os to within 5 cm of external urinary meatus anteriorly. Row areas are sutured together, vagina is converted into two narrow channels parallel to each other.

Goodall–Power Modification

Here, instead of removing rectangular flaps, small triangular flaps are removed with their bases near the cervix. The vagina is single in lower portion and double in upper portion, so sexual function is preserved.

Anterior Colporrhaphy

Anterior vaginal wall is cut open by inverted T incision, bladder along with its fascia is dissected away from either side flap. Vesicovaginal fascia is reconstructed by purse string sutures. Redundant vaginal flaps are excised and cut edges are sutured with interrupted or continuous No. 1 chromic catgut stitches. For urethrocele repair original vaginal incision is extended up to 1 cm below the external meatus.

Posterior Colporrhaphy

As along with posterior repair, perineum is also repaired the operation is called colpoperineorrhaphy. Posterior vaginal wall is cut transversely between 2 Allis forceps applied on mucocutaneous junction. Rectum along with rectovaginal fascia is dissected away by sharp dissection. The dissection is done higher up to the apex of rectocele. Levator ani muscles are approximated in the midline by No. 1 Vicryl. Redundant vaginal flaps are excised and edges are sutured by continuous No. 1 Vicryl. One or two sutures for superficial perineal muscles and suturing of perineal skin completes the perineorrhaphy.

Enterocele Repair Operations

- Culdoplasty sutures internally or externally approximating two uterosacral ligaments and pouch of Douglas peritoneum at higher level serves the purpose
- Along with Manchester and extended posterior repair operation after opening the sac it is obliterated at its neck by purse string sutures. The portion of the peritoneum below the suture is cut-off.
- *Moschcowitz operation*: Through abdominal route 3–4 successive purse string sutures are taken by non-absorbable or delayed absorbable material starting from the bottom of the cul-de-sac so as to, obliterate it. Sutures pass through the peritoneum, serosa of rectum and uterosacral ligaments.

Vault Prolapse Operations

- *Colposacropexy*: Mattingly described it in 1982. Two cm wide strips from anterior rectus sheath or Marlex mesh is used to suspend the vaginal vault to the anterior sacral ligament in front of the third sacral vertebra
- *Sacrospinous fixation*: Richter and Nichols recommended fixation of vaginal vault to the sacrospinous ligament vaginally. It is now increasingly done operation for vault prolapse. It can be done along with vaginal hysterectomy in case of procidentia to prevent vault prolapse in future.
- *Laparoscopic sacrocolpopexy*: It is described by Nezhat, et al. It is same as open sacrocolpopexy but done by laparoscopic technique. Synthetic mesh is either sutured or stapled.

Following operations are **not commonly** done.
- *Iliococcygeus fixation:* Fixation of the vault to iliococcygeus fascia anterior to the ischial spines done by vaginal route. It is reported by Shull and colleagues. Results are same as sacrospinous fixation.
- *Posterior intravaginal slingoplasty (infravaginal sacropexy):* It is described by Petros and utilizes a multifilament prolene tape introduced by using the IVS (infravaginal sacropexy) tunneler. A new ligament similar to uterosacral ligament is thus created.
- *High uterosacral ligament suspension:* It can be done by abdominal or vaginal route. Nonabsorbable suture are used anchor vaginal vault to the tied uterosacral ligaments. Vaginal vault thus gets elevated to the hollow of sacrum.
- *Levator plication-vault fixation:* It was suggested by Zacharin and Hamilton. First levator ani muscles are repaired strongly by vaginal route and then from abdominally route vaginal vault is fixed to levator plate. It is complex procedure and has a lower success rate than abdominal Sacrocolpopexy.
- *Williams–Richardson's operation:* Same as Purandare's cervicopexy, but here the strips of anterior rectus sheath are fixed to the angles of the vagina as the uterus is already removed.
- *Shaw's operation:* Instead of transverse strips longitudinal strips of rectus sheath are made. They are cut from upper ends and brought down and tied to the angles of vagina.
- *Le Fort's partial colpocleisis and Goodall-Power modification:* Already described before. Le Fort operation is done when patient is no longer sexually active. There is as high as 30% chances of postoperative stress urinary incontinence. It can be performed under local anesthesia.
- *Complete colpocleisis:* It is total vaginectomy by complete dissection of anterior and posterior vaginal walls. The raw areas are then sutured together obliterating the space completely.

CHAPTER 10

Bony Pelvis and Fetal Skull

Bony pelvis is a bony passage through which the fetus passes during the normal labor. Any abnormality of pelvis can modify the mechanism of labor or may lead to obstructed labor.

It is made up of 4 bones and 4 joints.

Bones: Two innominate (hip) bones, the sacrum (5 sacral vertebrae) and the coccyx (4 coccygeal vertebrae).

Joints: Two sacroiliac joints (synovial), symphysis pubis (secondary cartilaginous) and sacrococcygeal joint.

Classification: Caldwell and Moloy in 1933 developed a classification of female pelvis on the basis of shape of inlet and other anatomical features. They divided the female pelvis in four parent types:
1. Gynecoid (Gyne = Woman): 50%
2. Android (Ander = man): 20%
3. Anthropoid (Anthropos = human): 25%
4. Platypelloid (Platy = flat, Pelis = Pelvis): 5%

However pure (parent) forms are rarely found. Mixed types are common which are described by combined nomenclature, e.g., gyne-android or andro-gynecoid. First term refers to the features of posterior segment and second term refers to the anterior segment.

This classification is not very useful as for outcome of labor exact size (capacity) of the pelvis is more important than shape.

The pelvis is anatomically divided into a **false pelvis** above and a **true pelvis** below by the boundary line called pelvic brim. False pelvis is of little importance. Its anterior and posterior walls are deficient. Laterally the iliac bones are its main components. It supports the gravid uterus in latter half of pregnancy.

Differences between female and male pelvis

Female	Male
Inlet—transversely oval	Tringular
Sacrum—short, wide and smoothly curved	Long, narrow flat and abruptly curved in lower part
Sacral angle 90 to 100°	<90°
Symphysis pubis—short	Long heavy
Sacrosciatic notches—wide and shallow	Long and prominent
Ischial spines—not prominent	Heavy and prominent
Side walls—parallel	Convergent
Subpubic angle - 85 ± 5°	75 ± 5°
Bituberous diameter—wider	Narrow
Ischial tuberosities everted	Inverted

TRUE PELVIS

It is the important bony canal through which the fetus must pass during the labor. For descriptive purposes it is divided into **inlet, cavity and outlet**.

Pelvic Inlet

It is also known as **pelvic brim** or **upper pelvic strait**.

Boundary

From before backwards, it is bounded on each side by the upper border of symphysis pubis, pubic crest, pubic spine, ileopectineal eminence, ileopectineal line, sacroiliac articulation, anterior border of ala of sacrum and sacral promontory.

Plane

It is imaginary flat surface bounded by the bony points as those of inlet.

Shape

It is almost round with slight anteroposterior flattening.

Inclination

In the erect posture the place makes an angle of 55° with the horizon. This is called the angle of inclination.

Diameters

Anteroposterior (true conjugate, anatomical conjugate, conjugate vera): It is the distance between the midpoint of the inner margin of the upper border of symphysis pubis in front to the midpoint of the sacral promontory behind.

Clinically it cannot be measured, so it is derived from measuring the diagonal conjugate.

Diagonal conjugate: It measures from the lower margin of symphysis pubis in midline to the midpoint of sacral promontory. It is measured clinically by pelvic examination by palpating the promontory with the tip of middle finger while keeping flush contact of radial border of index finger to the lower margin of symphysis pubis. (Normally the promontory is not palpated easily so examining hand is depressed slightly to reach it and point of lower border of symphysis is marked on the gloved hand by index finger of left hand).

Deducting 1/2" (1.25 cm) from diagonal conjugate usually gives true conjugate. Actual deduction depends upon the height, thickness and the inclination of symphysis pubis.

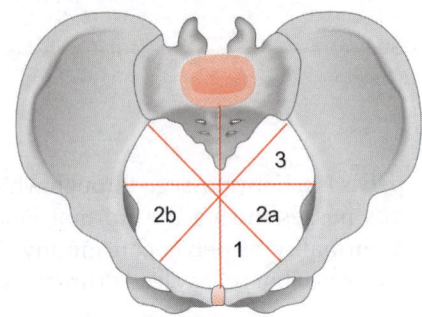

Fig. 10.1: Pelvic inlet diameters. 1. Anteroposterior; 2a and b. Oblique; 3. Transverse.

Obstetric conjugate: It is the distance between the midpoint of the sacral promontry behind to the nearest point in the midline on the posterior surface of symphysis pubis near upper border. It is slightly below the upper border. As it is the narrowest anteroposterior diameter through which head has to pass near the inlet it is called obstetric conjugate.

Oblique diameters: They are 2—right oblique and left oblique, each measuring from one sacroiliac joint to opposite iliopectineal eminence. It is named according to the sacroiliac joint from which it starts, i.e., left or right.

Transverse diameter: It is the distance between the two farthest apart points on the iliopectineal lines. It passes slightly behind the center of the plane, so truly speaking it is not a diameter.

Posterior sagittal diameter (inlet): It is the part of the anteroposterior diameter lying behind the transverse diameter of the inlet.

Measurements

Inlet
- True conjugate   – 10.8 cm
- Oblique diameter   – 12.0 cm
- Diagonal conjugate – 12.0 cm
- Transverse diameter – 13.2 cm
- Obstetric conjugate – 10.0 cm

Axis: It is an imaginary perpendicular line passing through the center of the plane of the inlet. Its direction is downward and backward and usually passes from the umbilicus to the tip of the coccyx.

Cavity

Boundary

It is a curved canal bounded above by the pelvic inlet and below by the plane of the least pelvic dimension.

Plane

Reference plane for the cavity is taken at the level of midpoint of symphysis pubis on the posterior surface in front to the junction of second and third sacral vertebra behind. It is called **plane of greatest pelvic dimension**.

Shape

It is round in shape. The plane is also called the plane of greatest pelvic dimension.

Axis

It is an imaginary perpendicular line passing through the center of the plane. It passes almost vertically downwards.

Measurements

Cavity
Anterior wall	– 3.75 cm (1.5")
Posterior wall	– 11.25 cm (4.5")
Lateral wall	– 7.5 cm (3.0")
Anteroposterior diameter	– 12 cm
Transverse diameter	– 12 cm
Oblique diameter	– 12 cm

(As such transverse and oblique are not measured as the points lie over the soft tissues.)

Outlet

Anatomical Outlet (Bony Outlet)

It is anatomically the lowermost (outermost) bony landmarks.

Boundary: It extends from the lower border of symphysis, inferior pubic rami, ischial tuberosity, sacrotuberous ligament and tip of the coccyx.

Plane: It is not a single plane, but there are 2 triangular planes with common base formed by 2 ischial tuberosities, i.e., bituberous diameter.

Shape: Lozenge shape or diamond shape.

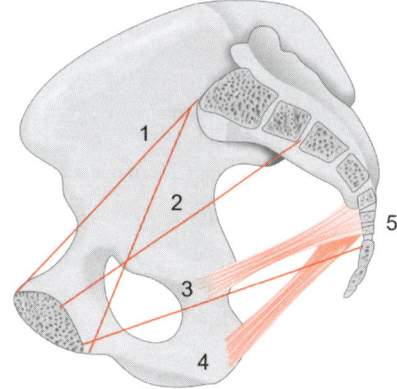

Fig. 10.2: Planes of pelvis. 1. Inlet; 2. Cavity; 3. PLPD; 4. Anatomical outlet and oblique line—DC.

Diameters

Anteroposterior: It measures from lower border of symphysis pubis to the tip of coccyx.

Transverse (bituberous): It measures between the inner borders of ischial tuberosities.

Oblique: Not adequately defined.

Posterior sagittal: It is the part of the anteroposterior diameter lying behind the bituberous diameter. Clinically it can be measured by the distance between the sacrococcygeal joint and anterior margin of anus.

Axis: It is an imaginary perpendicular line passing through the center of anteroposterior diameter. It is downwards and forward.

Obstetrical Outlet

Slight narrowing of the pelvis occurs at a level above the bony outlet, i.e., at the plane of least pelvic dimension. Obstetrically it is important for the head to negotiate this plane. So, obstetrical outlet is three-dimensional structure. It is the segment between the plane of least pelvic dimension above and the anatomical outlet below. Its anterior wall is deficient at the pubic arch. Its lateral walls are formed by ischial bones and the posterior wall consists of the whole coccyx.

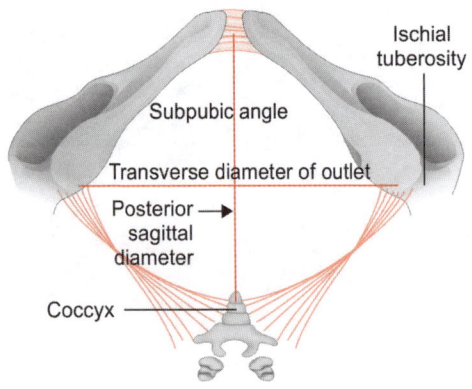

Fig. 10.3: Pelvic outlet.

Plane of least pelvic dimension (PLPD, narrow pelvic plane): It is from the lower border of symphysis pubis to the tip of ischial spines, sacrospinous ligaments and the tip of the sacrum.

Shape: Anteroposteriorly oval.

Diameters

Anteroposterior: Lower border of symphysis pubis to the tip of the sacrum.

Transverse: It is the distance between the two ischial spines.

Oblique: Not adequately defined.

Postsagittal: It is the part of anteroposterior diameter lying behind the interspinous diameter.

Axis: It is obtained by joining the center of the plane with sacral promontory. It is almost vertical.

Measurements: Outlet:

	Anatomical outlet	Obstetrical outlet (PLPD)
Anteroposterior	– 13.2 cm	13.2 cm
Transverse	– 10.8 cm	10.5 cm
Postsagittal	– 8.5 cm	5.0 cm

The pelvic axis

- **Anatomical axis (curve of Carus):** It is an imaginary curved line formed by joining the axis of inlet, cavity and outlet, traversing the center of the canal of the bony pelvis. It roughly corresponds to the sacral curvature. It is of no clinical significance.
- **Obstetrical axis:** It represents the true path of the head through the pelvis. It is not uniformly curved. It is first downwards and backwards upto the level of ischial spines and then directed downwards and forwards abruptly.

Midpelvis: It is the segment of the bony pelvis bounded above by the plane of greatest pelvic dimension and below by the mid-pelvic plane.

Mid-pelvic plane: It is from the lower border of symphysis pubis, through ischial spines to the junction of S_4 and S_5 or tip of the sacrum depending upon the configuration of sacrum. If it meets the tip of the sacrum it is same as plane of least pelvic dimension.

Mid-plane: It is same as the plane of greatest pelvic dimension, i.e., from the center of the symphysis pubis to junction of S_2 and S_3.

Pubic arch: This is an arch formed by the descending pubic rami of left and right sides. It measures 6 cm in between the pubic rami at a level of 2 cm below the apex. Clinically it accommodates at least two fingers.

Morris's waste space: When a round disc of 9.3 cm is placed under the pubic arch, the distance between the apex of the arch and the circumference of the disc is called waste space of Morris. Normally it is 1 cm or less. In a narrow pubic arch this distance is increased and it leads to difficulty in delivery with more backward displacement of the head, perineal tears or obstructed labor.

High assimilation type of pelvis

In this type there is sacralization of 5th lumbar vertebra, i.e., incorporated in the body of the sacrum. It leads to high inclination of pelvic brim and some disadvantages: (1) Delay in engagement of the head due to uterine axis not coinciding with the axis of inlet, (2) Favors occipitoposterior position and (3) Difficulty in descent due to long sacrum.

Low assimilation: Here there is lumbarization of first sacral vertebra, i.e., sacrum consists of 4 pieces only. It leads to low inclination and short sacrum, so it has no disadvantages.

Sacral angle: It is the angle between the true conjugate of the brim and the line joining the first and second sacral vertebra. Normally it is more than 90⁰. Narrow angle suggests funneling of the pelvis.

Importance of ischial spines:
- It is used to refer the station of the presenting part.
- It marks the beginning of the forward curve of the pelvic axis.
- It corresponds to the site of the origin of levator ani muscles.
- Internal rotation occurs at this plane.
- Pudendal block is given at ischial spines.

THE FETAL SKULL

The fetal skull consists of vault, base and face. Facial part is relatively small, base is rigid and compressible, while vault is obstetrically important and made up of 5 pliable tabular bones, i.e., 2 frontal, 2 parietal and 1 occipital.

Sutures: An unossified membrane uniting the 2 neighboring bones of vault of skull are called sutures.
- **Frontal suture:** It lies between 2 halves of the frontal bones.
- **Sagittal suture:** It lies between 2 parietal bones.
- **Coronal suture:** It lies between the frontal and parietal bones on either side.
- **Lambdoid suture:** It lies between the occipital and parietal bones on either side.

Fontanelles: The wide spaces in the suture line between the corners of these bones are called fontanelles. Out of total 6 fontanelles, 2 are obstetrically important.
- **Anterior fontanelle:**
  - It is situated at the junction of the frontal, 2 coronal and sagittal sutures.
  - It is diamond or kite shaped.
  - It is bigger than posterior fontanelle (usually measures 3 cm anteroposterior × 2 cm transverse).
  - It is membranous and gets ossified at 18 months after birth.

  Importance of anterior fontanelle:
  - *During labor:* 1. It helps to determine the degree of flexion of the fetal head. 2. It helps in molding.
  - *During neonatal period:* 1. If depressed—suggests dehydration. 2. If tense—suggests raised intracranial tension. 3. Blood transfusion—when other sites are not available. 4. To collect blood sample. 5. It helps to accommodate the fast growing brain.
- **Posterior fontanelle:** It is at the junction of sagittal and 2 lambdoid sutures. It is smaller, triangular in shape. It is a bony depression rather than a defect and disappears at 6 months of age. It helps to determine the position of fetal head during labor.

The Regions of the Skull

- **Vertex:** It is the area of the fetal skull bounded anteriorly by the anterior fontanelle and coronal suture, posteriorly by the posterior fontanelle and lambdoid suture and laterally by the arbitrary lines passing through the parietal eminencies. In anatomy highest point on the vault of the skull is called vertex.

- **Face:** This is the area from the junction of the floor of the mouth with neck to the root of the nose and supraorbital ridges.
- **Brow:** It is the area between the route of the nose and supraorbital ridges to the anterior fontanelle and coronal sutures.
- **Sinciput:** It is the forehead region of the fetal head lying in front of the anterior fontanelle and it corresponds to the area of brow.
- **Occiput:** It is the area occupied by that bone, sometimes it is used for external occipital protuberance.

Circumferences: Circumference of the plane of girdle of contact varies according to the attitude of the head.

Vertex (fully flexed):
- Biparietal suboccipito-bregmatic
- 27.5 cm.

Deflexed vertex (occipitoposterior):
- Biparietal occipitofrontal
- 34.0 cm.

Face (fully extended):
- Biparietal submento-bregmatic
- 27.5 cm.

Diameters of Skull

Different engaging diameters present to the maternal pelvis depending upon the presentation and attitude of the presenting part as mentioned in below table.

Engaging Diameters	Length	Presentation
Suboccipito-bregmatic (from the nape of the neck to the center of bregma)	9.4 cm	Vertex
Suboccipito-frontal (from suboccipital region, i.e., nape of the neck to the center of frontal suture)	10.0 cm	Incompletely flexed vertex
Occipito-frontal (from occipital protuberance to the root of the nose)	11.5 cm	Deflexed vertex as in occipitoposterior
Submento-bregmatic (from the angle between neck and chin to center of the bregma)	9.4 cm	Completely extended face
Submentovertical (from angle between neck and chin to center of sagittal suture)	11.5 cm	Incompletely extended face
Mentovertical (from point of chin to the center of sagittal suture)	14.0 cm	Brow
Biparietal (between two parietal eminences)	9.4 cm	–

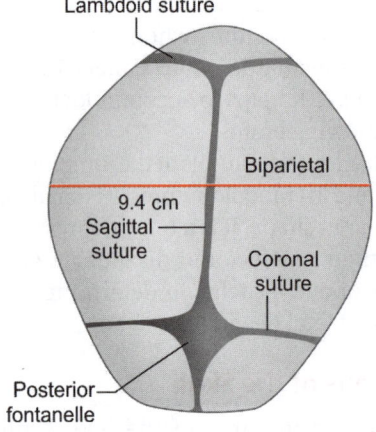
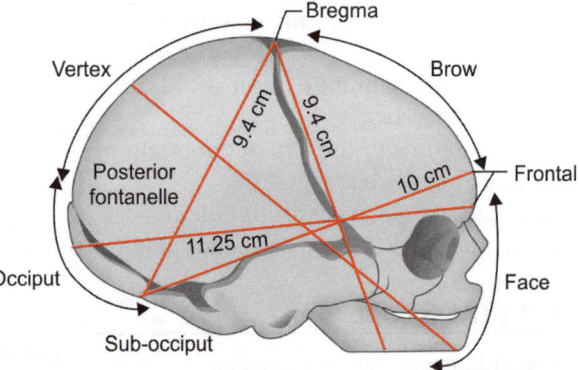

Fig. 10.4: Fetal skull.

Lie: It is relation of the long axis of the fetus to the long axis of the centralized maternal uterus. It can be longitudinal (99%), transverse or oblique.

Attitude: It is the relation of the various fetal parts to each other. Common is flexion attitude, because in flexion attitude fetus occupies the smallest possible space in the uterus.

Presentation: It is the part of the fetus which lies at the lower pole of the uterus and faces the pelvic brim.

Different presentations are:
- Cephalic – 96%
- Breech – 3.5%
- Shoulder – 0.5%

Presenting part: It is the particular area of the fetal presentation which first enters the pelvic brim. (It is felt through cervix by pelvic examination). In cephalic presentation depending upon the degree of flexion there are 3 presenting parts.
1. Fully flexed - Vertex
2. Fully extended - Face
3. Neither flexed nor extended - Brow

Position: It is the relation of the denominator to the various quadrants of maternal pelvis. In vertex presentation occiput is the denominator. Different positions in decreasing frequency are LOA (V_1), ROA (V_2), ROP (V_3) and LOP (V_4).

Denominator: It is an arbitrary fixed bony part, specific for each presentation and used to indicate position.

Engagement: When the maximum transverse diameter of the presenting part (i.e., BPD for vertex) crosses the pelvic brim, it is called engagement.

In pelvic examination if head is at zero station it is definitely engaged.

Presentation	Denominator
Vertex	Occiput
Breech	Sacrum
Face	Mentum
Brow	Frontum
Shoulder	Dorsum

Station: It is the relation of the lowermost bony part (without caput and molding) in cm to the plane of ischial spines. If presenting part is 2 cm above ischial spies it is –2 station and if 1 cm below it is +1 station. At ischial spines it is '0' (zero) station.

Caput succedaneum: It is formation of swelling on fetal head during normal labor. This is caused by edema of the subcutaneous layers of the scalp due to obstruction to venous return and lymphatic drainage at the level of girdle of contact which may be cervical rim or introital ring or bony pelvis. It is diffuse in nature and disappears spontaneously within 24 hours of birth.

Molding: The change in the shape of the head during labor is molding. It helps the head to pass through the pelvis during labor. It is formed due to pressure at girdle of contract by pelvic bones. The base of the skull is incompressible but the bones of the vault of the skull are compressible as the suture lines allow some movement between the individual bones. Occipital and frontal bones go beneath the parietal bones and one parietal bone overlaps the other.

Obliteration of suture lines is + molding, reducible overlapping is + + and irreducible overlapping is + + + molding. Excessive molding suggests cephalopelvic disproportion and is harmful. It disappears within few hours after birth.

CHAPTER 11

Obstetric Cases Performa: Antenatal and Postnatal

ANTENATAL CASE HISTORY PORFORMA

Basic Data

Mrs ABC (full name of the patient) .... gravida ....para, a Hindu (caste) patient of .... years (age) old, residing at.............., coming from............socioeconomic (U/M/L) class, a homemaker (if working mention about her job) was admitted in .... hospital, since .... days with .... months amenorrhea and chief complaints of: ....since..........days
.....................since..........days (etc. in chronological order)

(Patient may not have any complaints and may be admitted on obstetric grounds after checkup in antenatal OPD, e.g. IUGR, malpresentation, anemia, PIH.)

Origin, Duration and Progress

Patient is having..............................months amenorrhea. She developed..................... (all complaints in detail).
- Mention in detail about any abnormalities, if she had during her present pregnancy.
- Mention about antenatal visits, she has attended in this pregnancy, including tetanus toxoid immunization.
- Inquire about exposure to irradiation, teratogenic drugs or viral infection in first trimester of this pregnancy.

Menstrual History

Past MP: $\dfrac{\text{No of days of bleeding}}{\text{Interval}}$ regularity, Amount, pain

Example: $\dfrac{3-4}{30}$ RMPL

Last menstrual period (LMP): First day of last menstrual period.

Expected date of delivery/Expected due date (EDD): It is calculated by **Naegele's formula,** i.e. add 9 months and 7 days to LMP, e.g. if LMP is 16-8-2014, EDD will be 23-5-2015.

This formula is for 28 days menstrual cycle:
- If interval of cycle is more than 28 days then add this difference (number of days) days in calculating EDD. If interval is less than 28 days, deduct this difference (number of days) in calculating EDD.
- In patients with irregular cycles EDD is difficult to calculate. Average of last 6 cycles may be taken to calculate EDD.
- Some patients do not remember their LMP at all, while some may able to correlate their LMP with some important religious

festival. So knowledge of the calendar dates of common festivals (e.g. Diwali, Holi, Janmashtami, Ganesh Chaturthi, Idd Makar Sankranti, Mahashivaratri, Onam, Ugadi, Pongal, etc.) of the current or last year might help in calculating the EDD.

Obstetric History

- It is taken in detail.
- It is described as G3, P1, A1, L1 (Gravida 3, Para 1, Abortion 1, Live 1)
- All pregnancy events are described in chronological order, e.g.

First is .... full term normal delivery in hospital 4 years back, a live male child of 3.0 kg and no antepartum, intrapartum or postpartum complications.

Second is .... spontaneous abortion 2 years back of 2½ months gestation, Dilation and Evacuation (D&E) was done and no post-abortal complications.

Deliveries

- Date and year
- Full term/Preterm
- Home delivery/Hospital delivery
- Normal delivery/Abnormal and operative deliveries with indication of operation
- Any antepartum, intrapartum or post-partum complications
- Newborn—alive/stillbirth, gender, weight and neonatal period.

Abortions

- Date and year
- Spontaneous/Induced
- Complete/Incomplete
- Gestational age at abortion
- Any post-abortal complications.

Gravidity: No. of conception irrespective of its outcome, i.e. it might be abortion, MTP, vaginal delivery, cesarean section, ectopic pregnancy or vesicular mole.

Parity: No. of children delivered after the age of viability (even if they are delivered dead). Current pregnancy even if it has crossed the age of viability is included in gravida not parity.

- Twin pregnancy is single gravida and twin delivery is considered single parity.
- In primigravida patient, mention duration of active married life.
- Whether patient has conceived after infertility Rx, is also asked.
- History of use of any contraceptive measures before pregnancy. Whether pregnancy is due to failure of contraception or not, is also asked.
- Whether it is consanguineous marriage or not, is asked.

Past History

- Diabetes, tuberculosis, hypertension, jaundice, rheumatic fever in childhood, rickets or osteomalacia and syphilis
- History of any pelvic surgery or h/o accidents affecting pelvic bones before this pregnancy
- Any major hospitalization or h/o blood transfusion.

Family History

Diabetes, hypertension, tuberculosis, hemoglobinopathies, twins, postmaturity and genetic disorders if any in the family.

Personal History

Diet: Vegetarian/Nonvegetarian (mixed)

Adequate/Inadequate (daily caloric requirement of 45 kg weighing woman during pregnancy is 2500 kilocalories, i.e. 2200 nonpregnant requirement +300 due to pregnancy from second trimester onwards. In lactation, 200 more calories are required). One gram or

Appetite: Pica, dyspepsia (dyspepsia is due to gravid uterus causing venous congestion in bowel wall due to pressure)

Bowel: Constipation is common in second and third trimesters. It may be due to: (1) relaxation of smooth muscles due to progesterone effect, (2) gravid uterus pressing over large bowel, (3) patient taking iron tablets and (4) physical inactivity and stretching of muscles of expulsion

Bladder: Simple frequency is common in last 2 months. It is due to pressure of presenting part on the bladder but frequency with element of pain indicates infection. It is also due to increased glomerular filtration rate (GFR) during pregnancy

Habits: Smoking, tobacco chewing. [It is common in low socioeconomical group. Because of effects of nicotine, it can lead to intrauterine growth restriction (IUGR) and premature labor]

History of any allergies particularly to drugs is important.

General Examination

Build: Well-built /fairly built /poorly built

Nutrition: Well-nourished/fairly nourished/malnourished

Height: It is measured at first visit. If height is < 4' 10" (145 cm) then there are more chances of contracted pelvis

Weight: It is measured at every visit (each time it should be measured on the same weighing machine, before meals, with same ornaments but no footwears worn by patient)

From second trimester onwards increase in weight is ½ kg per week. More than 1 kg per week and less than ½ kg in 15 days, suggests some abnormality.

Exact Body Mass Index (BMI) should be calculated BMI $\geq$ 30 at first antenatal consultation is considered obesity.

Vital Data

- Pulse
- BP
- Temperature
- Respiration
- Tongue, Conjunctiva, Nails
- Pink (no pallor)
- Pallor present—mild/moderate/severe
- Sclera → for jaundice
- Teeth and gums → for septic focus
- Thyroid, Neck veins, Lymph nodes → for any abnormalities
- Edema over legs—over medial malleolus or lower part of the shin of the tibia. It may be physiological or pathological.

Systemic Examination

For any abnormality:
RS: Liver and Spleen:
CVS: CNS:

Obstetric Examination

Per Abdominal Examination (P/A)

Inspection
- Uterine enlargement—longitudinal, undue distension if any. Fullness in flanks suggest near term gestation as bowels are displaced laterally at term
- Umbilicus stretched, flattened or everted
- Stria gravidarum, stria albicans, linea nigra, any operative scar.

Palpation
In obstetric palpation following precautions are observed:
- It should be done in the presence of any female attendant (for male candidate).
- Palpation is done by standing on the right side of the patient.

- Patient lies in supine position with both lower limbs semi-flexed at both joints.
- Palpation is done when uterus is relaxed and abdominal muscles are relaxed.
- Palpation is done with palmer surface of the fingers and not with the fingertips.
- Before palpation patient is informed about what you are going to do.

Fundal height

It is taken by ulnar border of left hand kept over the fundus. Uterus becomes just palpable per abdomen (i.e. symphysis pubis) at 12 weeks. Fundus reaches umbilicus at 24 weeks and reaches xiphisternum at 36 weeks. From 36 to 40 weeks fundal height decreases to 32 weeks size.

Then fundal height is measured in cm from the upper border of the symphysis pubis, along the uterine contour with legs extended.

McDonald's rule

Fundal height in cm × 8/7 = gestational age in weeks.

Obstetric grips (Leopold)

First grip (fundal grip): First centralize the uterus, then keep both hands over the fundus nearly parallel to the costal margins. Palpate with the pulp of the fingers and not with the fingertips. In cephalic presentation breech is felt at fundus, i.e. soft to firm, larger, irregular, nonballotable mass is felt suggestive of the buttocks.

Second grip: Lateral grip (umbilical grip)
- *Left lateral grip:* Push with left hand and palpate with right hand. In LOA or LOT positions, smooth firm curve is felt suggestive of the back of the fetus.
- *Right lateral grip:* Push with right hand and palpate with left hand. In LOA or LOT positions, irregular feeling is there or knobs like structures are felt suggestive of the limbs of the fetus.

Third grip (second pelvic grip): Ulnar border of right hand is kept on the upper border of symphysis pubis, uterus is steadied by left hand over the fundus. Presenting part is palpated between four fingers and the thumb of the right hand and ballottement is also tried. This is also known as *Pawlik's grip*.

Fourth grip (first pelvic grip): Both hands are kept on the lower abdomen, parallel to both inguinal ligaments. Palpate the presenting part. Note which pole is lower, try to ballot and try to push the hands below the presenting part in the pelvis to see that the hands diverge or converge.

Hard, smaller as compared to fundal grip, regular and ballotable (non-engaged) mass is felt suggesting of the head of the fetus. If the hands converge (or diverge) below the presenting part, head is not engaged (or engaged).

Degree of flexion of fetal head can be judged by relation of occipital and sincipital prominences to each other, occipital prominence is sharp and lies on the side of the back.

Some authorities consider third grip as fourth grip and vice versa:
- First, second and third grips are done by facing towards the face of the patient while fourth grip is done by facing towards the feet.
- In less than 24 weeks pregnancy only external ballottement is carried out instead of obstetric grips.
- Mention about amount of liquor, i.e. normal, excessive (hydramnios) or redued (oligohydramnios). In oligohydramnios fundal heights is less, uterus is full of fetus and fetus is in more flexed (crowding).

Johnson's formula (for fetal weight estimation):
- Fundal height in cm: 11 (engaged head) x 155 = fetal weight in grams
- In nonengaged head: 12 is deducted from fundal height in above formula
- If patient is > 91kg, 1 cm more is subtracted from fundal height

This formula is applicable in cephalic presentation only.

Auscultation
Fetal heart sounds—present/absent. When present, mention exact site, rate and rhythm of FHS.

They are best heard at the site of anterior shoulder/back.

Breasts Examination

It is done to look for retracted or cracked nipples. If present, they are treated in the antepartum period, so that there is no problem in breastfeeding after delivery. In primigravida, breast changes are noted.

Per Vaginal Examination (P/V)

It is not routinely done during antenatal period. It is indicated in following situations:
- At first visit to confirm the pregnancy, uterine size and to see if there is any abnormal mass in the fornices
- For clinical pelvimetry in all primigravida patient after 37 weeks and in parous patients with h/o prolonged and difficult labors
- Before induction of labor (Bishop's score)
- For diagnosis of incompetent os and preterm labor.

Diagnosis

Mrs ABC .... gravida................ para with .... weeks pregnancy with .... (disease) with single fetus, vertex presentation, V1 (LOA) position, engaged head and FHS present at................. (site) 140/min (rate) and regular.

Investigations

- Urine is tested for albumin, sugar and pus cells
- Hb estimation is done at first visit and then repeated at 28 and 36 weeks or as necessary. Usually complete blood count (CBC) is done
- Blood grouping (ABO-Rh) is done at first visit if it is not known
- Serum VDRL test is done in indicated cases (e.g. bad obstetric history)
- Postprandial blood sugar (PPBS) estimation: Standard screening test involves glucose determination in blood after 1 hour of 50 g oral glucose. If it is > 140 mg/dL full GTT should be performed
- Indirect Coombs test is done if mother is Rh –ve and father is Rh +ve
- Pap's smear once during antenatal visits is advisable
- HIV testing, HbsAg testing are now routinely advocated to prevent vertical transmission to baby. Consent of the patient for HIV testing must be obtained after pretest counseling
- Serum thyroid-stimulating hormone (TSH) is also now routinely advocated.

Schedule of Antenatal Visits

First visit → First trimester then
At every 4 weeks → up to 28 weeks
At every 2 weeks → up to 36 weeks
Weekly → up to EDD, i.e. 40 weeks
Twice a week → up to 41 (42) weeks
Then admission and induction of labor

WHO recommends minimum 4 antenatal visits during pregnancy: First in first trimester ideally before 12 weeks, no later than 16 weeks, second <26 weeks and third at 32 weeks and last between 36 and 38 weeks.
First
Second
Third
Last

Importance of Basic Data

Name
- Identification
- Communication
- Record purpose
- Developing rapport with the patient.

Age
- *Teenage:* Anemia, preeclampsia, eclampsia, IUGR, traumatic delivery, preterm labor, emotional upset, contracted pelvis, if very young.
- *Elderly:* Abortion, preeclampsia, chromosomal anomaly (trisomy 21), placental insufficiency, diabetes, hypertension, obesity, occipitoposterior, preterm labor, breastfeeding problems.

Residence
- Record purpose
- Endemicity of some diseases
- Epidemics if any
- Future correspondence
- Distance from the hospital.

Caste and religion
Muslim: Consanguineous marriages, *burkha* system leads to vitamin D deficiency and osteomalacia → contracted pelvis, low SE class (see below), less practice of contraception and MPTs

Sindhi: Thalassemia (also in Lohana community in Gujarat)

Tribal: Sickle cell disease.

Occupation
Laborer: IUGR, preterm labor, anemia, malnutrition

Officer: Obesity, diabetes, hypertension, preterm labor if mental stress, post-term

Working in factories: Exposure to teratogens

Medical and paramedical: Radiology department—radiation hazards. Anesthesia department—exposure to gases-teratogenicity

Socioeconomic (SE) status: Kuppuswamy classification is commonly used in low SE status illiteracy, poor hygiene, malnutrition, anemia, frequent pregnancies and infections are commonly found.

Modified Kuppuswamy scale 2019: It is based on occupation and education of the head of the family and monthly family income as follows:

Occupation of the head	Score
Legislators, senior officials and managers	10
Professionals	9
Technicians and associate professionals	8
Clerks	7
Skilled workers, shop and market sales workers	6
Skilled agricultural and fishery workers	5
Craft and related trade workers	4
Plant and machine operators and assemblers	3
Elementary occupation	2
Unemployed	1

Education of the head of the family	Score
Profession or Honors	7
Graduate	6
Intermediate or diploma	5
High school certificate	4
Middle school certificate	3
Primary school certificate	2
Illiterate	1

Updated monthly family income in Rs	Score
$\geq 78{,}063$	12
39,033–78,062	10
29,200–39,032	6
19,516–29,199	4
11,708–19,515	3
3,908–11,707	2
$\leq 3{,}907$	1

Total score of above three parameters is calculated and socioeconomical classes are divide according to this score:

SE class	Total score
Higher	26–29
Upper middle	16–25
Middle	11–15
Upper lower	05–10
Lower	< 5

Modified BG Prasad classification: It was originally formulated in 1961. Per capita income is recalculated frequently to take inflation and depreciation of rupee into account.

Recalculated per capita income per month for Prasad's scale.

Social class	Per capita monthly income in Rs
Upper class	7008 and above
Upper middle class	3504–7007
Middle class	2102–3503
Lower middle class	1051–2102
Lower class	Below 1050

POSTNATAL CASE HISTORY PORFORMA

Mrs XYZ (full name of the patient) .... gravida .... para .... a Hindu (caste) patient of .... years (age) old, residing at .... (address) of .... SE class (U/M/L), a homemaker (occupation) has delivered normally a _____ child on _____ (date) and today is her fourth postpartum day.

Origin, Duration and Progress

Patient was having 9 months amenorrhea and she started labor pains at .... (time) on .... (date) and was admitted to labor room at...... (time). She had blood stained discharge (i.e. show if present) and no leaking per vagina. At the time of admission, she was in first stage of labor with mild labor pains (mention details of contractions and P/V findings if available). She was given routine first stage management (shaving, enema, bladder care, reassurance, analgesia if used, ambulatory and monitoring). She progressed normally in labor.

She delivered at .... on .... a full-term female child with episiotomy. Baby cried soon after birth. Apgar was 6 at 1 min and 9 at 5 min. Weight of the newborn was 3.0 kg and there was no external congenital anomaly. Active management of third stage of labor (AMTSL) was done and she had no postpartum complications. (Mention duration of labor and any medications given during labor by asking the patient or from available records.)

Today is fourth postpartum day and she has normal lochial discharge and she c/o pain (e.g. perineal pain, after pains, backache).

(If patient is delivered by cesarean section indication of operation and type of anesthesia is asked and other operative details are taken from operative notes.)

Menstrual History

PaMP
LMP
EDD

Obstetric History: G4 P3 A1 L3

- First full-term normal hospital delivery of male child 3.0 kg 6 years back no antepartum, intrapartum or postpartum complication.
- Second spontaneous abortion of 2½ months gestation 4 years back and D & E was done.
- Third full-term normal home delivery of female child 2 years back no complication.
- Fourth full-term normal hospital delivery (present one) of female child 4 days back.

Past History

As mentioned in antenatal case OR NAD (nothing abnormal detected).

Family History

As mentioned in antenatal case OR NAD (nothing abnormal detected).

Personal History

Diet:

Appetite:

Bowel: Constipation is common due to lack or tone of abdominal muscles, perineal stitches, bed rest and less food intake during labor.

Bladder: Frequency is common due to diuresis in 2nd, 3rd, 4th day. Retention is common due to bladder atony and trauma during labor.

Sleep: Disturbed due to baby care and feeding.

General Examination
As mentioned in antenatal case.

Vitals
Pulse: Tachycardia if anemia or infection

BP: Hypertension

Temperature: > 38.4°C after first 24 hours suggest infection

Respiration: Normal

Tongue, Conjunctiva, Nails: No pallor OR Pallor—mild/moderate/severe

Edema legs: Present in cases of PIH, anemia, hypoproteinemia

Per Abdominal Examination
Uterus firm, contracted _____ weeks size fundal height _____ cm
  (Uterus involutes rapidly in first 7–10 days by about 1 to 1.5 cm/day. At the end of 2nd week it becomes a pelvic organ).

Local Vulval Examination
Lochia: Healthy, amount normal
Episiotomy stitches: Normal (no edema, induration, discharge, wound gap)

Breasts Examination
Nipples: Normal (no cracked nipples, fissures or retracted nipples)
Colostrum/milk—present
  (In UG examination vulval and breasts examination are usually not allowed to the students)
Newborn on 3rd day
- Weight _____
- Reflexes: Normal
- Temperature: Normal
- Cry: Normal
- Feeding: Taking breastfeeding normally
- Skin: No jaundice, no erythema toxicum
- Eyes: Normal, no conjunctivitis/jaundice
- Umbilical cord stump: Dry, no infection
- Urine: Passing urine 4–8 times per day
- Stool: Passed at least once after birth

Diagnosis
Patient is gravida 4 para 3, a case of normal delivery on 4th pastpartum day with female child of 3.0 kg weight on breastfeeding. Both mother and baby are normal.

Postnatal Advices
To mother
- Adequate rest
- Early ambulation
- Good hygiene, perineal care
- Nutrition diet with plenty of water
- Postnatal exercises
- Hematinic supplements
- Breastfeeding
- Contraception
- Abstinence for six weeks

For baby
- Breastfeeding
- Immunization
- Regular pediatric follow-up
- Immediate consultation if any problem.

Minor Complaints in Puerperium and Rx
- Afterpains due to uterine contractions—Rx by analgesics antispasmodics
- Perineal pain due to stitches—Rx by sitz bath, cold compresses, analgesics
- Backache—Rx by analgesics, hotwater bag, local ointment.

Breastfeeding Problems
- *Cracked nipples:* Rx by salt water rinse, applying breast milk on nipples, using emollients, e.g. lanolin ointment, Nipcare ointment.

- *Retracted nipples:* Rx by manual pull out, using nipple shield, breast pump.
- *Breast engorgement:* Rx by frequent manual expression, proper feeding, tight breast support.
- *Inadequate lactation:* Rx by nutritious diet, plenty of water, proper sucking and ayurvedic preparations (leptaden, lactare, promolact, etc.)
- *Lactation inhibition:* Discontinue sucking, tight breast support, vitamin B_6 (pyridoxine), cabergoline. Mixogen (estrogen + androgen) tablets were used in past.

Bladder Problem

Retention of urine—Rx by motivation, simple catheterization.

Bowel Problem

Constipation—Rx by laxatives.

Lochia

Lochia is vaginal discharge after delivery. It lasts for 2–3 weeks. It contains blood, bits of decidua, membranes, leucocytes, bacteria, cholesterin crystals, mucus and epithelial cells.
- Lochia rubra: Red—2 to 5 days
- Lochia serosa: Light brown—5 to 10 days
- Lochia alba: Pale white—10 to 12 days
- Excessive lochia suggests retained placental bits or infection
- Offensive (foul smelling) lochia suggests infection
- Scanty lochia is found in anemia and lochiometra.

Common Minor Problems of Newborn

In first week include skin rashes, vomiting, feeding problems, constipation, diarrhea, physiological jaundice, dehydration fever, excessive crying or excessive sleeping and superficial infections.

Rarely neonate can have vaginal bleeding, vaginal mucous discharge (female newborn) or mastitis neonatorum or cephalhematoma.

Baby is given vitamin K (1 mg IM) to prevent hemorrhagic complications and vaccination is started (BCG + Polio).

Features of premature baby are—less weight, single or no deep crease in sole, genitals less developed, hair less and wooly, breast nodule < 5 mm, deficient ear cartilage, shiny skin with plenty of lanugo, less body fat, weak cry, poor muscle tone.

COMMON QUESTIONS: GENERAL

Q1. Definitions of normal labor, lie, attitude, presentation, position, denominator, engagement.

Ans. *Normal labor:* It is a process of spontaneous expulsion of live fetus with its afterbirth, presenting by vertex, at term, without any artificial aid (except episiotomy), without any complications in a normal time limit.

Definitions of lie, attitude, presentation, position, denominator and engagement are given in Chapter 10.

Q2. What are the various clinical methods for calculating gestational age?

Ans. Clinical methods of calculating gestational age are—from LMP, first trimester P/V examination, from ovulation date (infertility treatment), date of quickening, McDonald's rule and fundal height by palpation.

Q3. Why at 32 and 40 weeks, fundal height is same? How can you differentiate the two?

Ans. At 32 weeks and 40 weeks, fundal height is same because after 36 weeks fundal height decreases again to 32 weeks level due to: (1) decrease in liquor, (2) in some patients head engages and (3) formation of lower segment in some patients.

Clinically one can make out by shape of the abdomen (fullness in the flanks) and amount of liquor or engagement.

Q4. What are the signs and symptoms of onset of labor?

Ans. Two symptoms of onset of labor: (1) Onset of true labor pains and (2) Show blood stained, mucus discharge. Two signs are: (1) Cervical dilatation and (2) Formation of bag of waters.

Rupture of membranes is not a sign or symptom of labor, however labor follows soon in most of the cases at term.

Q5. What are the stages of labor? What is the duration of primi and multi?

Ans. There are four stages of labor:
1. First stage (stage of dilatation): From onset of true labor pains to full (10 cm) dilatation of cervix. Primi 6 to 14 hours and multi 4 to 10 hours
2. Second stage (stage of expulsion): From full dilatation to complete expulsion of fetus.
   Primi ½ to 2 hours and multi 15 minutes to 1 hour.
   If epidural analgesia is given in 1 hour, more is given both in primi and multi.
3. Third stage (stage of afterbirth, placental stage): From expulsion of the fetus to complete expulsion of the placenta.
   Primi and multi: 5 to 15 minutes
4. Fourth stage (stage of observation): From expulsion of the placenta till 1 hour in all.

Q6. What are the signs of separation of placenta?

Ans. The signs of separations of placenta are: (1) Apparent lengthening of cord, (2) uterus becomes hard, globular cricket ball-like, (3) fundal height slightly rises, (4) suprapubic bulge, (5) fresh gush of blood: Matthews Duncan method of separation, (6) negative cord traction test and (7) P/V examination—placenta felt in lower segment or cervix.

Q7. What are Braxton-Hicks contractions? What is its purpose?

Ans. Braxton-Hicks contractions are painless uterine contractions which occur infrequently throughout pregnancy. Its exact purpose is not known. Probably it helps in regulating (by preventing stagnation) the blood flow in the placenta.

Q8. Why is the head ballotable?

Ans. Because of good range of movement at atlantooccipital joint head appears to be ballotable. Because of it hard consistency and regular round shape it is appreciated better.

Q9. How can you differentiate true labor pains from false pains?

Ans. True labor pains are rhythmic, progressive (increasing in intensity, frequency and duration), grinding or colicky in nature, radiating from loin to groin, associated with cervical dilatation and not relieved by analgesics, antispasmodics or enema.

Q10. What are the causes of FHS not heard?

Ans. Causes of absent fetal heart (with fetus alive) are obesity, polyhydramnios, posterior vertex position, malpresentation, severe bradycardia and very premature fetus.

Q11. What are the signs of fetal distress?

Ans. Signs of fetal distress are fetal bradycardia < 110/min, fetal tachycardia >160/min, irregular fetal heart sounds, meconium-stained liquor and sometimes excessive fetal movements.

Q12. How can you say from distance that patient has entered in second stage of labor?

Ans. When the patient in labor starts bearing down and there is rupture of membranes, you can say that patient has entered in second stage of labor.

Q13. What is crowning? Why it occurs?

Ans. When scalp hair (head of the fetus) is seen at vulva during uterine contraction and if it does not go back (retreat) in between pains it is called crowning (crown of vulval soft tissue on fetal head). It occurs because Biparietal diameter

(BPD) gets fixed under the subpubic arch with pain (uterine contractions) and soft tissue resistance cannot now push it back in between pains.

Q14. Why LOA position is most common?

Ans. LOA position is most common because in both anterior positions resistance of maternal spine (lumbar lordosis) is avoided and in left anterior position long anteroposterior diameter of fetal head remains in right oblique diameter of inlet avoiding sigmoid colon of left posterior quadrant of maternal pelvis.

Q15. What is deep transverse arrest?

Ans. Deep transverse arrest (DTA) is one of the arrested occipitoposterior situation in labor. When the head is arrested in: (1) transverse position, (2) at '0' station, (3) in second stage of labor, i.e. full dilatation, (4) for half an hour and (5) inspite of good uterine contractions it is called DTA.

Q16. What do you mean by contracted pelvis?

Ans. Contracted pelvis means when any of the essential diameter of true pelvis is shortened so as to alter the normal mechanism of labor or leads to obstructed labor it is called contracted pelvis.

Q17. What is the difference between contracted pelvis and cephalopelvic disproportion (CPD)?

Ans. Contracted pelvis is described above. Cephalopelvic disproportion (CPD) means disproportion between fetal head and maternal pelvis leading to problem in labor. It is relative, so even if pelvis is normal very large size fetus can cause obstruction and even if pelvis is contracted very small size fetus can come out through it without problem.

Q18. Why cephalic presentation is most common?

Ans. Cephalic presentation is common because: (1) low of accommodation—smaller fetal head better accommodated in smaller lower pole of uterus and bulky buttocks better accommodated in wide fundus of uterus and (2) gravitational theory—heavy fetal head sinks to lower pole of uterus as it is free in fluid.

Q19. How will you locate the anterior shoulder? What is its importance?

Ans. Anterior shoulder is located by palpating from fetal head upwards on the side of back—first resistance you feel is anterior shoulder. It is useful: (1) To locate fetal heart sounds during pregnancy and labor and (2) To assess the progress of labor—downwards and medial shifting suggest progress of labor.

Q20. Why FHS are heard best at the anterior shoulder or over the back?

Ans. FHS are heard best at anterior shoulder or back because sound conduction is best in solid media and fetal lungs are relatively solid in intrauterine life (after birth lungs have air) and these fetal parts are readily accessible and relatively fixed.

Q21. Why head engages at > 37 weeks in primigravida?

Ans. Head engages at 37 weeks in more than half of the primigravida because uterus and abdominal muscles are stretching for the first time, so their tone is good and they offer resistance and as fetus continue to grow with no space at fundus, formation of lower segment occurs and head engages.

Q22. What are the causes of non-engaged head at term in primi?

Ans. Causes of non-engaged head at term in primi include occipitoposterior position (deflexed head), contracted pelvis, placenta previa, polyhydramnios, large fetal head (CPD) and rarely soft tissue pelvic tumors. It can be idiopathic in some cases.

Q23. Which are the different methods to confirm the presence of FHS?

Ans. Different common methods to confirm the fetal heart sounds are ultrasonography, ultrasound Doppler, auscultation by medical stethoscope or Pinard's fetal stethoscope. It can also be detected by fetal ECG, fetal echocardiography and phonocardiography.

Q24. What do you mean by antepartum fetal surveillance? How it is done?

Ans. Antepartum fetal surveillance means various methods to evaluate fetal well-being. In early pregnancy for chromosomal defects USG (11–14 weeks scan) and biochemical marker studies (Double, Triple, Quadruple) are done. Chromosomal defects once suspected are confirmed by chromosomal analysis of fetal cells obtained by chorionic villous biopsy, amniocentesis or fetal blood sampling. At 18–20 weeks fetal structural anomaly scan is done by USG and at 22 weeks fetal echo can be carried out. In late pregnancy growth abnormalities are detected by daily fetal movement count (DFMC), nonstress test, biophysical profile scoring (BPS), modified BPS, fetal Doppler study. (Contraction tress test was done in past).

Q25. What is nonstress test (NST)?

Ans. Nonstress test is described in Chapter 15.

Q. Define vertex.

Ans. Vertex is an area bounded anteriorly by anterior fontanelle and coronal suture on either side, posteriorly by posterior fontanelle and lambdoid sutures and laterally lines passing through parietal eminencies.

Q26. How can you differentiate anterior fontanelle from posterior fontanelle?

Ans. Anterior fontanelle is differentiated from posterior fontanelle as follows:

Anterior fontanelle	Posterior fontanelle
Large size	Small size
Quadrangular of lozenge shape	Triangular
Connected with 4 suture lines and 4 bones	Connected with 3 suture lines and 3 bones
It is a bony defect	It is bony depression
Closes at 18 months	Closes at 6 months

Q27. What are the complications of 1st stage of labor?

Ans. The complications of first stage of labor are prolonged first stage, early rupture of membranes, cord prolapse, fetal distress, fetal death and obstructed labor.

Q28. What are the complications of second stage of labor?

Ans. Complications of second stage of labor are prolonged second stage, obstructed labor, fetal distress, maternal distress, fetal death and rupture uterus.

Q29. What are the complications of third stage of labor?

Ans. Complications of third stage of labor are retained placenta, postpartum (third stage hemorrhage), inversion of uterus, amniotic fluid embolism and shock.

Q30. What are the ways to cut short the second stage of labor?

Ans. Ways of cutting short the second stage of labor are artificial rupture of membranes (ARM), oxytocin drip, episiotomy and instrumental delivery, i.e. forceps delivery or vacuum extraction.

Q31. How will you manage the first stage of labor?

Ans. First stage is managed under the following headings: (1) Reassurance-psychological support, (2) strict asepsis, (3) posture, (4) bladder care, (5) bowel care, (6) pain relief and (7) most important—monitoring of mother, fetus and progress of labor.

Q32. How will you actually conduct the delivery? (Second stage)

Ans. Delivery is conducted in lithotomy position with proper asepsis. Head is delivered slowly after giving episiotomy (if required) with good bearing down efforts of mother and giving perineal support with sterile pad.

Q33. What are the components of active management of third stage of labor?

Ans. Components of active management of third stage of labor as recommended by WHO are:
- Injection oxytocin 10 units IM immediately after the delivery of the baby
- Delayed cord clamping for at least 1–3 minutes after birth
- Controlled cord traction
- Postpartum vigilance: Check uterine tone every 15 minutes for 2 hours.

Q34. How will you confirm leaking?

Ans. Leaking can be confirmed by per speculum examination and if required asking the patient to cough or strain or fundal pressure during examination. Other tests confirming leaking are nitrazine paper test (yellow to blue) or slide test (secretion on slide turns white on heating) or ferning (vaginal fluid seen under microscope) or by AmniSure (detection of amniotic fluid protein PAMG-1 by test strips).

Q35. What is the normal time of rupture of membranes? Why?

Ans. Normally membranes rupture after full dilatation, i.e. in beginning of second stage of labor because in first stage round cervical rim supports the membranes equally from all around during uterine contraction, but when cervix is fully dilated membranes are exposed to vagina which has anterior and posterior walls so middle portion of membranes (being not well supported) balloons out during contraction and ruptures.

Q36. What do you mean by PROM, PPROM, EROM, and ARM?

Ans. PROM (Premature rupture of membranes): Rupture of membranes before onset of labor.
PPROM (Preterm premature rupture of membranes): Rupture of membranes before onset of labor and before 37 weeks.
EROM (Early rupture of membranes): Rupture of membranes before full dilatation, i.e. during first stage.
ARM (Artificial rupture of membranes): By instruments.

Q37. What do you mean by early deceleration, late deceleration and variable deceleration in fetal heart rate patterns?

Ans. Deceleration means transient decrease in fetal heart rate below the baseline by 15 bpm or more and lasting for >15 seconds.

Early deceleration: Here the FHR begins to slow with beginning of uterine contraction and onset, nadir and recovery exactly coincides with onset, peak and ending of uterine contraction. It is because of vagal stimulation due to head compression.

Late deceleration: Here deceleration begins near the height of uterine contraction and FHR returns to normal after the contraction is over. This is seen in uteroplacental insufficiency.

Variable deceleration: Here the decelerations are variable in all aspects, i.e. onset, peak, duration and frequency and are independent of uterine contractions. It is thought to indicate cord compression.

Q38. What do you mean by saltatory fetal heart rate pattern? What do you mean by sinusoidal fetal heart rate pattern?

Ans. *Saltatory fetal heart pattern:* Saltatory baseline heart rate pattern consists of rapidly recurring couplets of accelerations and decelerations causing relatively large oscillations of the baseline fetal heart rate. It is associated with umbilical cord compression.

Sinusoidal fetal heart rate pattern: Smooth sine-like pattern of fetal heart rate. There is stable baseline heart rate of 120 to 160 beats/min with regular oscillations above or below a baseline. There is fixed short-term variability and absence of accelerations. It is found in severe fetal anemia, fetomaternal hemorrhage and fetal hypoxia.

Q39. What is asynclitism? What is its importance?

Ans. *Asynclitism means parietal obliquity:* It is due to lateral tilting of head of fetus in labor. Anterior asynclitism (Naegele's obliquity) means anterior parietal bone is lower down than posterior parietal bone. It is found commonly in parous patient and does not cause many problems. Posterior asynclitism (Litzman's obliquity) means posterior parietal bone is lower than anterior one. It is common in primigravida and can cause obstruction.

Q40. What is caput succedaneum? How can you differentiate it from cephalhematoma?

Ans. Caput succedaneum is described in Chapter 10.

It is differentiated from cephalhematoma by: (1) not limited by suture lines, (2) present at birth, (3) more soft and (4) disappears spontaneously within 24 hours after birth.

Q41. What is molding?

Ans. Molding is described in Chapter 10.

Q.42 What is asphyxia neonatourm? What is Apgar score?

Ans. Asphyxia neonatorum is defined as failure of establishment of satisfactory respiration in newborn at birth. Apgar score is described in Chapter 15.

Q43. Which cases are included under high risk pregnancy?

Ans. Any pregnancy which carries increased risk to mother or fetus is included in high risk pregnancy. It includes medical disorders, obstetric complications in past or present pregnancy, fetal abnormalities and previous OB-GYN surgeries, e.g. CS, myomectomy.

Q44. What is rate of involution of uterus?

Ans. The rate of involution of uterus is 1–1.5 cm/day. It becomes a pelvic organ by the end of second week.

Q45. What are the causes of subinvolution?

Ans. The causes of subinvolution are infection, retained placental tissues, anemia, fibroid of uterus, multiple pregnancy, hydramnios, prolapse of uterus and some cases of lower segment cesarean section (LSCS).

Q46. Define puerperal pyrexia.

Ans. Puerperal pyrexia is defined as pyrexia of 100.4°F (38°C) on two separate occasions 24 hours apart, excluding first 24 hours within 10 days of delivery.

Q47. What are the causes of puerperal pyrexia?

Ans. Causes of puerperal pyrexia are genital tract sepsis, urinary tract infection, mastitis, septic thrombophlebitis, malaria or other intercurrent infections.

Q48. What do you mean by rooming in? What are its advantages?

Ans. *Rooming in* means soon after the birth baby is kept in a cot by the bedside of the mother. Mother and baby remain together 24-hour a day.

Q49. What are the 10 steps in promoting breastfeeding under baby friendly hospital initiative?

Ans. The 10 steps in promoting breastfeeding under baby friendly hospital initiative are: (1) Written breastfeeding policy, (2) Trained health care staff, (3) Mothers motivated to initiate breastfeeding within half an hour of birth, (4) Mothers informed about the benefits of breastfeeding, (5) Mothers are taught the best way to breast feed, (6) Newborns are given no other food or drink, (7) To practice rooming in, (8) To encourage demand breastfeeding, (9) No artificial teat should be given, (10) Mothers are referred to breastfeeding support groups.

Q50. What are the advantages of breast-feeding?

Ans. The advantages to mother are: (1) helps in involution of uterus 2) mother-child bonding, (3) prevents ovulation so helps in contraception and (4) decreases risk of breast cancer in future.

The advantages for baby are: (1) ideal food, (2) sterile, (3) cheap, (4) readily available, (5) easily digestible, (6) contains all required nutrients, (7) increases immunity and (8) child-mother bonding.

Q51. What contraceptive advices will you give to your patients?

Ans. Patients who have completed child bearing are advised permanent method, i.e. postpartum tubal ligation operation. Patients who want laparoscopic tubal ligation (Lap TL) are advised to come back after 6 weeks.

For those who wish temporary methods are advised CuT 380A insertion either immediately in first 48 hours postpartum or after 6 weeks. Progesterone only pills can be advised but combined pills are contraindicated. Lactational amenorrhea method requires 3 criteria to be fulfilled, i.e. first 6 months postpartum, babies on exclusive breastfeeding and patient does not get menstruation.

Common Antenatal Cases

1. Anemia
2. Hypertension in pregnancy
3. Previous cesarean section
4. Intrauterine growth restriction
5. Breech
6. Twins
7. Rh negative mother
8. Postdate pregnancy
9. False labor pains
10. Polyhydramnios, oligohydramnios
11. Bad obstetric history
12. Pregnancy with pyrexia [malaria, urinary tract infection (UTI), respiratory tract infection]
13. Medical diseases like heart disease, diabetes, respiratory diseases.

Cases of preterm labor and placenta previa (APH) are either not kept or when kept, P/A examination is not allowed.

Usually antenatal cases in second half of pregnancy are asked but sometimes cases in first half of pregnancy or postnatal cases are kept in exam. In early pregnancy, cases will be of abortion, hyperemesis gravidarum and rarely ectopic pregnancy or gestational trophoblastic disease, e.g. hydatidiform mole.

Common Postnatal Cases

1. Normal delivery
2. Cesarean section
3. Instrumental delivery—forceps/vacuum
4. Preterm delivery
5. Twins delivery
6. Delivery of IUGR fetus
7. Delivery of high risk cases, e.g. anemia, pregnancy-induced hypertension (PIH), vaginal birth after cesarean (VBAC)
8. Post-abortal case.

MECHANISM OF NORMAL LABOR

The series of movements which the fetal head undergoes during its passage through the birth canal is described as mechanism of normal labor.

- **Engagement:** It is the first mechanism. As already described before when biparietal diameter crosses the inlet of pelvis it is called engagement. Diameter of fetus is suboccipitobregmatic and diameter of engagement (of pelvis) is right oblique diameter in case of left occipitoanterior (V_1) position. In nearly half of the primigravida head engages in last few days or pregnancy before the labor actually starts. This is because good tone of the anterior abdominal wall and the uterine wall, which is stretching for the first time offers resistance and as the fetus continuously grows it has to descend in pelvis as there is no space up in the abdomen. In remaining of the primigravida and most of the parous patients head engages after labor pains start.

- **Descent:** Descent of the head is second movement and it continues with other movements till head delivers by extension. Descent occurs due to downward force of the uterine contraction which coincides with axis of inlet which is directed downward and backward. Retraction of upper uterine segment (little shortening with each contraction) also helps in descent. Active pushing by mother (bearing down) in second stage of labor also helps in descent.
- **Flexion:** It is the next movement on fetal head. As described earlier, it is occurring with descent. Explanation given for flexion is "lever theory". The fetal head moves on atlantooccipital joint. Now considering joint as the fulcrum, sinciptal arm is longer than occipital arm as the joint is situated more posteriorly in the head. Now when the contraction comes sinciptal arm will meet with more resistance (longer arm—more area of contract) than occipital arm. As per Newton's law forces are equal and opposite, more thrust back will happen to sinciput than occiput, so flexion occurs.
- **Internal rotation:** Next movement with descent is anterior internal rotation of the occiput. This is because of gutter-like slope of pelvic floor which is directed downward, forward and medially. Pelvic floor is made of levator ani which has 3 components—pubococcygeus, iliococcygeus and ischiococcygeus. Occiput touching the pelvic floor first will be guided actively and passively downward, forward and medially towards the symphysis pubis and this is called internal rotation.
- **Crowning:** It is the next thing happening on the fetal head. It is not the special movement of mechanism of labor but occurs before delivery of the head by extension. When fetal head (scalp hair) is visible at vulva during contraction and it does not retreat back in between contraction, that stage is called crowning. Literally it is the crown of maternal soft tissue of vulva on fetal head.
- With every contraction head is pushed down and scalp is seen at vulva. When contraction passes of elastic recoil of maternal soft tissue pushes the head back. With continuous retraction of upper uterine segment little advancement occurs with each contraction. At the stage, when BPD of the fetal head negotiates subpubic arch, it cannot go back after contraction passes of by elastic recoil of the soft tissue which cannot overcome the bony resistance of subpubic arch and head is continuously seen at vulva even in between contraction and this is crowning.
- **Extension:** After crowning, head delivers by extension. This is because the downward force of uterine contraction is meeting the resistance of pelvic floor obliquely, so resultant reflected force is also oblique and this is at outlet anteriorly directed. As the head is fully flexed with occiput anterior this anterior movement is extension for fetal head.
- **Restitution:** This is occurring to relieve torsion at the neck which has occurred during internal rotation. During internal rotation only head has rotated and not the whole body so there is twisting at the neck which gets automatically relieved when head has delivered out and free. This movement of head is called restitution and it is opposite to internal rotation, i.e. on left side in LOA position.
- **External rotation:** Further ⅛ of circle or so, rotation of head on the direction of restitution is called external rotation. This is due to internal rotation of the shoulders, which is transmitted to the head outside as external rotation.

Mechanisam of Labor in Occipitoposterior Position

Occipitoposterior position is malposition not malpresantation. Presentation is vertex only.

But as it can cause problems in labor it is descried here.

At the beginning of labor 10–15% can be occipitoposterior position. Right occipitoposterior (ROP) is 3 to 4 times more common than left occipitoposterior position (LOP).

Mechanism of Labor in ROP Position

The head engages in right oblique diameter of inlet engaging diameter is suboccipitofrontal (10 cm) due to deflexion associated with occipitoposterior positions.

Favorable Outcome

In 90% cases descent occurs with completion of flexion and long internal rotation of head occurs (nearly ⅜ of circle) with ½ of circle rotation of shoulders. So now it is converted exactly into right occipitoanterior position and the remaining mechanism is same, i.e. crowning, extension of head, restitution and external rotation.

Unfavorable Outcome

In 10% of cases long internal rotation does not occur or it occurs incompletely. The reasons for failure of internal rotation are: (1) Deflexion of head, (2) abnormal pelvis, (3) poor uterine contraction, (4) PROM or early rupture or membranes (i.e. during first stage), (5) poor pelvic floor and (6) large fetal head. Different types of arrests can be explained on the basis or degree of deflexion.

1. If there is mild deflexion, occiput is still little lower down than sinciput and touches the pelvic floor first and so guided anteriorly first for internal rotation. But by the time it reaches in transverse position (45° rotation) sinciput also start touching pelvic floor and also tries to rotate anteriorly. Both will not allow each other to go anteriorly and thus head gets arrested in transverse position, i.e. deep transverse arrest (DTA). Criteria of DTA include: (1) transverse position of head, (2) '0' station, (3) good uterine contractions, (4) second stage of labor and 5) half to one hour.
2. If head does not rotate at all as in case of moderate deflexion due to both occiput and sinciput touching pelvic floor simultaneously head remains in posterior original position in second stage of labor leading to arrest of labor, it is called oblique occipitoposterior arrest.
3. If head rotates to posterior position, i.e. severe deflexion (sinciput lower down than occiput, touching the pelvic floor first so guided anteriorly and occiput rotates posteriorly) then it gets arrested it is called occipito-sacral arrest.

All above 3 arrests are also described together as POP (persistent occipitoposterior).

In last variety, i.e. occipito-sacral arrest, if pelvis is of good capacity, delivery can still occur as face to pubis delivery. Here root of the nose gets fixed under the subpubic arch, first posterior part of the head delivers by flexion and then face delivers by extension. Here there are chances of perineal tears as bulky parietal and occipital area of the head delivers from posterior aspect.

Course of labor is altered (labor prolonged) in occipitoposterior position due to: (1) delayed engagement of head due to deflexion presenting larger diameter, (2) weak uterine action due to poor stimulation, (3) long internal rotation and (4) early rupture of membranes.

Management of arrested occipitoposterior in modern times is mainly by cesarean section. Although instrumental delivery or manual rotation can be done due to decreasing skill of such maneuver, this is rarely practiced.

Induction of Labor

INTRODUCTION

Induction of labor (IOL) is defined as artificial initiation of uterine contractions before spontaneous onset of labor for maternal or fetal indications to have successful vaginal delivery.

It is common obstetric practice in present times. Its incidence has increased in last two decades and currently it varies from 20% to 40% at different places.

Indications

It is done in conditions where continuation of pregnancy is either harmful to mother or fetus.

Maternal:
- Postdate pregnancy (41st week)
- PROM, PPROM
- Hypertensive disorders of pregnancy
- Medical conditions: Diabetes, renal disease, liver disease
- Abruptio placenta
- Chorioamnionitis.

Fetal:
- IUFD
- Major fetal malformation incompatible with life
- IUGR
- Oligohydramnios
- Rh-isoimmunization.

Prerequisites for IOL

- There should be clear maternal or fetal indication for IOL.
- Benefits and risks must be explained to patients and relatives.
- Written consent should be taken.
- Gestational age should be clearly established.
- Assessment of fetal size, presentation and maternal pelvis.
- Cervical assessment by Bishop's score.
- Facility for emergency cesarean section should be available.

Contraindications

Induction of labor (IOL) should not be done if there is any contraindication to labor or vaginal delivery.

- Fetal malpresentation
- CPD
- Placenta previa
- Previous two or more CS
- Previous classical CS or rupture uterus
- Active genital herpes
- Precious pregnancy (Direct CS is usually preferred).

Elective Induction of Labor

It is defined as induction of labor in absence of acceptable fetal or maternal indications. So

by definition it does not provide any benefits. It is done for logistic reasons:
- History of precipitate labor
- Patient staying at far off place
- Unexplained IUFD in previous pregnancy
- Psychological or astrological reasons.

Many times it is done for doctor or patient's conveniences.

Preinduction Cervical Ripening

- Modified Bishop's score is used for predicting success of induction.
- If it is 5 or less, it suggests poor response to induction or failure.
- If it is 9 or more, it predicts successful induction.

Cervical ripening can be done by all of the above methods but usually prostaglandins (Pharmacological) are used for the purpose, as such ripening and induction is continuous process in most of the patients. Bishop's score is described in Chapter 15.

Methods of Inductions of Labor

- Pharmacological
- Mechanical
- Natural.

Pharmacological Methods

- **Prostaglndin E2 (Dinoprostone) gel:**
  - It is used as endocervical gel.
  - Proper full endocervical insertion is must.
  - Maximum 3 insertions at the interval of 6 hours are recommended.
  - The drug should be stored in refrigerator between 2°C and 8°C.
  - It is useful both for ripening as well as induction.
- **Dinoprostone vaginal pessary:**
  - It is available as 10 mg vaginal insert. It releases 0.3 mg/hour of the drug.
  - It is stored in freezer at –10° to –25° C.
  - It is inserted transversely in the posterior fornix.
  - The pouch forms one end a long of tape remains outside, so it can be removed easily.
  - It is removed after 24 hours or if pains start or leaking occurs.
  - Its advantages are: 1. It is easy to insert, 2. retrievable if hyperstimulation occurs.
  - Its disadvantages are: 1. High cost, 2. cold chain maintenance.
- **Misoprostol (PG E1):**
  - It is not yet approved for induction of labor by CDSCO, Government of India. It is only approved for MTP purpose as Combikit along with mifepristone.
  - It is permitted for IOL by WHO in the dose of 25 µg vaginally 6 hourly. Cochrane review in 2014 suggested that oral misoprostol (preferably in solution) 20–25 µg 2 hourly is as effective as vaginal misoprostol and with less risks.
  - Off label use of misoprostol in India is common. It is not to be used in previous cesarean section cases and in PROM. More than 25 µg dose results in hyperstimulation and meconium stained liquor.
- **Oxytocin:**
  - It is more used for augmentation rather than induction.
  - Two dose regimens are there:
    - Low dose: 1–2 mIU/min, increased by 1–2 mIU/min every 15–40 min.
    - High dose: 4–6 mIU/min, increase by 4–6 mIU/min every 15–40 min.
  - Adding 5 units (1 ampoule of oxytocin) in 1 liter makes 5000 mIU in 1000 mL, i.e., 5 mIU/1 mL. Considering 16 drops = 1 mL. When you give IV fluid with pitocin 16 drops /min you are giving 5 mU/mL.
  - When oxytocin is used after prostaglandins it is administered 6 hours after the last dose of PGE2 gel and 4 hours after the misoprostol tablet.
  - Maximum dose of oxytocin is 36–48 mIU/min.

– Optimum uterine activity is 200 Montevideo units.

Mechanical Methods

- **Sweeping of membranes:** It is done by per vaginal examination. Finger is introduced in the cervix and 360° rotation of finger is done twice as high as possible above the internal os, stretching the lower uterine segment.
- **ARM**
  - It is called British method or induction.
  - It is done by keeping the presenting part fixed with suprapubic pressure. It is done using either long needle held in swab holder or straight Kocher's clamp or special amniotome.
  - Due to risk or infection, cord prolapse or abruption and unpredictable response, it is less favored purely for induction. It is now used for augmentation usually after 5 cm cervical dilatation and always coupled with oxytocin.
- **Balloon:**
  - Foley's catheter
  - Atad double balloon catheter.

  Foley's catheter is introduced through the cervix and bulb is inflated. Its efficacy is similar to prostaglandins and it is of relatively of low cost. There is less uterine hyperstimulation and less fetal heart rate variability.

Natural

These include Nipple stimulation, Acupuncture/acupressure, herbs, homeopathy, soap water enema sexual intercourse and castor oil. Strong evidence is lacking for each one of these methods and success is unpredictable, so it is not recommended.

Complications of Induction of Labor

- Failure leading to cesarean section. Incidence of cesarean section almost doubles due to failure of induction. Also there is increased risk of operative vaginal delivery.
- Uterine hyperstimulation, precipitate/dysfunctional labor
- Fetal distress. Rarely fetal death
- Rupture uterus
- Intrauterine infection, sepsis
- Increased risk of PPH—atonic as well as traumatic.

Failure of Induction

Failure of induction is not yet well defined. It is considered when there is failure to establish labor after one cycle of treatment with any agent. For endocervical gel (0.5 mg PGE2) 2 doses at 6 hourly. interval and for PGE2 controlled release pessary (10 mg) over 24 hours is considered one cycle.

Some authorities consider failure as failure to achieve vaginal delivery.

Prevention of Induction of Labor

As recommended by WHO sweeping of membranes from 37 weeks onward reduces formal induction of labor. However, due to its associated problems of discomfort to the patient, PROM and infection, it is not commonly practiced.

IOL in Special Situations

- *IUFD:* Prostglandins are preferred. Prior treatment with mifepristone tablet 200 mg Orally 36-48 hours prior to induction increases success rate.
  50–100 μg misoprostol 3–6 hourly orally or vaginally is given. Foley's catheter is also good option.
- *PROM:* Endocervical PGE2 gel followed by oxytocin is recommended after 12–24 hours.
- *Previous CS:* There is increased risk or cesarean section as well as rupture of uterus by any method. Misoprostol is not recommended. Foley's catheter is better option.
- *Twins:* Induction of labor is recommended after 37 weeks.
- *Breech presentation:* Vaginal breech delivery at term is controversial, so IOL is not favored in breech presentation.

CHAPTER 13

Ultrasonography and X-rays

ULTRASONOGRAPHY

Ultrasonography (USG) is very important and commonly used diagnostic procedure in current obstetrics and gynecological practice. Diagnostic ultrasound was first introduced in medical field by Professor Ian Donald from UK in 1958. Ultrasound is defined as the sound above the range of human hearing, i.e., 20,000 Hz (one Hz = one cycle per second).

Ultrasound equipment consists of the following:
1. *Transducer or probe*: This is applied to the patient's body. It contains piezoelectric crystals which generate ultrasound. According to the arrangements of crystals, the probe can be linear, sector or curvilinear (convex).
2. *Central processing unit (CPU)*: Probe is connected to CPU by means of a cable. It passes high voltage AC current to the crystals in the probe and also receives electrical signals from the crystals. These signals are processed, amplified and converted into visual signals to produce an image on the screen. CPU has an operating panel on it to control the functions.
3. *Viewing monitor:* The screen on which the display occurs.

All ultrasound machines are real-time scanners. This is done by replacing each B mode image in rapid sequence, i.e., >20 frames per second to produce actual movements like fetal movements, cardiac pulsations, etc.

Mechanism of Production of Ultrasound

Piezoelectric (PZE) crystals are quartz, barium titanate and lead zinconate titanate. They have a unique property of interconverting various forms of energy. When an electric current is applied to such a crystal, it changes its width and in doing so it produces mechanical vibration, i.e., soundwaves. More thinner the crystal, higher the frequency of ultrasound produced. These soundwaves travel into the body tissue from the site of probe contact and strike back the same crystal (in resting phase) after being reflected back from various tissues depending upon the difference in the sound properties of different tissues and its distance (depth) from the probe. This produces electric current which is processed by the machine as mentioned earlier.

Piezoelectric phenomenon of PZE crystal is as shown below :
- Electrical energy → Machanical energy → Vibration → Sound wave
- Reflected sound (echo) → Vibration of crysal → Mechanical energy → Electrical energy converted to visual signal

In medical field ultrasound frequency of 2–10 MHz is used, which is not in any way harmful to the body (1 MHz = 1 million Hz).

Sonography in obstetrics and gynecology is done by transabdominal route (TAS) and transvaginal route (TVS) using respective probes.

TAS is mainly for obstetric evaluation from second trimester onwards, while TVS is better for all gynecological cases (except big tumors) and early pregnancy evaluation (first trimester).

TAS and TVS are compared as below:

	TAS	TVS
Frequency	3–5 MHz	5–7 MHz
Resolution	+	+++ (very good)
Field of view	12–14 cm	6–8 cm
Bladder	Full	Empty
Orientation	Better	Slightly difficult
Maneuverability	Free	Limited
Magnification	+	+++
Obesity	Difficult	Comparatively easy
Big tumors	Better studied	Less
Palpation	Nonspecific	Tenderness elicitable
Infection	None	Possibility exists
Material used	Only gel used	Gel + condom used

Obstetric Uses

For TAS examination full bladder is must, because full bladder displaces gas-filled intestinal loops and helps in making out the relation of different pelvic organs. It provides a medium that enhances the transmission of sound thus it acts as an ultrasonic window. For TVS examination bladder should be empty.

Early Pregnancy Evaluatuion

A. **Diagnosis:** White ring of gestational sac surrounding a sonolucent area is diagnostic. Double decidual sac (DDS) sign is also confirmatory. Gestational sac and other early pregnancy features appear as follows:

	TVS
Gestational sac	5th week
Yolk sac	5 weeks
Embryo	6th week
Cardiac activity	6 weeks

B. **Viability:** Early pregnancy failure and blighted ovum (anembryonic pregnancy) are diagnosed from following criteria:
   - Thin irregular or interrupted echogenic ring.
   - Failure to grow after 1 week. Normal increase is at least 75% in size after 1 week.
   - The absence of fetal pole in gestational sac with a volume of 2.5 mL or more
   - No yolk sac when MSD is >8 mm
   - Mean sac diameter >18 mm with no embryonic echoes by TVS confirms the diagnosis.

C. **Nuchal translucency:** Increased nuchal translucency is associated with chromosomal defects and other abnormalities.
   Fetal Medicine Foundation (FMF) criteria:
   - Measured between 11 and 13 weeks 6 days.
   - Crown-rump **length** (**CRL**) must be between 45 and 84 mm.
   - Fetal head and thorax should occupy the whole screen.
   - Fetal head should be in neutral position neither flexed nor extended.
   - Midsagittal veiw of the face is taken.
   - Calipers should be placed on the inner borders of the nuchal fold.
   - Care must be taken to distinguish between fetal skin and amnion.
   - Widest part of translucency measured. More than 1 measurement taken and maximum one should be recorded in data base.

   Other features checked during NT scan (11–14 weeks) are presence of nasal bone, no

tricuspid regurgitation and normal ductus venosus waveform.

Abortion

A. **Threatened abortion:** USG help in diagnosis, prognosis and follow-up
   - Fetal cardiac activity confirms the viability but rate <85/min suggest bad prognosis.
   - Subchorionic or retroplacental hemorrhage may be seen as hypoechoic area. Hematoma size of <25% of sac size has good prognosis. Fundal and corporeal hematomas (usually retroplacental) have bad prognosis than supracervical hematoma.
   - If MSD-CRL = ≤5 mm also suggest bad prognosis.
B. **Inevitable abortion:** Low level sac, cervical dilatation and sac in process of expulsion may be seen.
C. **Incomplete abortion:** Gestational sac in various stages of collapse and evacuation, amorphous echogenic material surrounded by disrupted choriodecidual tissue and pockets of fluid or hemorrhage.
D. **Complete abortion:** Uterine cavity empty with endometrial surfaces well opposed.

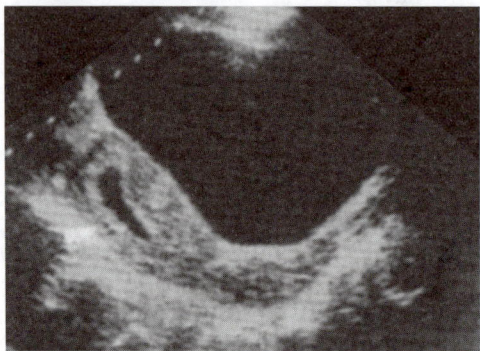

Fig. 13.1: Gestational ring of early pregnancy.

E. **Missed abortion:** Identification of embryo/fetus with no cardiac activity. Amniotic fluid reduced or absent, irregular mixed echogenic tissues inside the cavity.

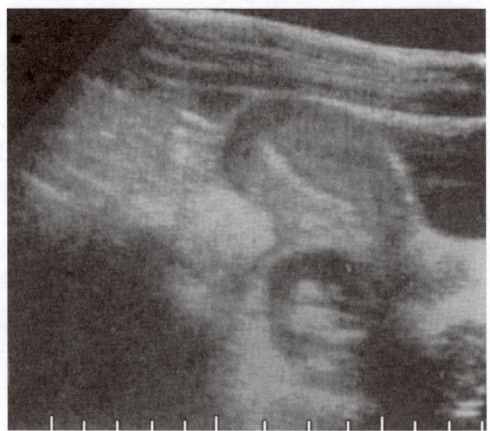

Fig. 13.2: Ectopic pregnancy.

Hydatidiform Mole

A characteristic **snow-storm** appearance of uterine cavity. A large uterus filled with multiple sonolucent spaces. No fetal element seen in case of complete mole. Lutein cysts of the ovary if present (20–30%), can be visualized. In partial mole, fetus may be visualized along with cystic spaces.

Ectopic Pregnancy

Uterine cavity empty with uterus normal size or slightly enlarged and pregnancy test positive.
- Pseudosac in the uterus may mimic gestational sac but yolk sac is absent.
- A mixed echogenic adnexal mass.
- Actual gestational sac with or without an embryo may be occasionally visualized outside the uterus.
- Free fluid in the pouch of Douglas or adnexal region. If in doubt evaluate the case by serial beta human chorionic gonadotropin (hCG) testing (doubling every 2 1/2 days in normal pregnancy) and follow-up USG.
- The color Doppler of adnexal region showing increased vascularity (ring of fire) may be helpful.

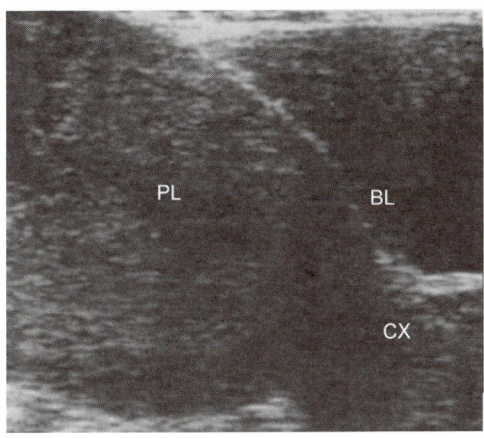

Fig. 13.3: Placenta previa.

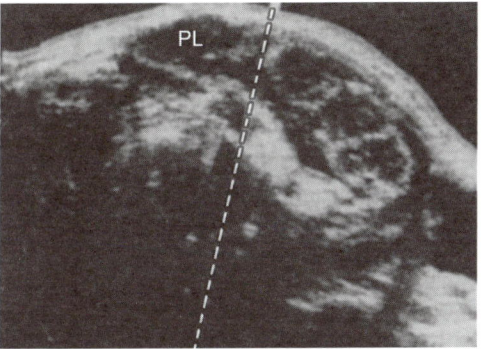

Fig. 13.4: Grade III placenta.

Placental Study

A. **Localization of placental site:** Before amniocentesis, amnioinfusion and external cephalic version.
B. **Placenta previa:** It can be easily diagnosed by USG by checking its relation to internal cervical os. Transvaginal sonography (TVS) is better than transabdominal sonography (TAS). TAS may be less accurate when there is—(1) posterior placenta previa and fetal head is in between, (2) in obese patients, and (3) with underfilling or overfilling of bladder.
   - During a myometrial contraction the wall of the uterus may thicken and imitate placental tissue. To avoid this pitfall, a contraction is suspected if the myometrium is thicker than 1.5 cm and repeat imaging is performed after 30 minutes.
   - In TVS distance from the internal os is measured and documented. If low-lying placenta is diagnosed in early pregnancy, scan should be repeated after 28 weeks to recheck the position of placenta. With increase in gestational age upward migration is common.
   - If placental edge is 2 cm away from internal os at 18 weeks almost 100% will migrate. If placenta crosses the internal os by 2 cm almost 100% sensitivity for placenta previa at term.
C. **Diagnosis of abruption placenta:** Unlike placenta previa USG is less helpful. Sonographic appearance of retroplacental hemorrhage is variable. Usually it is characterized by bizarre echoes between placenta and myometrium. Initially it is hyperechoic than myometrium, after 48 hours it becomes isoechoic and after few days it becomes hypoechoic.

   Sensitivity and specificity of USG for diagnosis of placental abruption 24% and 96%, respectively.
D. **Placental grading:** It reflects maturational changes of placenta and it correlates with gestational age in normal pregnancy but may be altered in medical or obstetric diseases complicating pregnancy. They are as follows:

   Grade 0: Smooth chorionic plate and placenta without any echogenic density.

   Grade 1: Chorionic plate shows subtle undulations and there are linear or comma-shaped echogenic densities in substance of placenta.

   Grade 2: Presence of basal echogenic density in linear fashion, markly indented chorionic plate, increased comma like densities.

   Grade 3: Indentations of chorionic plate reach up to basal plate and there is appearance of sonolucent areas in the substance of the placenta giving a "Swiss-cheese pattern".

Placental grading is not used for fetal wellbeing assessment.

Fetal Maturity

A. **Crown rump length (CRL):** It is useful in the first trimester of pregnancy only because after that flexion of fetal spine renders the measurement less accurate.
   - Longest measurement is taken
   - Fetal limbs are excluded
   - York sac is excluded
   - Measurement is made from the cephalic pole to the outer edge of the rump
   - Fetus in neutral position

   Formula:
   - Gestational age in weeks = CRL in cm + 6.5.
   - Gestational age in days = 0.6 x CRL in mm + 51.

   It predicts gestational age within 5 days in 95% of cases.

B. **Biparietal diameter (BPD):** It is useful after first trimester of pregnancy. Single BPD measurement between 12 and 28 weeks is quite accurate in pregnancy dating. It predicts gestational age within 7 days. But in third trimester it is less accurate parameter.
   - It is measured from outer edge of proximal skull to inner edge of distal skull (outer to inner measurement).
   - Standard plane of measurement includes the thalamus and the cavum of septum pellucidum.
   - It is measured perpendicular to midline echo, which is generated by interhemispheric fissure.
   - The head shape must be oval.

   Formula:
   (BPD in cm x 4) + 2 = Gestational age in weeks. This formula is used in clinical practice but the most precise calculation of gestational age can be obtained by referring the standard BPD charts for different populations.

C. **Femur length:** It is useful in third trimester of pregnancy and it is as reliable as BPD measurement.

   Criteria:
   - It is measured from the greater trochanter to the lateral condyle of the femur.
   - Only diaphyseal length is taken. Epiphysis are not included in measurement.
   - Golf club-like appearance is characteristic.
   - Bone image should be parallel to the top of the screen.

   Formula:
   - Gestational age in weeks = Femur length in mm/2.
   - At 40 weeks femur length is 80 mm.

D. **Head circumference (HC):** It is useful in second half of pregnancy. Unlike BPD, HC is independent of the shape of the head.
   - Fronto-occipital diameter is measured along the axis of the skull at the level of BPD.
   - It is outer edge to outer edge measurement.
   - Inbuilt software gives direct measurement of HC from the measurements of BPD and fronto-occipital diameter.

   Formula:
   - HC = (BPD + Occipitofrontal diameter) × π/2
   - The gestational age is obtained from the standard growth curve charts for the HC. It is reliable up to 40 weeks. At 40 weeks, it is 34.5 cm.

E. **Abdominal circumference (AC):** It is useful in second half of pregnancy.
   - Measurement is at the level of fetal liver.
   - Cross section of the fetus should be as round as possible.
   - Umbilical part of the left portal vein must be visualized. The vein should be short, not elongated and perpendicular to fetal spine.

Formula:
- AC = (Anteroposterior diameter + Transverse diameter) × π/2.
- It should only be used when there is no maternal condition which can modify fetal liver or spleen growth, i.e., diabetes, Rh isoimmunization, congenital viral infection.

Note: Estimation of fetal gestational age from multiple fetal measurements (i.e., BPD, HC, AC, FL) is more accurate than that obtained from single measurement alone.

Intrauterine Growth Retardation

Intrauterine growth retardation (IUGR) can be symmetrical or asymmetrical.

In asymmetrical variety fetal brain is spared so BPD is not altered. Multiple sonographic parameters, such as serial BPD, head circumference (HC), abdominal circumference (AC), HC/AC ratio, femur length (FL), FL/AC ratio, are used to diagnose and differentiate between two types of IUGR. Correct knowledge of gestational age is important for diagnosis of IUGR.

Two Important ratios for differential diagnosis of types of IUGR are HC/AC and FL/AC
1. *HC/AC ratio:* Normally pattern is:
   - HC > AC up to 32 weeks
   - HC = AC from 32 to 36 weeks
   - AC > HC after 36 weeks
   If HC is >AC after 32 weeks it suggests asymmetrical IUGR
2. *FL/AC ratio:* Normally it is 0.22 + 0.02
   - 0.24 suggests asymmetrical IUGR
   In symmetrical IUGR all parameters are reduced equally.

Doppler waveform studies: Absent end-diastolic flow in umbilical artery suggest fetal jeopardy and reversal of flow suggests fetus in imminent danger. Pulsatility index in middle cerebral artery (MCA) decreases as there is centralization of blood flow in initial stages of IUGR so as to maintain good circulation to brain. Pulsations in large veins, i.e., inferior vena cava and reverse flow in ductus venosus suggest severe fetal jeopardy and imminent death. Cerebroplacental ratio (CPR) is the ratio between MCA and umbilical artery PI or S/D ratio. A CPR below 1 is considered as abnormal. It has high sensitivity and specificity.

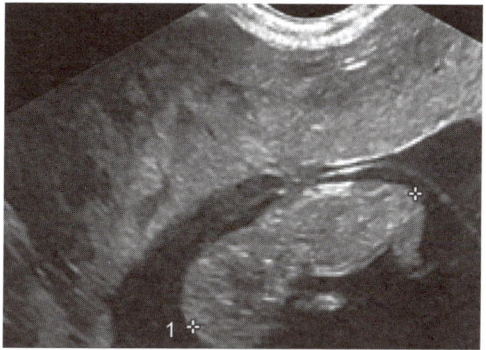

Fig. 13.5: Crown rump length (CRL).

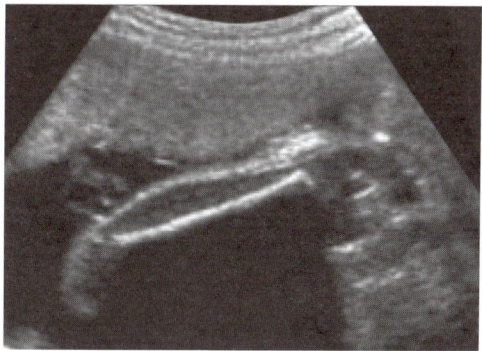

Fig. 13.6: Femur lenth (FL).

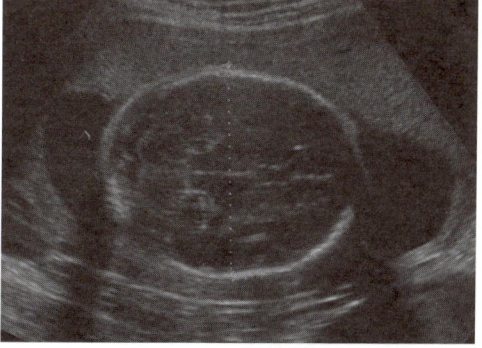

Fig. 13.7: Biparietal diameter (BPD).

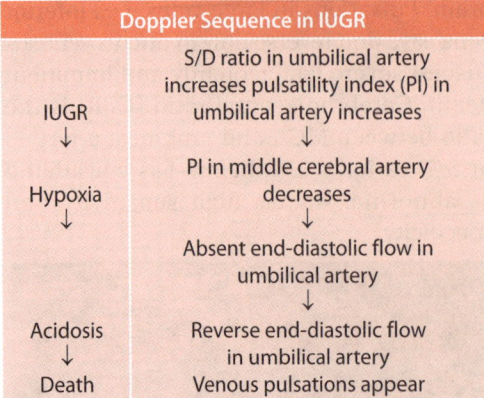

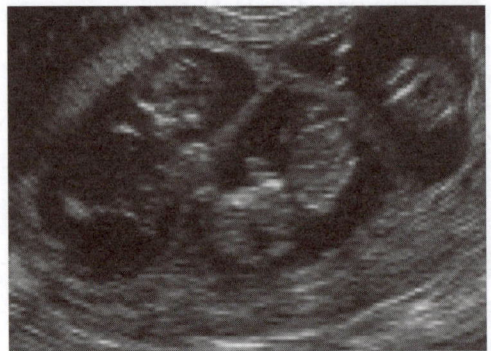

Fig. 13.8: Triplets—USG.

Other sonographic evidence of IUGR is presence of oligohydramnios or congenital anomaly.

Multiple Pregnancy

Earliest diagnosis can be made at 6th or 7th week of pregnancy by finding two gestational sacs in the uterus. Later on demonstration of two embryos and then fetuses confirms the diagnosis.

- Sonography is now crucial for management of twin pregnancy. Apart from diagnosis it helps in following: Fetal maturity
- Type of twins monochorionic or dichorionic
- Fetal presentation
- Fetal malformation
- Fetal growth
- Placental localization
- Hydramnios
- Intrauterine device (IUD) of one fetus
- Twin-twin transfusion syndrome (TTTS)

Fetal Malformations

Anencephaly can be diagnosed as early as 10–12 weeks. Hydrocephalus can be diagnosed as early as 16–18 weeks. Microcephaly can be diagnosed as early as 20–22 weeks. Many malformations are readily diagnosed by USG in antenatal period, e.g., limb reduction deformities, renal tract anomalies, congenital cardiac anomalies, fetal tumors, conjoined twins, fetal ascites, duodenal atresia, exomphalos, spina bifida, menigocele, encephalocele, etc.

Biophysical Profile Score

It is very useful for fetal well-being assessment in IUGR and high-risk pregnancy. It is discussed in Chapter 15.

Abnormality of Amniotic Fluid

Large cystic areas surrounding the fetus or blob-like echo complexes of the floating limbs suggest polyhydramnios. Vertical pockets of ≥8 cm or AFI >24 is diagnostic.

Oligohydramnios is diagnosed by amniotic fluid pockets of ≤2 cm length or AFI <5 cm. Amniotic fluid index (AFI) is the sum of largest vertical pockets of AF in each of the four quadrants.

Other Uses

- *IUFD:* Absence of fetal heart and fetal movements confirms the diagnosis.
- *Diagnosis of malpresentation:* Breech, shoulder.
- *Diagnosis of pregnancy with pelvic tumors:* Fibroid, ovarian tumor.
- *LSCS scar integrity:* It is discussed in Chapter 8.
- *Cervical incompetence:* It is discussed in Chapter 8.
- *Puerperium:* For diagnosing retained placental tissue—white echoes.

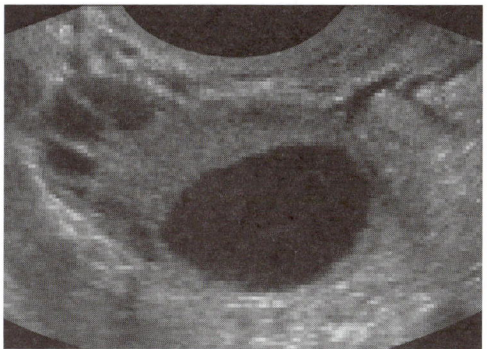

Fig. 13.9: Mature follicle.

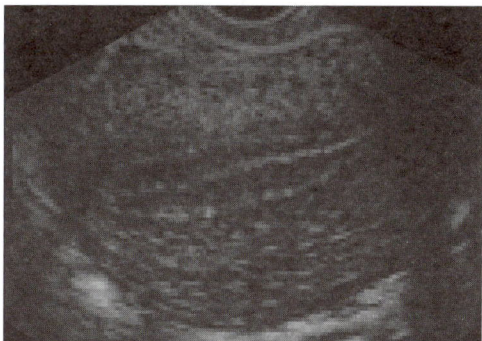

Fig. 13.10: Tripel line endometrium.

Gynec Uses

Infertility

It is useful as follows:
- Follicular study and detection of ovulation
- Timing of intrauterine insemination (IUI)
- To retrieve ovum for assisted reproductive techniques
- To study endometrial thickness
- Other condition related to infertility, i.e., polycystic ovary syndrome (PCOS), ovarian hyperstimulation syndrome (OHSS), congenital anomalies.
  Ovulation is sonographically characterized by any of the following features:
    - Partial or total collapse of the follicle
    - Development of internal filling in echoes, giving the follicle a more solid than cystic appearance
    - Appearance of or increase in free fluid in cul-de-sac.

Fibroid

- Well-defined **hypoechoic** areas
- Echogenicity depends upon type of degeneration and ratio of muscle tissue to connective tissue. More muscle tissue → Hypoechoic, calcification → Hyperechoic.
- It is usually echodense lesion with shadowing distal to fibroid.

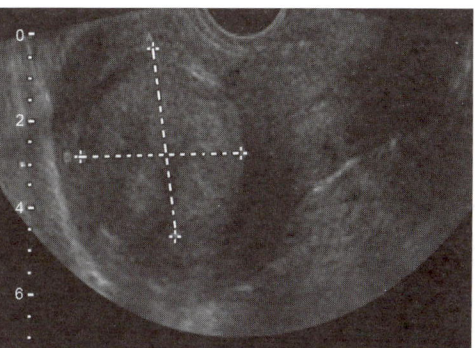

Fig. 13.11: Uterine fibroid.

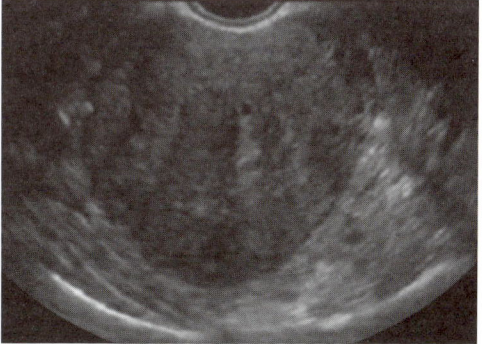

Fig. 13.12: Adenomyosis.

Adenomyosis

It is less echodense lesion as compared to fibroid and do not shadow. Disordered echogenicity, small cystic areas in inner myometrium, salt and pepper appearance, diffuse nature with more involvement of posterior wall are quite characteristic.

Physiological Cyst (Functional) of Ovary

- Anechoic
- Smooth walled
- Well defined
- Unilocular with strong posterior wall
- Acoustic enhancement

They are >3 cm in size and usually <6 cm. Corpus luteal cysts are larger than follicular cysts and thick walled.

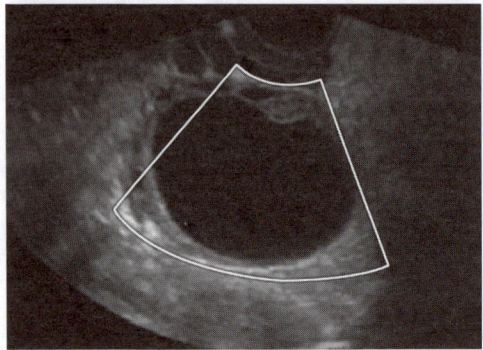

Fig. 13.13: Functional cyst of ovary.

Dermoid Cyst

A cystic mass containing a core of solid tissue with highly echogenic focus and posterior shadowing is a pathognomonic finding, although appearance depends upon the internal contents.

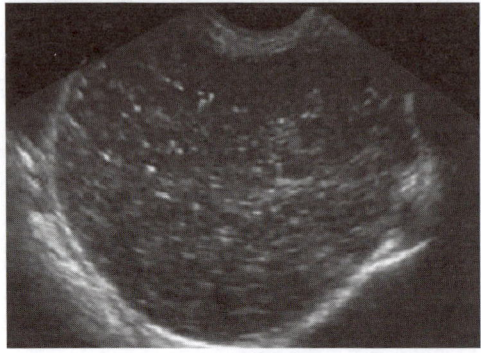

Fig. 13.14: Dermoid cyst.

Endometriosis (Ovary)

It can be anechoic or complex with evenly disbursed echoes, nodules due to clot or fluid debris levels. Ground glass appearance is characteristic. The walls are typically irregular and thickened.

Tubo-ovarian Mass

Complex hypoechoic adnexal mass with variable septations, irregular thick margins, scattered internal echoes and fluid debris levels. Ovarian tissue may be demonstrated incorporated within the abscess wall forming a rim of compressed tissue.

Ovarian Neoplasm

Wall thickness, tumor volume, septations, inner wall structure (papillae) are the various parameters used by different authors to device morphological scores to differentiate benign from malignant tumor (Depriest score, Sassone score et al.). More complex the tumor appears on sonography more the chances of malignancy.

Sonosalpingography

It is a procedure to detect tubal patency in cases of infertility. Isotonic saline is injected transcervically through No. 8 Foley's catheter and fluid collection in pouch of Douglas (POD) confirms patency of one or both tubes. This is done without anesthesia. It is safe, cost effective and more convenient to conventional methods. TVS probe can actually detect fluid movement from the outer end of the tubes, i.e., water fall sign (Sion test). In sonohysterosalpingography echogenic ultrasonic contrast media (Echovist) may be used.

Other Uses

Transvaginal sonography (TVS) is also useful in diagnosis of endometrial hyperplasia (≥5 mm in postmenopausal patient requires evaluation), polyp and displaced IUCD.

Invasive Procedures

Therapeutic uses: Various procedures which can be done under USG guidance are:
- Intraperitoneal or intravascular transfusion for Rh incompatibility
- Ventriculoamniotic shunt in hydrocephalus
- Vesicoamniotic shunt in obstructive uropathy
- Surgery for diaphragmatic hernia
- Amnioinfusion for oligohydramnios
- Fetal abdominal paracentesis, thoracocentesis

Diagnostic procedures:
- Amniocentesis
- Chorion biopsy
- Fetoscopy
- Fetal blood sampling (cordocentesis)
- Fetal skin or liver biopsy
- Fetal urine sampling in obstructive uropathy to know renal function.

X-RAYS

Gynecologic X-rays
- Various hysterosalpingograms (HSG)
- X-rays for displaced IUCD
- X-ray with radiopaque shadow in pelvis

HSG

Radiological procedure for visualization of uterus and fallopian tubes by injection of radiopaque dye.

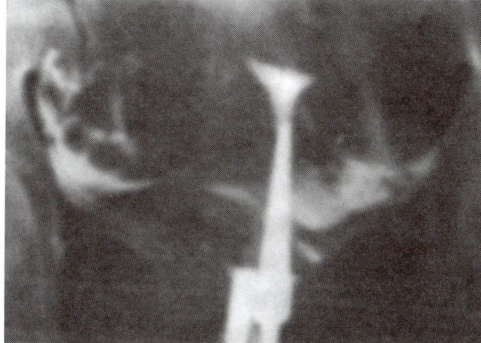

Fig. 13.15: Normal HSG showing bilateral free peritoneal spill.

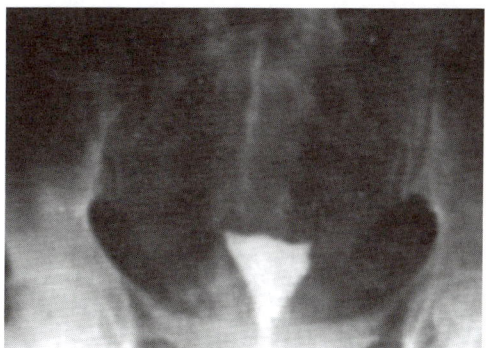

Fig. 13.16: HSG showing bilateral cornual block.

Indications:
- Evaluation of tubal factors in infertility: Complete or partial tubal block, site of block, hydrosalpinx, peritubal adhesions.
- Determination of size and shape of uterine cavity: Congenital malformations, hypoplastic uterus, fibroid, intrauterine synechiae.
- In follow-up evaluation tuboplasty and after metroplasty operations.
- Chronic pelvic tuberculosis: Features seen on HSG are small uterine cavity with irregular surface, intravasation of dye. Tubes—blocked, beaded, shortened or hydrosalpinx.
- Visualization of sinus tract communicating with female genital tract.

Due to increased use of ultrasonography (TVS) and endoscopy (laparoscopy and hysteroscopy), indications of HSG are decreasing.

Contraindications:
- Suspected intrauterine pregnancy
- Acute or subacute pediatric infectious disease (PID)
- Local infection
- Sensitivity to dye
- Abnormal uterine bleeding
- Recent curettage

Instruments:
- Cannula, 20 cc syringe, radiopaque dye and routine vaginal instruments.

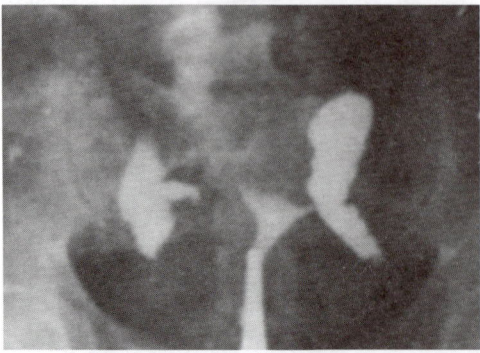

Fig. 13.17: HSG showing bilateral hydrosalpinx.

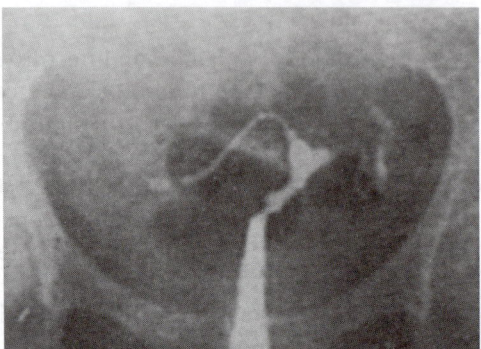

Fig. 13.18: HSG in case of genital tuberculosis. Note small irregular uterus, blocked tubes with beading.

- Dye may be oily, i.e., lipiodol or water soluble, i.e., urografin 60% or 76%, available as 20 mL ampoule. Nonionic dye, e.g., iopamiro is better but costly. Only water-soluble dye is used nowadays.
- Oily media can create adhesions, salpingitis, parametritis, granuloma and oil-retention cysts. So they are **not** used at present. They have value in cases of delayed tubal patency or in cases of tubal adhesions. Because of slow absorption they permit 24 hours follow-up study in such cases.

Procedure:
- Time: From 2 to 7 days after completion of normal menstrual period.
- Premedication: Injection atropine 0.6 mg 1/2 an hour before procedure. It reduces the tubal spasm and viscero-peritoneal shock is prevented.

Steps:
- Emptying of bladder
- Patient lies in dorsal position at the edge of the X-ray table.
- Patient should be fully covered and given as much privacy as possible so as to promote relaxation.
- No anesthesia is required.
- Aseptic and antiseptic measures.
- Expose the cervix, clean it and catch it with tinaculum.
- Sounding of the uterus
- Cannula is filled with radiopaque dye from the syringe attached to its proximal end.
- Cannula is introduced in the cervix and firmly pressed at external os. Tinaculum pulls the cervix to give tight fitting. Other instruments are removed.
- Patient shifted upwards with cannula in position, so that pelvis comes to lie over the X-ray source.
- When radiologist gives signal 5–10 mL of dye is slowly injected in the uterus and it is watched on the X-ray screen. Skiagram is taken when satisfactory visualization of uterus occurs. Second plate may be taken soon after within 10 minutes.
- Cannula is kept in place till wet plates are examined and found satisfactory.
- Total screening time must not exceed 45 seconds.
- Maximum 3 X-ray plates exposures are permitted.
- Patient is routinely given antibiotics and analgesics.

Complications:
Infection
Pelvic pain
Adhesions
Endometriosis
False positive → 4%
False negative → 15%

Ultrasonography and X-rays

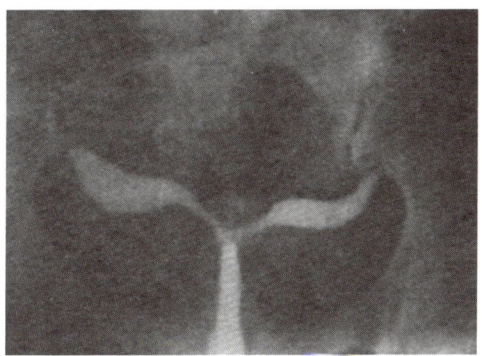

Fig. 13.19: HSG showing bicornuate uterus.

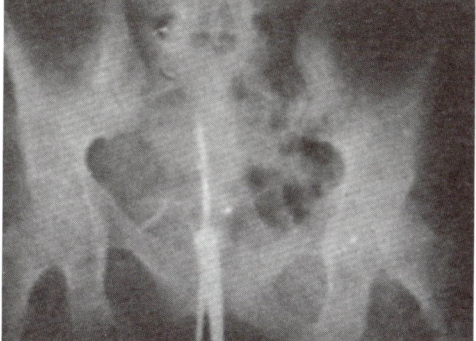

Fig. 13.20: X-ray with sounding of uterus showing displaced Cu-T.

Normal HSG Report:
X-ray PA view of lower abdomen and pelvis with special investigation of hysterosalpingography. Uterus is visualized by radiopaque dye, it is of normal size and shape. Both tubes are visualized and are without any abnormality and there is free peritoneal spill on both sides indicating that both tubes are patent.
- Normal size of uterine cavity is 5–6 cm length and 3–4 cm intercornual width, shape is triangular with side walls slightly concave.
- Normal tubes are seen as long, thin, wavy shadow passing from each cornu laterally.
- Free spill is seen as irregular multiple concave shadows due to small bowels coating.

- HSG has some therapeutic value also, because it removes some delicate adhesions and clears out inspissated mucus, pregnancy can follow HSG in some cases.
- If on HSG tubes appear blocked, it can be false in 15% of cases (false negative due to spasm or other reasons. It should be confirmed by other method (laparoscopy) before planning treatment.

X-rays for Intrauterine Contraceptive Device

They may be any of the following:
- Intrauterine contraceptive device (IUCD) seen in pelvis (may be intrauterine or extrauterine).
- IUCD seen outside the true pelvis (always extrauterine).
- Displaced IUCD checked by sounding.
- Displaced IUCD confirmed by AP and lateral views (rare at present).

Radiopaque Shadow in Pelvis

- Tooth of dermoid cysts
- Calcified fibroid
- Foreign body in uterus—IUCD
- Foreign body in vagina
- Calcified tuberculous lesion
- Lithopedion
- Fetal skeleton of early pregnancy
- Bladder stone
- Calcified lymph node
- Phlebolith

Obstetric X-rays

- As such obstetric X-rays for any indication has become the **investigation of past.** Hazards to the fetus attributable to radiation are those of: (1) malformation of the fetus and (2) childhood neoplasia (carcinoma and leukemia).
- Natural incidence of severe congenital defects is 1–3% (without exposure to any teratogens) while incidence of major

defects due to diagnostic radiation (up to 5 rads) is under 1 per 1,000 live births, i.e., negligible.
- Natural rate of leukemia and carcinoma in childhood is between 0.5 and 1 per 1,000 live births. A dose of >5 rads might increase the incidence 10 fold.
- Maximum danger to the fetus is in the first trimester of pregnancy.
- X-rays kept in examination: Breech, twins, intrauterine death, anencephaly, hydrocephalus, normal vertex for maturity, and rarely oblique/transverse lie, face presentation.

Normal Vertex Presentation (For Maturity)

With sonography freely available X-ray is not done for maturity anymore on X-ray maturity of the fetus was judged by detecting epiphyses.

Time of appearance of epiphyses:
- Lower end of femur—36 weeks
- Upper end of tibia—38 weeks
- Cuboid bone—40 weeks (but variable)

Variation in appearance of epiphyses:
- Twins, spina bifida, congenital hypothyroidism—delay in appearance.
- Anencephaly, diabetic mothers—early by 1–2 weeks (acceleration of bone development).

Common questions:
1. Questions about pre-maturity.
2. Questions about post-maturity.
3. Questions about normal labor.
4. Which are the clinical criteria to judge maturity?
5. How can you judge maturity by USG examination?
6. What are the hazards of X-ray during pregnancy?
7. What is intrapartum radiography? What is its advantage?

Breech

Plain X-ray AP view of the abdomen showing single fetus with breech presentation.

Following information can be gained from the X-ray:
- Confirmation of diagnosis
- The type of breech
- Fetal congenital anomalies
- Maturity of the fetus
- Size of fetal head and its hyperextension
- Pelvic capacity

Common questions:
1. What is the incidence of breech presentation?
2. What are the types of breech presentation?
3. Which type is the best for fetus?
4. What are the prerequisites, contraindications and complications of external cephalic version?
5. Why episiotomy is required in breech delivery? When it should be given?
6. What are the first stage (labor) complications in breech delivery?
7. What are the fetal complications in vaginal breech delivery?

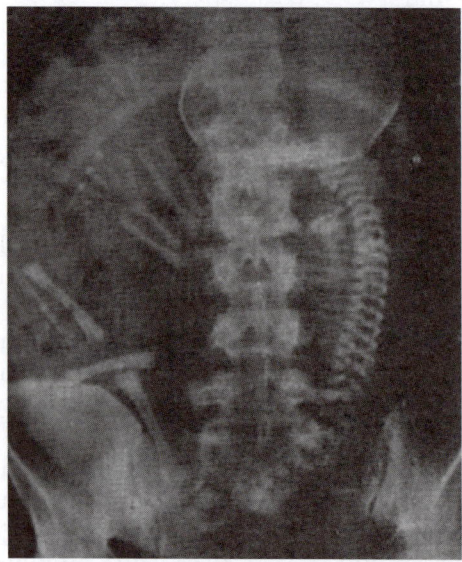

Fig. 13.21: Breech presentation (X-ray).

8. In what time the aftercoming head should be delivered? Why?
9. What are the different methods to deliver the aftercoming head? Which is the best method? Why?
10. How can you differentiate breech from face by p/v (per vaginal) examination?
11. What is breech extraction? What are its indications?
12. Which things are kept ready while conducting assisted breech delivery?
13. What are the indications for cesarean section in breech presentation?
14. What is Lovest's maneuver? How it is done?

Twins (or Triplets)

Plain X-ray abdomen showing 2 (or 3) fetuses (Describe the presentation of all).

Following information can be gained from the X-ray:
- Confirmation of diagnosis (rare possibility of triplets)
- Presentation of both fetuses
- Congenital anomalies
- Fetal maturity
- Intrauterine fetal demise (IUFD) of one fetus

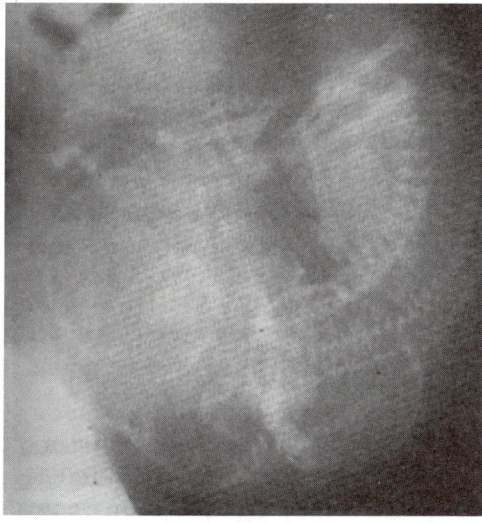

Fig. 13.22: Triplet (X-ray).

Common questions:
1. How can you diagnose twins clinically?
2. What are the common causes of undue enlargement of uterus?
3. What are the characteristics of monozygotic twins?
4. What are the antenatal complications of twin pregnancy?
5. What are the intranatal complications?
6. What are the causes of postpartum hemorrhage (PPH) in twins?
7. Why there should be active management for second fetus?
8. What is the only indication of internal podalic version in modern obstetrics?
9. How will you conduct twin delivery?
10. In which conditions cord is clamped immediately?
11. Indications of lower segment cesarean section (LSCS) in twins.
12. What is Hellin's law for multiple pregnancy?
13. What is superfecundation? What is superfetation?
14. What is fetus compressus? Fetus papyraceus?
15. What is Siamese twins? Why are they so named?
16. What is twin transfusion syndrome? What is Quintero's five stages of twin-to-twin transfusion syndrome (TTTS)?
17. What do you mean by vanishing twin?
18. What is embryo reduction? Why it is done in multiple pregnancy?

Intrauterine Fetal Death

With USG facility available, X-ray for diagnosis of intrauterine fetal death (IUFD) is **not done** now.

Radiological signs of IUFD:
- **Spalding sign:** Overriding of cranial bones at suture lines in absence of active labor. It develops 4 days after the death. It is due to negative intracranial pressure produced by shrinkage of brain due to its autolysis after fetal death.

- Hyperflexion of the fetal spine **(Ball sign)**: Due to softening of supporting ligaments after death fetal vertebral column collapses under gravity effect after few days.
- **Robert's sign**: Gas shadow in fetal heart and large blood vessels (aorta, vena cava). It occurs within 12 hours. It is due to liberation of bound gases (O_2, CO_2) from red blood cell (RBC) during their disintegration.
- **Duel's Halo sign**: Frequently present. It is due to elevation of pericranial fat by underlying soft tissue edema. In case of severe degree hydrops fetalis it is present even in living fetus.
- Constancy of fetal position: Two X-rays taken at an interval. There is no change in position or attitude.

Common questions:
1. What are the fetal causes of IUFD?
2. How can you clinically diagnose a case of IUFD?
3. What is rare but dangerous complication in a case of IUFD?
4. What are intrapartum complications in cases of IUFD?
5. How will you confirm the diagnosis of IUFD?
6. How will you induce the labor in IUFD?
7. How will you investigate a case of IUFD in reference to future obstetric carrier of your patient?

Anencephaly

It is one of the major congenital malformations of fetus grouped under the neural tube defects. There is partial or complete absence of vault of skull with cerebral hemispheres absent or rudimentary.

Incidence: 1–2 per 1,000 births. It is more common in white people than blacks or orientals. There is recurrence risk of 5% (1 in 20) in the same couple. With history of previous 2 children malformed risk increases to 1 in 8 next pregnancy.

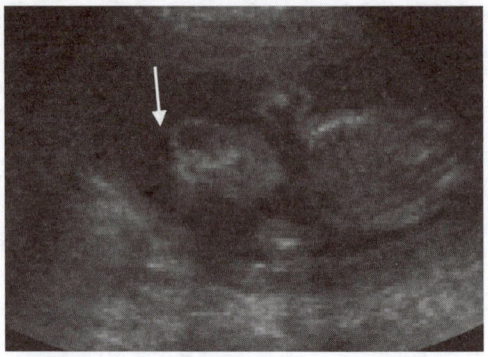

Fig. 13.23: Anencephaly (USG—froghead appearance).

Etiology: Exact etiology is not known. Genetic and environmental factors are probably responsible. No specific gene is identified. But ethnic variation, high recurrence rate in the same couple and increased risk in first degree relatives suggest that there is polygenic predisposition (multifactorial disorder). Geographical and seasonal variation is commonly found suggesting environmental factors also responsible.

Folic acid deficiency: Valproic acid, maternal hyperthermia in early pregnancy and insulin-dependent diabetes can cause this defect.

Fetus: Many fetuses are still born and eventhough born alive they cannot survive for more than few hours. More than 2/3rd babies are female. Apart from cervical defect other features are prominent eyes, protruding tongue and very short neck gives the fetus a peculiar **frog-head** appearance. Fetal pituitary is either absent or rudimentary. Adrenals are also hypoplastic with absent fetal cortex. Weight of adrenal is less than 1 g (normal is about 5 g). Fetal shoulders may be bigger than normal.

Clinical features: It is more common in first babies and babies of very young or old mothers. Hydramnios is found in 70–90% of cases. Causes of hydramnios in anencephaly include: (1) Swallowing defect (anatomical, i.e., esophageal anomalies or duodenal atresia may be present in these babies or physiological, i.e., swallowing reflex is absent because higher centers are not developed; (2) Transudation of fluid from open meninges or neural tissue; (3) Lack or ADH (posterior pituitary absent), and (4) Lack of aldosterone leading to excessive urine formation.

Gross hydramnios may give rise to pressure symptoms and there is tendency for preterm labor. Cases without hydramnios may go for postmaturity. Face and breech presentations are common.

Diagnosis:
- *Clinical:* Positive past or family history, gross hydramnios, small head or difficulty in palpation of fetal head per abdomen and per vaginal examination in labor are helpful but definite diagnosis is either by X-ray or sonography.
- *USG:* It can be diagnosed as early as 11–12 weeks by TVS. The head instead of being seen as a well-defined circular structure presents as an amorphous mass. At later gestational age USG easily diagnoses anencephaly by absence of vault of skull leading to incomplete head outline and inability to get BPD. Incordinated jerky limb movements (due to severely defective CNS) may help in diagnosis.
- *X-ray:* There is absence of vault of skull with irregular bony shadows (of sphenoid bones). There may be foggy appearance due to excessive liquor. With USG available this is **not done** now.
- *Alpha fetrofrotein (AFP):* It is estimated in amniotic fluid (AF) or maternal serum. This fetal protein is in high concentration in fetal serum. Normally, it comes in amniotic fluid from fetal kidney through urine. In AF it has peak values at 10–14 weeks and gradually decreases steadily thenafter up to term. From AF it diffuses across the fetal membranes (some amount transported across the placenta) to reach maternal serum (MS). The level in MS in contrast to AF increases steadily throughout pregnancy up to 32 weeks.

In anencephaly more AFP diffuses from fetal serum or CSF into the amniotic fluid through the open defect. So more amount also reaches the maternal serum. Thus abnormal high level of AFP in AF or MS for the corresponding gestational age is helpful for diagnosis. But AFP may increase in many other conditions, so it is nonspecific. High level of AFP + acetylcholine esterase in AF always indicate open neural tube defect.

- *Urinary estriol:* Low level of urinary estriol <10 mg/24 hours urine (because there is no precursor of estrogen from fetal adrenal which is hypoplastic).

Management

If diagnosed before 20 weeks, MTP is done. After 20 weeks induction of labor is the treatment. Prostaglandins, i.e., dinoprostone gel for cervical ripening and induction of labor followed by oxytocin drip is commonly used. As compared to other cases in anencephaly response to induction is less. Nowadays misoprostol 25–100 µg tablet depending upon the gestational age is inserted vaginally every 3–4 hourly for induction. Low ARM is never done as it may lead to abruptio placentae. Tablet mifepristone given 24–48 hours prior to induction increases success rate. Slow abdominal amniocentesis and removal of 1–3 liters of amniotic fluid as the case may be, helps in induction.

- **Open neural tube defects:** These include anencephaly, inencephaly, spina bifida (occult and open), encephalocele, meningocele, meningomyelocele.
- **Increased levels of alpha fetoprotein:** In amniotic fluid are found in neural tube defects, congenital nephrosis, esophageal anomalies, ventral wall defects and other fetal malformations, multiple pregnancy,

oligohydramnios, placental anomalies, fetomaternal haemorrhage, etc.
- **Breech presentation**: It is advantageous than cephalic presentation because progress of labor is better and arrest of shoulders, i.e., shoulder dystocia does not occur.
- **Shoulder dystocia:** It may be due to big shoulders or incomplete dilatation of cervix. As there is no fetal concern one can wait and watch initially, oxytocin drip is continued and even after full dilatation if delivery does not occur or if there is maternal distress cleidotomy may be done.

Hydrocephalus

In this malformation of head there is abnormal enlargement of cranium due to excessive accumulation of cerebrospinal fluid (CSF) in the ventricles. Hydrocephalus can be: (1) Non-communicating or internal obstruction to fluid flow within the ventricular system or at its outlets, and (2) Communicating or external type where there is free escape of fluid from the ventricular system but obstruction is sited more peripherally or absorption is impaired.

Its incidence is 1 in 2,000 deliveries. There is 2-5% chance of recurrence in the same patient. Various **etiological factors** for congenital hydrocephalus include:
- Atresia of foramina of Luschka and Magendie (Dandy–Walker syndrome).
- Atresia or stenosis of aqueduct of Sylvius (recessive sex-linked or autosomal recessive gene inheritance).
- Obstruction to subarachnoid pathway (Arnold–Chiari syndrome).
- Congenital aneurysm of vein of Galen.
- Congenital platybasia, achondroplasia— causing obstruction by causing deformity of the base of the skull.
- Congenital cysts in the region of midbrain.
- Toxoplasmosis, cytomegalovirus, mumps and congenital syphilis causing ependymitis and aqueductal stenosis.

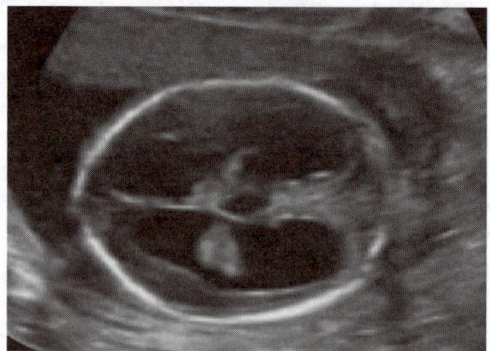

Fig. 13.24: Hydrocephalus (USG—lemon sign).

Lie is logitudinal but more than 1/3rd cases have breech presentation. There may be associated other congenital malformation, such as spina bifida in 1/3rd cases. In untreated cases fetal prognosis is very poor. It may be still born or dies early in neonatal period or if survived, they are mentally defective. Maternal prognosis is only affected when it remains undiagnosed even in labor. Gross cephalopelvic disproportion and severe dystocia is the rule.

Diagnosis
- **Clinical:** On per abdominal examination there is cephalic or breech presentation. In cephalic presentation head is high, large, not hard and cannot be pushed in. Lower segment is stretched and vertically head may be felt up to umbilicus. There is obvious disproportion between the size of the head and the size of rest of the fetus. Fetal heart sound (FHS) are heard at higher level.
    - On per vaginal examination particularly during labor wide sutures and large fontanelles are felt. It has been described as "Island of bones in a sea of membranes". Cranial bones are soft indentable or there is crackling sensation on pressure.
- **Ultrasonography:** USG has a major role in the management of hydrocephalus now. Large echo-free head with dangling of choroid plexus on USG is very peculiar.

- Atria of lateral ventricle >10 mm confirms ventriculomegaly.
- Separation of choroid plexus from the wall of lateral ventricle of >3 mm is abnormal.
- In communicating hydrocephalus there is overlapping of frontal bones **(lemon sign)** and downward displacement of cerebellum **(banana sign).**
- Marked difference between the size of thorax/abdomen and the head.
- Apart from diagnosing hydrocephalus USG also helps in assessing associated other congenital defects, exact cortical thickness for prognosis and exact site of obstruction in the ventricular system. USG is also helpful for the antepartum treatment of hydrocephalus, i.e., in selected cases intrauterine ventriculoamniotic shunt may be done under USG guidance.

- **X-ray:** Radiological features are:
  - Disproportion between the large size of cranium and normal facial bones (face shadow small)
  - Cranial vault is poorly calcified and may even be difficult to see, with widening of the sutures
  - Cranial shadow is globular (normal head is ovoid)
  - There may be small rarefied areas in the skull bones—craniolacunae
  - If there is associated spina bifida of severe degree it can be identified by: (a) Pedicles are widely separated at the defect and (b) There is often a local kyphosis.

With USG available X-ray is not done in present times.

Management

A. **Antenatal:** Antenatal management depends upon maturity of the fetus, cortical thickness on sonography and associated other defects.
  - If associated defects, such as spina bifida is present or cortical thickness is less than 1 cm then fetal prognosis is extremely poor. In such case pregnancy is terminated by induction of labor. Proper documental evidence and consent of the patient and relatives is must to avoid medicolegal problem.
  - If there is no other defect and cortical thickness is more than 1 cm then management depends upon fetal maturity. If on serial USG hydrocephalus is increasing and baby is more than 34 weeks it should be delivered by cesarean section and neonatal shunt (e.g. ventriculo- jugular) is carried out to relieve the compression. This is practised where good neonatal facilities are available.
  - If fetus is very premature and hydrocephalus is progressive on USG, to relieve compression on the remaining brain tissue intrauterine shunt can be carried out. Ventriculoamniotic shunt with one-way valve can be done under USG guidance.

  The results have shown that extrauterine shunts (i.e., after birth) are better than intrauterine shunts.

B. **In labor:** Labor may be spontaneous or induced or hydrocephalus may be first time diagnosed in labor. Whatever is the case, important thing is decompression of the head. In cephalic presentation labor may be induced by slow guarded oxytocin drip and when the cervix is about 3 cm dilated membranes are ruptured and head is punctured from vaginal route by a wide bore (16–17 gauze) long needle through the gapping sutures or wide open fontanelles, under guidance of 2 fingers in the vagina.
  - 500–1,500 mL fluid is the usual amount, but can be more. Once the head is decompressed there is no much problem in delivery, but if it is delayed, a vulsellum or long Allis may be applied to the head for traction.

- Alternatively head may be decompressed by PA route, suprapubically after emptying the bladder. Blood stained thick fluid with tissue flakes coming out and decreased flow of fluid indicates the end of procedure.
- In breech the delivery is allowed up to the head then the after coming head can be decompressed by any of the following ways: (a) spinal needle through suprapubic route and (b) metal catheter through the spinal defect (if present) or after doing laminectomy.
- In breech presentation head can also be decompressed before delivery while it is lying at fundus, under USG guidance.
- In whatever way, the delivery is accomplished, the uterus must be explored to rule out rupture uterus.
- In cephalic presentation rupture of uterus may occur in first stage of labor if labor is allowed to progress and if one waits till second stage of labor for decompression. In fact cervix may never get fully dilated.

CHAPTER 14

Specimens

Following Specimens are usually asked in following:

OBSTETRIC TABLE

- Anencephaly
- Hydrocephalus
- Twin fetuses
- Placenta of twin pregnancy
- Hydatidiform mole (vesicular mole)
- Ectopic pregnancy
- Rupture uterus
- Normal placenta
- Abortus fetus or complete abortion
- Placenta with retroplacental clot (abruptio placentae).

GYNECOLOGICAL TABLE

- Fibroid—single or multiple, subserous, submucous or intramural sessile or pedunculated (myomatous polyp), cervical fibroid.
- Adenomyosis.
- Ovarian tumors—simple serous cyst, dermoid cyst, pseudomucinous cysts, solid ovarian tumor.
- Cervical elongation (for prolapse)
- Carcinoma cervix—cauliflower or ulcerative growth
- Carcinoma body uterus
- Hydrosalpinx, pyosalpinx
- Intrauterine contraceptive device (**IUCD**) perforating the uterus.

On viva table the student is first asked to identify the specimen. He or she should examine the specimen from all sides and then start describing it to reach the diagnosis. Many times the diagnosis is asked straightaway and relevant questions are asked.

In any specimen following three questions are commonly asked:

1. **How will the patient with this disease come to you?**
   (Complaints—symptoms related to that particular specimen only).
2. **How will you diagnose such a case?**
   (Symptoms, signs and investigations related to that particular specimen only).
3. **How will you manage such a case?**
   (Confirmation of diagnosis, treatment and follow-up).

In some of the specimens one more question commonly asked is whether the specimen is **antemortem or postmortem**? It is judged from following points:

a. The risk of death in that disease, whether it is increased or death is uncommon.
b. The structures removed as seen in specimen whether adequate, inadequate or more than required.
c. The normal line of treatment of that disease, whether it is surgical or conservative.

OBSTETRIC TABLE

Anencephaly
Discussed fully in previous chapter.

Hydrocephalus
Discussed fully in previous chapter.

Twin Foetuses or Placenta of Twin Pregnancy

Description
Specimen consists of 2 fetuses of approximate 6–8 months gestation (as per the specimen). Appearance of both fetuses is described, i.e., any malformation if seen is narrated.

Placenta: Specimen consists of single large placenta (monochorionic or dischrionic but fused placenta) or 2 separate placentas. On fetal surface membranes and cut umbilical cords are seen. If both placentas are separate it is diamniotic dichorionic twin pregnancy.

1. **How will the patient with twin pregnancy come to you?**
   Patient may have family history of twin pregnancy or she has taken treatment for infertility. Patient will have undue enlargement of abdomen, exaggerated all symptoms of pregnancy and excessive weight gain. Some patients will have anemia and hypertension.

2. **How will you diagnose twin pregnancy?**
   Earliest diagnosis is by **ultrasonography** (**USG**). Transvaginalsonography (TVS) not only diagnose twin pregnancy but also helps in finding out type of twin pregnancy. Later on clinical examination helps, i.e., edema legs, undue enlargement, multiple fetal parts palpable, 3 poles palpable, auscultation of 2 fetal heart sounds simultaneously with difference of 10 heart beats per minute.

3. **How will you manage twin pregnancy?**
   Since it is high-risk pregnancy more antenatal visits are advised. Proper diet and bedrest are ensured. Growth monitoring of both fetuses is done by frequent USG examinations. Prophylactic cervical cerclage has no role. Steroids administration at 30–32 weeks is done as there are increased chances of preterm delivery.

   If first fetus is presenting by vertex vaginal delivery can be done otherwise elective cesarean section (CS) after 37 completed weeks is done. One should be careful to prevent and treat **postpartum hemorrhage** (PPH) if it occurs.

Hydatidiform Mole

Description
Specimen consists of uterus filled with small **grape-like** grayish black vesicles. Some necrotic tissue or hemorrhagic collection may also be seen in uterus. In partial mole fetus may be seen but in complete mole fetus is absent.

1. **How will the patient of hydatidiform mole present?**
   Patient will have amenorrhea, **hyperemesis gravidarum**, vaginal bleeding, and sometimes pain. There may be history of (h/o) passage of grape—like vesicles in bleeding. Patient appears sick and few patients can have symptoms of hypertension and rarely **thyrotoxicosis**. Patient may have past history/of hydatidiform mole. Patient may be from high-risk ethnic group or from geographic region with high incidence, i.e., oriental countries.

2. **How will you diagnose hydatidiform mole?**
   It is diagnosed by clinical features, ultrasonography and quantitative serum beta-hCG estimation.
   On per abdomen (P/A) examination uterus is large for gestational age, consistency is doughy, and fetal features are absent, i.e., no fetal parts palpable, no fetal movements felt, no fetal heart sounds heard. USG by TVS/TAS shows uterus filled with small cystic areas, i.e., typical show strom appearance and embryo or fetus is not

seen. There may be theca leutein cysts in the ovaries in 1/3rd cases. So beta-hCG is in high titer compared to gestational age.

3. **How will you manage this case?**

   Suction evacuation under anesthesia with oxytocin drip and keeping blood ready is done. Cervix may be primed with Dinoprostone gel. Check curettage after 1 week is done if required. What is important is proper follow-up to detect development of **choriocarcinoma**. In follow-up clinical examination, So, beta-hCG estimation and transvaginal sonography are done.

1. How do you classify gestational trophoblastic disease?
2. What is the difference between partial mole and complete mole? Which is more dangerous? Why?
3. What is the chromosomal basis for the development of mole?
4. What is the pathogenesis of hydatidiform mole?
5. What is the highest incidence of hydatidiform mole? Where is it?
6. What are the changes in ovary in cases of trophoblastic disease? What is its treatment?
7. What are the causes of pain in case of mole?
8. What is the consistency of uterus in case of mole? Why it is so?
9. How will you treat a case of perforating mole?
10. What are the complications of vesicular mole?
11. Which are the risk factors for the development of choriocarcinoma?
12. What contraception is advised to the patient after **evacuation** of mole? For how much time?
13. How will you evaluate the patient completely on follow-up?
14. What is the role of prophylactic chemotherapy? How will you treat toxicity of methotrexate?
15. When beta-hCG level comes to normal after evacuation of benign complete mole?
16. What are the chemotherapy regimes for choriocarcinoma?

Ectopic Pregnancy

Description

Specimen consists of tube which is enlarged and thickened bluish in color. Rupture site of the tube may be visible with clots inside. Embryo or tiny fetus may be mounted alongside the tube in the specimen.

1. **How the patient with ectopic pregnancy will present?**

   Patient has amenorrhea, lower abdominal pain and little bleeding per vagina. History of fainting attack if present is pathognomonic. Ruptured ectopic pregnancy presents with features of shock and severe internal hemorrhage, i.e., rapid thready pulse, hypotension. perspiration and cold clammy skin.

2. **How will you diagnose ectopic pregnancy?**

   In patients of reproductive age group presenting with amenorrhea and pain in abdomen. Ectopic pregnancy should always be suspected. In ruptured ectopic care patient is pale and there is distension of lower abdomen and tenderness. In unruptured ectopic pervaginal (P/V) examination may be helpful which shows slightly enlarged uterus with tenderness and fullness in fornix. Cervical movement tenderness is peculiar. Ectopic pregnancy is diagnosed by TVS examination coupled with urine pregnancy test. Empty uterus with adnexal mass and free fluid in pelvis help in diagnosis. In case of doubt serial beta-hCG estimation is done. Beta-hCG doubles even 2 and 1/2 days in normal pregnancy but not in ectopic. Single beta-hCG estimation value of 1500 **mIU** /mL with no gestational sac in uterus on TVS confirms the diagnosis.

3. **How will you treat a case of old unruptured ectopic?**

   In small unruptured ectopic pregnancy (<8 weeks gestation) in a stable patient with beta-hCG <10,000 mIU/mL medical management is done, i.e., injection methotrexate 1 mg/kg body weight is given I/M. Beta-hCG is repeated on day 4 and if value decrease by 15% or more the treatment is effective. Otherwise in all cases of unruptured ectopic pregnancy **laparoscopic salpingostomy** is gold standard treatment. In ruptured ectopic with severe internal **hemorrhage**, resuscitation of the patient immediately followed by **laparotomy** and unilateral salpingectomy is done.

1. Why the incidence of ectopic pregnancy is increased at present?
2. How PID leads to ectopic pregnancy?
3. Why ampullary tubal pregnancy is the most common?
4. What is the difference between cornual pregnancy, angular pregnancy and interstitial pregnancy?
5. What are the causes of bleeding per vaginam in first trimester?
6. What are the characteristics of bleeding PV in ectopic pregnancy?
7. What are the causes of pain in ectopic pregnancy? What is the reason for fainting attack?
8. Why the tube ruptures in tubal ectopic pregnancy? What are the usual times of rupture in different types of tubal ectopic pregnancy?
9. What is the role of colpopuncture in diagnosing ectopic pregnancy?
10. Why the blood in ruptured ectopic does not clot?
11. What is Cullen's sign? What is Arias–Stella reaction?
12. What is the medical management of ectopic pregnancy?
13. What is the role of conservative surgery in the treatment of ectopic pregnancy?
14. Will you do total salpingectomy or salpingo-oophorectomy?
15. In which type of ectopic pregnancy hysterectomy is indicated?
16. What is autotransfusion? How it is given?? What are its risks?
17. What is the risk of isoimmunization in Rh-negative mother having ectopic?
18. What advice will you give to the patient of ectopic pregnancy on discharge?
19. What are **Spiegelberg** criteria for ovarian ectopic pregnancy? What are **Studdiford's** criteria for primary abdominal pregnancy?
20. What are Rubin's criteria for cervical ectopic?

Rupture Uterus

Description

Specimen consists of enlarged postpartum uterus (approximate 18–20 weeks pregnant uterus size). There is rent in lower segment (previous LSCS scar) or irregular tear in lateral wall (rupture after obstruction or manipulation). The edges of tear are necrotic and black in color, There may be broad ligament hematoma (bluish black mass) present. Usually **adnexa** and cervix are not seen as it is subtotal hysterectomy.

1. **How the patient will present to you?**
   Patient is having history of previous LSCS and this time trial of labor (TOLAC) might have been tried with no success or patient has not reached the institute after labor has started. In case of rupture due to obstructed labor patient might present with history of prolonged labor or some manipulations done. The pains might have subsided and there are features of shock. There is abdominal tenderness, irregular contour of uterus and fetus may be easily palpable and dead. On PV examination there may be **malpresentation** of loss of presenting part and bleeding.

2. **How will you diagnose this condition?**
   Rupture uterus is diagnosed from history and clinical features and if there is doubt USG abdomen may be carried out.

3. **How will you manage such a case?**
   Resuscitation of the patient with emergency **laparotomy** is carried out. On laparotomy there are three options:

a. Obstetric hysterectomy (usually subtotal) if childbearing is completed and/or uterus is severely damaged and patient is in shock.
b. Freshening of the necrotic margins and repair of the tear is done in previous CS scar rupture.
c. If patient is not severely ill freshening of the margins with tubal ligation is carried out if child-bearing is complete.

1. Why rupture uterus is more common in multipara?
2. Which are the most common causes of rupture uterus at present?
3. What is the difference between scar dehiscence and incomplete rupture?
4. What do you mean by triple rupture?
5. What are the signs of obstructed labor?
6. What is silent rupture of uterus? When does it occur? How can you diagnose it?
7. What do you mean by threatened rupture of uterus? How will you treat it?
8. Which are the iatrogenic causes of rupture? How will you prevent them?
9. How will you resuscitate the patient with rupture uterus?
10. How will you manage a patient with rupture uterus in subsequent pregnancy?
11. Which are the different risk factors in case of previous cesarean section for scar to rupture in next pregnancy?
12. What are the options for treatment in a case of rupture uterus at laparotomy?

Abortus Fetus

Description

Specimen consists of small fetus which may be normal looking with part of umbilical cord or umbilical cord with complete placenta. The approximate length of the fetus is ___ cm so gestational age is ___ months (Haase **rule** is up to 5 months total length of the fetus in cm = square of months, e.g., 9 cm = 3 months, 16 cm = 4 months. After 5 months length will be months of gestation × 5.)

1. **How the patient will present?**
Patient will present with amenorrhea followed by pain in abdomen and bleeding p/v which has resulted in spontaneous abortion. Or it may be the case or MTP (up to 20 weeks) for any legally valid indication and fetus is preserved and mounted for academic purpose.
2. **How will you diagnose abortion?**
Abortion is diagnosed by history and clinical features, i.e, per speculum(PS) and per vaginum (PV) examinations. USG features of different degrees of spontaneous abortion are described in Chapter 13.
3. **How will you manage abortion?**
In threatened abortion conservative treatment is given, i.e., reassurance, rest and progesterone support. In inevitable abortion process is accelerated by oxytocin drip and suction evacuation is done if <12 weeks. In incomplete abortion suction **evacuation**/check curettage is done with antibiotic cover. In complete abortion only prophylactic antibiotics are indicated.

1. Define abortion.
2. What are the causes of first trimester abortion?
3. What are the causes of second trimester abortion?
4. What is the difference in process of abortion in first trimester and second trimester?
5. What are the complications of spontaneous abortion?
6. How will you differentiate between threatened abortion, inevitable abortion and incomplete abortion?
7. What is missed abortion? How will you manage it?
8. How will you manage a case of septic abortion?
9. What do you mean by habitual abortion? What are the uterine causes of it?
10. How will you investigate a case of recurrent abortions?
11. What is the role of USG in case of abortion?
12. What is the effect of abortion on patient's future obstetric carrier?

Placenta with Retroplacental Clot

Description

Specimen consists of placenta with depression on the maternal surface having bluish black clot. So it is specimen of placental abruption.

1. **How the patient will present?**
   Patient may have history of hypertension or some manipulation done. Patient complains of pain in abdomen which is continuous in between uterine contractions. Uterus is tender and tense on palpation not relaxing well in between contractions. There may be fetal distress and death. Except in pure concealed hemorrhage there is bleeding PV and if membranes are ruptured liquor is blood stained.

2. **How will you diagnose placental abruption?**
   It is a case of antepartum hemorrhage and while in placenta previa there is painless, causeless recurrent bleeding, in this case there is painful bleeding and usually some cause for abruption. Abruption is diagnosed clinically. USG features are diagnostic only in 1/4th cases of abruption (USG features are described under Chapter 13). Abruption is confirmed at delivery or at cesarean section.

3. **How will you manage such a case?**
   Once abruption is diagnosed the plan of treatment is to **expedited** delivery. If cervix is favorable induction of labor is done. If cervix is already dilated (patient in labor) augmentation is carried out. It is done by artificial rupture of membranes (**ARM**) and oxytocin drip. If delivery appears to be delayed cesarean section should be carried out for maternal interest even if the fetus is dead or very premature. Dangerous complications of **acute renal failure** (ARF) and **disseminated intravascular coagulation** (**DIC**) occur if abruption delivery interval is prolonged. **Packed cell volume (PCV) and fresh frozen plasmas** (**FFPs**) are transfused as necessary.

1. Why is accidental hemorrrhage a misnomer?
2. What is Page's classification for abruptio placentae?
3. What is etiology of abruptio placentae?
4. What are the indications for cesarean section in abruptio placentae?
5. What is the difference in bleeding of placenta previa and revealed accidental hemorrhage?
6. What are the fetal complications of abruptio placentae?
7. Which are the two dangerous maternal complications of abruptio placentae?
8. Which are the obstetric causes of pain in abdomen in late pregnancy?
9. How will you manage a case of mixed accidental hemorrhage?
10. What is **couvelaire uterus**? What is its treatment?
11. What do you mean by indeterminate APH?

GYNECOLOGICAL TABLE

Fibroid

Description

Specimen consists of uterus with cervix. Uterus is enlarged, nodular and approximately $A \times B \times C$ cm in size. There is well-circumscribed mass at _____ of about $M \times N$ cm in size cut surface.

1. **How will the patient with this disease present to you?**
   Patient may have family history of fibroid. She is mostly from reproductive age group. She may be asymptomatic. Her symptoms will be menstrual (menorrhagia, metrorrhagia, polymenorrhea), dysmenorrhea (congestive or spasmodic), lump in abdomen (in big fibroid), pressure symptoms, infertility and recurrent pregnancy loss (This symptom may not be in patient having this pathology as uterus is not removed in infertile or recurrent pregnancy patient).

2. How will you diagnose such a case?

By clinical features (symptoms and signs) fibroid is suspected and then confirmed by USG. On PA and PV examination fibroid uterus is felt as firm, nodular, nontender and transmitted movements are present. On USG (TAS + TVS) fibroid usually appears as hypoechoic (black) well defined lesion on USG. In old fibroids with calcification echogenic sports are seen. MRI is superior to fibroid but costly. Fibroids produces low or medium signal intensity (SI) as compared to adjacent myometrium. Small sized fibroids are better detected by MRI, differentiation from adenomyosis and adnexal pathology is better.

3. How will you manage such a case?

The definitive treatment of fibroid is surgical. Myomectomy by different ways is done if infertility is the complaint or at least uterus is to be preserved. If child-bearing is completed age is >35 years hysterectomy by different ways is done. If age is >50 years **panhysterectomy** is day.

Conservative: Small asymptomatic fibroid may not require any treatment. Follow-up every 6 months till menopause is done as >99% fibroids are benign.

Medical treatment: Progesterones, GnRh **analogue**, **ulipristal**, mifepristone. They all have temporary effects.

Uterine artery embolization, magnetic resonance guided focused ultrasound (MRgFUS), high-intensity focused ultrasound (**HIFU**) and mirena insertion are other minimally invasive treatment

1. What is the etiology of fibroid?
2. What do you mean by the capsule of fibroid? Are all types of fibroid capsulated?
3. Describe the cut section appearance of fibroid.
4. How can you diagnose fibroid on sonography?
5. What are the causes of menorrhagia in fibroid?
6. What are the causes of pain in case of fibroid?
7. Which are the secondary changes in fibroid?
8. What is the risk of malignancy in fibroid? How can you diagnose it?
9. What is red degeneration? How will you manage it?
10. What are the effects of fibroid on pregnancy?
11. What are the effects of pregnancy on fibroid?
12. How will you manage a case of fibroid with pregnancy?
13. What is medical management of fibroid?
14. What do you know about uterine artery embolization for the treatment of fibroid?
15. What are the indications of myomectomy?
16. What is laparoscopic myomectomy?
17. What are the indications of hysterectomy in fibroid?
18. What is MRI-guided focused ultrasonic treatment?

Adenomyosis

Description

Uterus is uniformly enlarged (usually <14 weeks size). Cut surface shows diffuse altered echogenicity with tiny cystic areas in the myometrium. Posterior myometrium is commonly involved. Unlike fibroid there is no capsule or whorled appearance.

1. How the patient will present with this disease?

Patient is usually parous and in 3rd or 4th decade of life. Patient presents with heavy menstrual bleeding and severe dysmenorrhea (progressive congestive dysmenorrhea). There is pain in lower abdomen and may be dyspareunia.

2. How will you diagnose adenomyosis?

Diagnosis is suspected from symptoms and signs. On PV examination there is enlarged tender uterus, more evident **immediately** after menstruation. Transvaginal sonography is diagnostic and final confirmation is by histopathological examination of uterus.

3. **How will you treat adenomyosis?**
   Definitive treatment of adenomyosis is hysterectomy nondescent vaginal **hysterectomy** (**NDVH**) or total laparoscopic **hysterectomy** (**TLH**). When uterus is to be preserved debulking surgery is suggested. In rare case of localized adenomyosis excision of adenomyoma may be carried out. Medical treatment by analgesics or hormones only help temporarily.
   1. What is the difference between adenomyosis and endometriosis (externa)?
   2. What are the various etiological theories for endometriosis?
   3. What is the etiology for adenomyosis?
   4. How will you diagnose adenomyosis on sonograpy?
   5. How can you differentiate adenomyosis from fibroid macroscopically?
   6. How can you differentiate it clinically?
   7. What are the causes of menorrhagia in adenomyosis?
   8. What are the symptoms of patients with adenomyosis?
   9. What is the treatment of adenomyosis?
   10. What is the role of conservative surgery in localized adenomyosis?
   11. Why medical management is not much successful in adenomyosis?

Ovarian Tumors

Description

Specimen consists of thin walled enlarged cystic structure (unilocular or **multilocular**) grayish white in color. Contents are clear (tooth or hair may be seen in dermoid). Malignant tumors have thick walls, solid areas and papillary projections.

1. **How the patient will present?**
   Simple benign cyst of ovary is usually asymptomatic detected on routine clinical examination or USG. Patient may have dull aching pain in abdomen or menstrual irregularities. Complications of cyst, such as torsion, haemorrhage, etc., produces severe pain.
2. **How will you diagnose ovarian tumor?**
   It is easily diagnosed by USG-TVS. They are anechoic, unilocular, thin walled <8 cm in size (functional cyst) with acoustic enhancement. For malignant tumor apart from sonography, MRI and CT scans are indicated. In case of doubt frozen section during laparotomy is carried out.
3. **How will you treat?**
   Functional cyst is treated simply by follow-up TVS examination or OC pills for 3 months. For benign cyst laparoscopic cystectomy is carried out. For solid ovarian tumors staging laparotomy followed by **panhysterectomy** or radical hysterectomy is done as per frozen section report.
   1. What is the WHO classification of epithelial tumors?
   2. Which is the most common ovarian tumor? How does it origin?
   3. What is the difference between ovarian cyst and cystic ovary?
   4. Which are the functional ovarian tumors?
   5. Which ovarian tumors are common in adolescent girls?
   6. What is Krukenberg tumor? What are its characteristics?
   7. What is FIGO staging for ovarian tumors?
   8. What is the differential diagnosis (D/D) of any pelvic tumor?
   9. Which are the clinical features suggestive of malignancy in ovarian tumor?
   10. Which are the macroscopic features suggesting malignancy in ovarian tumor?
   11. What are the complications of ovarian tumor?
   12. What are tumor markers? What is their importance?
   13. How will you manage uncomplicated ovarian tumor during pregnancy?
   14. What is the role of second look operation in ovarian tumors?
   15. What is the most common cause of death in ovarian tumors?

Carcinoma Cervix

Description

Specimen consists radical hysterectomy (panhysterectomy + parametrium) with cervix showing ulcerative or cauliflower-like growth.

1. **How the patient with this disease present?**
   Patient is in 4th or 5th decade of life. Usually multiparous from low socioeconomical (SE) status. Symptoms include vaginal discharge (foul smelling) and abnormal vaginal bleeding. In late stage disease pain, cachexia, anorexia and loss of weight occur.
2. **How will you diagnose carcinoma cervix?**
   Early diagnosis of Ca cervix is by Pap smear colposcopy, **human papillomavirus (HPV)**—deoxyribonucleic acid **(DNA) testing**, visual inspection of the cervix with acetic acid (**VIA**), visual inspection with Lugol's iodine (**VILI**), etc. Definite diagnosis is by cervical biopsy and histopathological confirmation.
3. **How will you manage such a case?**
   Up to FIGO stage II A (nonbulky lesion) radical hysterectomy and **pelvic lymphadenectomy** is carried out. While for all stages radiotheraphy, i.e., full external and intracavitory radiation are the standard treatment.
   1. What do you know about the etiology of carcinoma cervix?
   2. What is differential diagnosis of ulcerative lesions of cervix?
   3. What is carcinoma in situ cervix? How will you diagnose it? What is its relation to invasive cancer of cervix? How will you manage it?
   4. What is Pap's smear examination? How it is done?
   5. What is FIGO classifications of carcinoma cervix?
   6. Which are the prognostic factors in carcinoma cervix?
   7. From where will you take the cervical biopsy for **histopathology** examination?
   8. How will you do colposcopy?
   9. What is the most common mode of death in carcinoma cervix?
   10. What is conization? What are its types?
   11. Which are the different techniques of internal radiation in carcinoma cervix?
   12. What is point A and point B in radiation treatment? What is their importance?
   13. What are the complications of radiation treatment?
   14. What structures are removed in **Wertheim hysterectomy**?
   15. What do you mean by **exenteration** operation?

Cervical Elongation (Prolapse)

Description

Specimen consists of uterus (may be menopausal atrophic) with cervix. Cervix appears elongated (supravaginal elongation).

1. **How the patient with this disease present?**
   Patient is in postmenopausal or perimenopausal age. Patient presents with typical symptoms of prolapse, i.e., something coming out PV, backache, leukorrhea, urinary or bowel symptoms. In reproductive age group patients there can be menstrual problems, infertility or sexual problems.
2. **How will you diagnose prolapse?**
   From the symptoms and clinical examination the diagnosis is evident. Cervix may be **hypertrophied** and edematous. There may be decubitus ulcer. There is supravaginal elongation of cervix. In associated **vaginal wall prolapse** there is loss of **rugosity**, pigmentation, keratinization and ulceration. There is descent of vaginal walls down from their normal position.
3. **How will you treat prolapse?**
   Treatment of prolapse is surgical, i.e., vaginal hysterectomy with repair. If uterus is to be preserved then abdominal sling operations or **laparoscopic sling operation** are done. In past **Manchester**

operation was carried out from vaginal route. Pessary treatment for prolapse is palliative only and for temporary purpose.

1. What are the causes of elongation of cervix?
2. What are the differences between congenital elongation and acquired elongation?
3. Why there is supravaginal elongation in case of prolapse?
4. What are the secondary changes in vagina in case of prolapse?
5. What do you mean by procidentia?
6. How will you explain prolapse in nulligravida patient?
7. What are the indications of pessary treatment?
8. Which are the conservative operations for prolapse of uterus?
9. What are the advantages of vaginal hysterectomy over abdominal hysterectomy in any gynec case?
10. What is **POP-Q** classification of prolapse?

Carcinoma Body Uterus

Description

Specimen consists of **panhysterectomy**, i.e., uterus with tubes and ovaries. Uterus is enlarged and on cut surface necrotic area may be seen in endometrial cavity invading surrounding myometrium.

1. **How the present will present to you?**
   Patient is in 4th or 5th decade of life either nulliparous or low parity. Patient may be obese, diabetic and hypertensive (corpus cancer syndrome). Patient has complaint of (c/o) irregular bleeding or prolonged heavy menstruation or postmenopausal bleeding.
2. **How will you diagnose carcinoma body uterus?**
   Carcinoma body uterus is diagnosed by endometrial cytology, endometrial biopsy or dilatation and curettage with histopathological confirmation. In advanced stage disease apart from USG, CT scan and MRI pelvis are required.
3. **How will you manage Carcinoma body uterus?**
   Depending upon the stage and characteristics of the cancer Ca body uterus is treated by surgery (panhysterectomy with lymph node dissection) or combination of surgery, radiation therapy, chemotherapy and hormone therapy.

1. Which are the etiological factors for carcinoma body uterus?
2. What is corpus cancer syndrome?
3. Which are the premalignant conditions for carcinoma body uterus?
4. What is the incidence of carcinoma body uterus as compared to carcinoma cervix in our country and in western countries?
5. What is the FIGO staging of carcinoma body uterus?
6. What are the causes of uterine enlargement other than pregnancy?
7. Which are the prognostic factors for carcinoma body uterus?
8. Which are the screening methods for carcinoma body uterus?
9. What are the common sites of metastasis in carcinoma body uterus?
10. What is the role of chemotherapy in the management of carcinoma body uterus?

Hydrosalpinx

Description

Specimen consists of thin walled elongated retort shaped swelling with grayish white in appearance.

1. **How the patient will present?**
   It may be asymptomatic or patient will have symptoms of chromic pelvic inflammatory disease (PID), i.e., pain, vaginal discharge, backache, menstrual irregularity and chronic ill health. Patient can have pelvic tuberculosis with infertility and oligomenorrhea as other symptoms.
2. **How will you diagnose it?**

Diagnosis is by clinical features and USG. TVS shows anechoic or hypoechoic structure related to uterine cornu and ovary of that side is separately seen. MRI and CT scan are superior but costly. Diagnosis is confirmed at laparoscopy or laparotomy.

3. **How will you manage?**
   Initially a course of antibiotics can be given. Usually surgical treatment by laparoscopy, i.e., salpingectomy is carried out. In case of TB full course of treatment is given.

1. What is the pathogenesis of hydrosalpinx?
2. Which are the mechanical factors in development of hydrosalpinx?
3. Why all tubal swellings are retort shaped?
4. What are the macroscopic differences between hydrosalpinx and pyosalpinx?
5. Which are the common organisms which cause hydrosalpinx and pyosalpinx?
6. How will you diagnose gonorrhea? How will you treat it?
7. How will you diagnose genital TB? How will you treat it?
8. What are the common symptoms in a case of chronic PID?
9. When surgery is indicated in case of chronic PID?
10. What is the conservative surgery in hydrosalpinx?

CHAPTER 15

Scores, Tests, FIGO Staging, and Classification

SCORES

Apgar Score

It was introduced by Virginia Apgar in 1953. It is used to assess neonatal oxygenation status at birth. It is calculated at 1 and 5 minutes after the birth of the baby. 1 minute score indicates need for immediate resuscitation of newborn, while 5 minutes score correlates well with long-term neurological sequelae.

Signs	Score		
	0	1	2
Heart rate	Absent	Slow	Over 100
Respiratory effort	Absent	Slow, irregular	Good, crying
Muscle tone	Limp (flaccid)	Some flexion of limbs	Active motion
Response to catheter in nostril (reflex irritability)	No response	Grimace	Cough sneeze
Color	Pale	Body pink extremities blue	Pink

Total score = 10
4–6: Mild depression
7–10: No depression
0–3: Severe depression

Bishop's Score

It was introduced by Bishop in 1964. It is practical method of predicting the success before induction of labor.

The score is calculated by checking five parameters on P/V examination. Cervical dilatation, cervical effacement, cervical consistency, position and fetal station. Total score is 13. Score 0–5 is unfavorable for induction while 6–13 is considered favorable for induction. Score of >8 suggests that induction is surely successful.

There are many modifications of Bishop score. Mainly cervical effacement is replaced by cervical length in cm. As per National Institute of Health and Care Excellence (NICE) Clinical Guidelines, 2008 it is as follows:

The modified Bishop score

Factor	Modified Bishop score			
	0	1	2	3
Dilation (cm)	<1	1–2	2–4	>4
Length of cervix (cm)	>4	2–4	1–2	<1
Station (relative to ischial spines)	–3	–2	–1/0	+1/+2
Consistency	Firm	Average	Soft	—
Position	Posterior	Mid/anterior	—	—

In another modification 1 point is added to the total score each for 1. Existence pre-eclampsia and 2. Each previous vaginal delivery. One point is subtracted from the total score each for 1. Nulliparity, 2. Post-term and 3. Preterm premature rupture of the membranes (PPROM).

Biophysical Profile Scoring

It was developed by Professor Frank A Manning from Canada in 1980. It is an important method of antepartum fetal surveillance. Recording of a number of acute biophysical variables is superior in predictive accuracy to that achieved by recording any single variable. Different variables are measured concurrently using a dynamic ultrasound imaging method as shown in Table 15.1.

Two major modifications are added to the original method (1) Nonstress test (NST) is not performed routinely now, if rest of the 4 variables are normal. The accuracy of 8 of 8 score is equal to 10 of 10. Only if other variables are abnormal NST is done. This has the advantage to limiting the test time. In 95% cases test is now completed within 8 minutes instead of full 30 minutes. (2) In the definition of oligohydramnios a fluid pocket of 2 cm or less as opposed to original 1 cm is used to define decreased amniotic fluid volume. The test is started after 25 weeks and usually repeated weekly.

Management: Fetal biophysical profile scoring (BPS or BPP) when normal (>8/10) is a direct accurate evidence of normal tissue oxygenation and absent central acidemia. When abnormal (6/10 or less) the score is a measurement of the probability of tissue hypoxia and central acidemia. Suggested management is as follows:

Score	Management
0 – 4	Deliver if gestational age is >26 weeks
6 (abnormal fluid)	
6 (normal fluid)	Deliver if fetus is mature
8 (abnormal fluid)	If not, repeat test in 24 hours and serially
8 (normal fluid)	Conservative management
10	No intervention

BPS is time consuming and requires a trained person in sonography. Clark and colleagues devised a **Modified biophysical profile.**

Table 15.1: Biophysical profile scoring.

Biophysical variable	Normal (Score = 2)	Abnormal (Score = 0)
Fetal breathing movements	≥One episode of ≥ 30 seconds in 30 minutes	Absent or one episode of ≥30 seconds in 30 minutes
Gross body movements	≥2 Discrete body/limb movements in 30 minutes (episodes of active continuous movement considered)	<2 episodes of body/limb movements in 30 minutes as single movement
Fetal tone	>One episode of active extension with return to flexion of fetal limb(s) or trunk. Opening and closing of hand is	Either slow extension with return to partial flexion movement of limb in full extension or absent fetal movement considered normal tone
Reactive fetal heart rate	≥ Two episodes of acceleration of ≥15 bpm and of >15 seconds associated with fetal movement in 20 minutes	<2 episodes of acceleration of fetal heart rate or acceleration of <15 bpm in 20 minutes
Amniotic fluid volume	≥ One pocket of fluid measuring 1 cm in vertical axis	Either no pockets or largest pocket <1 cm in vertical axis

Note: Total score is 10.

NST (VAST) is performed twice weekly, combined with amniotic fluid index (AFI). AFI <5 is considered abnormal. This testing requires 10 minutes to perform. If NST is not reactive and AFI is ≤5, full BPP scoring is performed.

Cervical Score

It is a score to assess the quality of cervical mucus in infertility cases. Cervical mucus greatly influences the sperm receptivity and migration, so it should be evaluated before a postcoital test (PCT) is performed. It was developed by Moghissi et al. (1977). Cervical mucus is collected by aspirating it with pipette or tuberculin syringe in preovulatory period and five properties of cervical mucus are studied. Each is given 0–3 score, 3 representing the optimum changes and total score is calculated.

Amount	Viscosity
0 = 0	0 = thick, highly viscous
1 = 0.1 mL	1 = intermediate viscosity
2 = 0.2 mL	2 = mildly viscous
3 = 0.3 mL or more	3 = normal
Ferning	**Cellularity**
0 = no crystallization	0 = 11 or more cells/HPF
1 = atypical pattern	1 = 6–10 cells/HPF
2 = primary and secondary stems	2 = 1–5 cells/HPF
3 = tertiary and quarterly stems	3 = 0 cells/HPF
Spinnbarkeit	**Total score**
0 = < 1 cm	>10 = normal
1 = 1–4 cm	5–10 = unfavorable
2 = 5–8 cm	<5 = hostile
3 = >9 cm	

TESTS

Nonstress Test

Nonstress test is now being increasingly used as primary method of antepartum fetal surveillance.

Principle

There is transient acceleration of fetal heart rate with each fetal movement. The exact cause of this is unknown but it indicates responsive central nervous system.

Methodology

It is ideally done with the use of electronic fetal monitor (cardiotocograph) but in absence of monitor, test performed with the use of Doppler or even stethoscope also gives quite reliable results. Mother is given semi-Fowler position with slight left lateral tilt to prevent supine hypotension. The fetal monitor is attached. Ultrasonic transducer detects the fetal heart rate and it is continuously recorded on moving strip, while fetal movement is recorded by mother by pressing a button which makes the mark on the strip. If there is no fetal movement in 20 minutes, fetus is stimulated manually or by acoustic stimulation using electronic artificial larynx (VAST) producing 100 db sound and test is further continued for 20 minutes.

Results

- *Reactive test*: NST is called reactive if there are at least 2 fetal movements in 20 minutes with acceleration of FHR by 15 beats/min for at least 15 seconds. The beat to beat variability should be > 5.
- *Nonreactive*: Anything that does not meet with the above criteria of reactive NST is called nonreactive NST.

Interpretation and Management

Reactive NST means fetus is well for at least a week to follow. So reactive NSTs are repeated weekly except in cases of postmaturity and diabetes, where they should be done twice a week.

Nonoccurrence of fetal movement, either spontaneous or induced makes the NST result **unsatisfactory.** It should be repeated in 24 hours.

Scores, Tests, FIGO Staging, and Classification

Nonreactive indicates fetal jeopardy. It is associated with poor fetal and neonatal outcome, but there is high incidence of false positive results also. This may be due to fetal sleep, sedative or narcotic drugs, congenital anomalies and premature fetus. So when NST is nonreactive it is repeated after 24 hours and if it still remains nonreactive BPPS is performed but direct intervention on the basis of NST result alone, is not advised.

Definitions of Fetal Heart Rate Patterns

Tachycardia: Baseline FHR >160 bpm

Bradycardia: Baseline FHR <110 bpm

Acceleration: Increase in FHR by ≥15 bpm above baseline, with a duration of >15 seconds but <2 minutes.

In prolonged acceleration it lasts ≥2 minutes but <10 minutes. If it lasts ≥10 minutes it is considered as baseline change.

Early deceleration: In association with a uterine contraction, a visually apparent, usually symmetrical, gradual onset to nadir ≤30 seconds—decrease in fetal heart rate (FHR) with return to baseline.

Nadir of the deceleration occurs at the same time as the peak of the contraction.

Late deceleration: In association with a uterine contraction, a visually apparent, gradual onset to nadir >30 seconds decrease in FHR with return to baseline.
Onset, nadir, and recovery of the deceleration occur after the beginning, peak and end of the contraction respectively.

Variable deceleration: An abrupt onset to nadir <30 seconds visually apparent decrease in the FHR below the baseline. The decrease in FHR is ≥15 bpm with a duration of ≥15 seconds but <2 minutes.

Prolonged deceleration: Deceleration is >15 bpm, lasting >2 minutes but <10 minutes from onset to return to baseline.

Baseline variability: Fluctuations in the baseline fetal heart rate due to the beat-to-beat changes (R to R interval differences).

Short-term variability: It reflects the beat-to-beat changes due to the interval differences between each successive R peak of the ECG signal or two successive signals from ultrasound transducer.

Long-term variability: It describes the cycling effect of the FHR over time. These changes are described in terms of frequency per minutes.

Three Tier Fetal Heart Rate Interpretation System (International Consensus)

Category I: Normal
Include all of the following:
- Baseline rate: 110–60/min
- Baseline FHR variability: Moderate
- Late or variable decelerations: Absent
- Early decelerations: Present or absent
- Accelerations: Present or absent

Category II: Intermediate
Include all FHR tracings not categorized as Category I or III

Category II tracings include any of the following:
- Baseline rate
  - Bradycardia not accompanied by absent baseline variability
  - Tachycardia
- Baseline FHR variability
  - Minimal baseline variability
  - Absent baseline variability not accompanied by recurrent decelerations
  - Marked baseline variability
- Accelerations: Absence or induced accelerations after fetal stimulation
- Periodic or episodic decelerations
  - Recurrent variable decelerations accompanied by minimal or moderate baseline variability
  - Prolonged decelerations >2 minutes but <10 minutes

- Recurrent late decelerations with moderate baseline variability

Variable decelerations with other characteristics, such as slow return to baseline, "overshoots", or "shoulders"

Category III: Abnormal
Include either:
- Absent FHR variability and any of the following:
  - Recurrent late decelerations
  - Recurrent variable deceleration
  - Bradycardia
- Sinusoidal pattern

Contraction Stress Test

In contraction stress test (CST) fetal wellbeing is tested by subjecting it to the stress of uterine contractions. Contractions may be spontaneous or induced by nipple stimulation or oxytocin infusion. When oxytocin is used the test is known as oxytocin challenge test (OCT).

Oxytocin Challenge Test

It is an invasive method of detecting antepartum fetal wellbeing.

Principle

During uterine contraction bloodflow through the placenta considerably decreases. This is tolerated well by a healthy fetus, but in a compromised fetus (uteroplacental insufficiency). This stress of contraction produces late deceleration of fetal heart rate.

Indications

For antepartum fetal surveillance in high-risk cases, e.g., postmaturity, intrauterine growth restriction (IUGR), pregnancy-induced hypertension (PIH) diabetes, Rh-isoimmunization.

Contraindications

- Patients at risk of premature labor, e.g., multiple pregnancy, hydramnios, past history of preterm labor, PROM
- Previous cesarean section
- Placenta previa

Methodology

Baseline FHR and uterine contractions are recorded initially and then continuously throughout the test. An infusion of dilute oxytocin is started at 0.5–1.0 miliunit/min. The rate is doubled every 15 minutes until uterine activity of 3 contractions per 10 minutes lasting for 40 seconds is achieved. The oxytocin is then turned off and fetal monitor tracing is observed until uterine activity returns to baseline level. The test usually takes 1–2 hours to complete.

Results

The test is interpreted under following headings:
- *Negative*: No late decelerations with a contraction frequency of 3 in 10 minutes lasting for 40 seconds.
- *Positive*: If late decelerations are present with >50% of such contractions the test is positive.
- *Suspicious*: Late decelerations are present but they are intermittent, do not persist and occur in <50% of the uterine contractions.
- *Hyperstimulation*: If uterine contractions are more frequent than 2 minutes or last longer than 90 seconds.
- *Unsatisfactory*: The frequency of contraction is < 3/10 minutes or duration of each contraction is <40 seconds or FHR tracing is not of readable quality.

Management

Negative OCT indicates good fetal conditions for at least a week to follow, so it is repeated weekly. Positive OCT indicates compromised fetus but there is high incidence of false positive result up to 25%.

Note:
As compared to OCT, NST is easier, noninvasive, less time consuming and it can be repeat-

ed as many times as required without risk. **So NST and BPP scoring have replaced OCT for antepartum fetal surveillance.**

However, it can be done intrapartum to screen the patients for continuous fetal monitoring as **an admission test (AT).**

Roll-over Test

It is simple clinical test to detect 'at risk' mothers particularly primigravida who are likely to develop PIH later on in the same pregnancy. However, due to high false positive rate it is not much used clinically.

Methodology

Usually it is done between 28 and 32 weeks of pregnancy but in cases of multiple pregnancy and other high-risk patients it is advisable to do test earlier, i.e., after 24 weeks.

The mother is asked to lie down in left lateral position and BP is taken in right upper limb after 15 minutes. Then the patient is turned to supine position and BP is again taken after 5 minutes.

Interpretation

Increase of 20 mm of Hg in diastolic pressure in supine position indicates positive "roll-over test" If the test is positive 60–70% patients develop pre-eclampsia later on. Negative test is more reliable, i.e., > 95% patients do not develop preeclampsia when it is negative. The exact mechanism by which supine position causes rise in BP is not clear but it may be due to intrinsic vascular hypersensitivity in such patients.

Amniotic Fluid "Shake Test"

As lecithin–sphingomyelin (L/S) ratio is not possible in most places in India this is a bedside test to detect fetal lung maturity.

Materials

Amniotic fluid recently collected 95% ethanol (19 parts of absolute alcohol mixed with 1 part of distilled water), 0.9% saline.and two glass tubes.

Steps of Test

1. Mix 1 mL of amniotic fluid and 1 mL of ethanol in one tube.
2. Mix 0.5 mL of amniotic fluid, 0.5 mL of saline, and 1 mL of ethanol in the second tube.
3. Shake both the tubes for 15 seconds and place tubes upright.
4. Wait for 15 minutes and look for a ring of bubble or foam at the air-liquid interface.

Results

- *Positive test*: Ring of bubble observed in both tubes
- *Negative test*: Ring of bubble not observed in either tube.
- *Equivocal test*: Ring of bubble observed only in first tube.

FIGO STAGING

FIGO (The International Federation of Gynecology and Obstetrics).

Carcinoma Cervix

Classifications

Stage I: The carcinoma is strictly confined to the cervix uteri (extension to the corpus should be disregarded)

IA: Invasive carcinoma that can be diagnosed only by microscopy, with maximum depth of invasion <5 mm[a]

    IA1: Measured stromal invasion <3 mm in depth

    IA2: Measured stromal invasion ≥3 mm and <5 mm in depth

IB: Invasive carcinoma with measured deepest invasion ≥5 mm (> stage IA), lesion limited to the cervix uteri[b]

    IB1: Invasive carcinoma ≥5 mm depth of stromal invasion and <2 cm in greatest dimension

IB2: Invasive carcinoma ≥2 cm and <4 cm in greatest dimension
IB3: Invasive carcinoma ≥4 cm in greatest dimension

Stage II: The carcinoma invades beyond the uterus, but has not extended onto the lower third of the vagina or to the pelvic wall

IIA: Involvement limited to the upper two thirds of the vagina without parametrial involvement
  IIA1: Invasive carcinoma <4 cm in greatest dimension
  IIA2: Invasive carcinoma ≥4 cm in greatest dimension
IIB: With parametrial involvement but not up to the pelvic wall

Stage III: The carcinoma involves the lower third of the vagina and/or extends to the pelvic wall and/or causes hydronephrosis or nonfunctioning kidney and/or involves pelvic and/or para-aortic lymph nodes[c].

IIIA: Carcinoma involves the lower third of the vagina, with no extension to the pelvic wall
IIIB: Extension to the pelvic wall and/or hydronephrosis or nonfunctioning kidney (unless known to be due to another cause)
IIIC: Involvement of pelvic and/or para-aortic lymph nodes, irrespective of tumor size and extent (with r and p notations)[c]
  IIIC1: Pelvic lymph node metastasis only
  IIIC2: Para-aortic lymph node metastasis

Note: When in doubt, the lower staging should be assigned.
a. Imaging and pathology can be used, where available, to supplement clinical findings with respect to tumor size and extent, in all stages.
b. The involvement of vascular/lymphatic spaces does not change the staging. The lateral extent of the lesion is no longer considered.
c. Adding notation of r (imaging) and p (pathology) to indicate the findings that are used to allocate the case to Stage IIIC. Example: If imaging indicates pelvic lymph node metastasis, the stage allocation would be Stage IIIC1r, and if confirmed by pathologic findings, it would be Stage IIIC1p. The type of imaging modality or pathology technique used should always be documented.

Stage IV: The carcinoma has extended beyond the true pelvis or has involved (biopsy proven) the mucosa of the bladder or rectum. A bullous edema, as such, does not permit a case to be allotted to stage IV

IVA: Spread of the growth to adjacent organs
IVB: Spread to distant organs

Endometrial Carcinoma (Ca Body Uterus)

FIGO Stage

Ia: Tumor confined to the corpus uteri[a]
  IAa: No or less than half myometrial invasion
  IBa: Invasion equal to or more than half of the myometrium
IIa: Tumor invades cervical stroma, but does not extend beyond the uterus[b]
IIIa: Local and/or regional spread of the tumor
  IIIAa: Tumor invades the serosa of the corpus uteri and/or adnexae[c]
  IIIBa: Vaginal involvement and/or parametrial involvement[c]
  IIICa: Metastases to pelvic and/or para aortic lymph nodes[c]
  IIIC1a: Positive pelvic nodes
  IIIC2a: Positive para-aortic nodes with or without positive pelvic lymph nodes
IVa: Tumor invades bladder and/or bowel mucosa, and/or distant metastases
  IVAa: Tumor invasion of bladder and/or bowel mucosa
  IVBa: Distant metastasis, including intra-abdominal metastases and/or inguinal nodes

Note:
a. Either G1, G2, or G3.
b. Endocervical glandular involvement only should be considered as Stage I and no longer as Stage II.
c. Positive cytology has to be reported separately without changing the stage.

Ovarian Cancer

FIGO staging classification for cancer of the ovary, fallopian tube, and peritoneum.

Stage I: Tumor confined to ovaries or fallopian tube(s)

IA: Tumor limited to 1 ovary (capsule intact) or fallopian tube; no tumor on ovarian or fallopian tube surface; no malignant cells in the ascites or peritoneal washings

IB: Tumor limited to both ovaries (capsules intact) or fallopian tubes; no tumor on ovarian or fallopian tube surface; no malignant cells in the ascites or peritoneal washings

IC: Tumor limited to 1 or both ovaries or fallopian tubes, with any of the following:
- **IC1:** Surgical spill
- **IC2:** Capsule ruptured before surgery or tumor on ovarian or fallopian tube surface
- **IC3:** Malignant cells in the ascites or peritoneal washings

Stage II: Tumor involves 1 or both ovaries or fallopian tubes with pelvic extension (below pelvic brim) or peritoneal cancer

IIA: Extension and/or implants on uterus and/or fallopian tubes and/or ovaries

IIB: Extension to other pelvic intraperitoneal tissues

Stage III: Tumor involves 1 or both ovaries or fallopian tubes, or peritoneal cancer, with cytologically or histologically confirmed spread to the peritoneum outside the pelvis and/or metastasis to the retroperitoneal lymph nodes

IIIA1: Positive retroperitoneal lymph nodes only (cytologically or histologically proven):
- **IIIA1(i):** Metastasis up to 10 mm in greatest dimension
- **IIIA1(ii):** Metastasis >10 mm in greatest dimension

IIIA2: Microscopic extrapelvic (above the pelvic brim) peritoneal involvement with or without positive retroperitoneal lymph nodes

IIIB: Macroscopic peritoneal metastasis beyond the pelvis up to 2 cm in greatest dimension, with or without metastasis to the retroperitoneal lymph nodes

IIIC: Macroscopic peritoneal metastasis beyond the pelvis > 2 cm in greatest dimension, with or without metastasis to the retroperitoneal lymph nodes (includes extension of tumor to capsule of liver and spleen without parenchymal involvement of either organ)

Stage IV: Distant metastasis excluding peritoneal metastases

IVA: Pleural effusion with positive cytology

IVB: Parenchymal metastases and metastases to extra-abdominal organs (including inguinal lymph nodes and lymph nodes outside of the abdominal cavity)

Cancer of the Vulva

FIGO Stage	Description
I	Tumor confined to the vulva
IA	Lesions ≤2 cm in size, confined to the vulva or perineum and with stromal invasion ≤1.0 mm, no nodal metastasis
IB	Lesions >2 cm in size or with stromal invasion >1.0 mm, confined to the vulva or perineum, with negative nodes
II	Tumor of any size with extension to adjacent perineal structures (lower third of urethra, lower third of vagina, anus) with negative nodes
III	Tumor of any size with or without extension to adjacent perineal structures (lower third of urethra, lower third of vagina, anus) with positive inguinofemoral nodes
IIIA	With 1 lymph node metastasis (≥5 mm), or with 1–2 lymph node metastasis(es) (<5 mm)
IIIB	With 2 or more lymph node metastases (≥5 mm), or with 3 or more lymph node metastases (<5 mm)

IIIC	With positive nodes with extracapsular spread
IV	Tumor invades other regional (upper 2/3 urethra, upper 2/3 vagina), or distant structures
IVA	Tumor invades any of the following: Upper urethral and/or vaginal mucosa, bladder mucosa, rectal mucosa, or fixed to pelvic bone, or fixed or ulcerated inguinofemoral lymph nodes
IVB	Any distant metastasis including pelvic lymph nodes

Classifications

Endometriosis: Revised American Fertility Society (RAFS) Classification (1985)

Endometriosis		<1 cm	1–3 cm	>3 cm
Peritoneum	Superficial	1	2	4
	Deep	2	4	6
Ovary	Right superficial	1	2	4
	Deep	4	16	20
	Left superficial	1	2	4
	Deep	4	16	20

Posterior cul-de-sac Obliteration			Partial 4	Complete 40
Ovary	Adhesions	<1/3	1/3–2/3	>2/3
	Enclosure		Enclosure	
	Right filmy	1	2	4
	Dense	4	8	16
	Left filmy	1	2	4
	Dense	4	8	16
Tube	Right filmy	1	2	4
	Dense	4*	8*	16
	Left filmy	1	2	4
	Dense	4*	8*	16

* If the fimbriated end of the fallopian tube is completely enclosed, change the point assignment to 16.

Stage I (Minimal): 1–5
Stage II (Mild): 6–15
Stage III (Moderate): 16–40
Stage IV (Severe): >40

Modified White's Classification

Priscilla White form Boston—USA first suggested it in 1965.

Class	Diabetes onset age (years)	Duration (years)	Vascular disease
Gestational diabetes			
A1* (FBS ≤105 PPBS ≤120)	Any	Any	0
A2 (FBS > 105 PPBS > 120)	Any	Any	0
Pregestational diabetes			
B	>20	<10	0
C	10–19	10–19	0
D	<10	>20 and or Background retinopathy	+
F (nephropathy)	Any	Any	+
R (retinopathy)	Any	Any	+
T (renal transplant)	Any	Any	+
H (ischemic heart disease)	Any	Any	+

* Class A1, diabetes is managed by diet alone while class A2 and pregestational diabetes cases require insulin.

Functional Grading of Heart Disease (New York Heart Association, NYHA)

NYHA Class	Symptoms
I	No limitation of physical activity. Ordinary physical activity does not cause undue fatigue, palpitation, dyspnea (shortness of breath)
II	Slight limitation of physical activity. Comfortable at rest. Ordinary physical activity results in fatigue, palpitation, dyspnea (shortness of breath)

NYHA Class	Symptoms
III	Marked limitation of physical activity. Comfortable at rest. Less than ordinary activity causes fatigue, palpitation, or dyspnea
IV	Unable to carry on any physical activity without discomfort. Symptoms of heart failure at rest. If any physical activity is undertaken, discomfort increases.

Page Clinical Classification for Placental Abruption

Grade 0: Clinical features may be absent. The diagnosis is retrospective by examining the placenta after delivery.

Grade I: (i) External bleeding is slight, (ii) Uterus is irritable. Tenderness may or may not be present, (iii) FHS are good.

Grade II: (i) External bleeding is mild to moderate, (ii) Uterine tenderness is always present, (iii) Fetal distress or even fetal death occurs, (iv) Shock is absent.

Grade III: (i) Bleeding moderate to severe, it may be concealed, (ii) Uterus tenderness is marked, (iii) Shock is pronounced, (iv) Fetal death is the rule, (v) Associated coagulation defect or anuria may be present.

Sher and Statland Grading:
Grade I: Not recognized before delivery and usually diagnosed by presence of retroplacental clot.

Grade II: The classical signs of abruption placenta are present whereas the fetus is alive.

Grade III: The fetus is dead.
III a: Without coagulopathy.
III b: With coagulopathy.

Types of Placenta Previa

Type I (Lateral, low lying)
When only part of the placenta is implanted in lower uterine segment and none of its margin reaches internal os.

Type II (Marginal)
The placental margin reaches the internal os but does not cover it. It can be anterior (II A) or posterior (II P).

Type III (Incomplete central)
The placenta covers the internal os when it is closed but does not cover it when it is fully dilated

Type IV (Complete central)
The placenta completely covers the internal os even after it is fully dilated

Type II P, type III and type IV are called major degrees placenta previa, while type I and type II A are called minor degrees placenta previa. However, bleeding is not always proportional to degrees of placenta previa.

Robson Classification

Robson MS in 2001 suggested classification of cesarean sections. Based on a few basic obstetric variables the system classifies all women admitted for delivery into one of ten groups that are mutually exclusive and totally inclusive. Every woman admitted to deliver in any facility can be classified into one, and only one, of the ten groups and no woman will be left out of the classification.

WHO in 2017 recommended "Robson classification system as a global standard for assessing, monitoring and comparing cesarean section rates within healthcare facilities over time, and between facilities".

The classification is simple, robust, reproducible, clinically relevant, and prospective.
- Nulliparous women with a single cephalic pregnancy >37 weeks gestation in spontaneous labor
- Nulliparous women with a single cephalic pregnancy >37 weeks gestation who either had labor induced or were delivered by cesarean section (CS) before labor
- Multiparous without a previous uterine scar with a single cephalic pregnancy >37 weeks gestation in spontaneous labor

- Multiparous women without a previous uterine scar with a single cephalic pregnancy >37 weeks who either had labor induced or were delivered by cesarean section before labor
- All multiparous women with at least one previous CS with a singleton cephalic pregnancy >37 weeks
- All nulliparous women with a single breech pregnancy
- All multiparous women with single breech pregnancy including women with previous uterine scars
- All women with multiple pregnancies including women with previous uterine scars
- All women with a single pregnancy with transverse or oblique lie including women with previous uterine scars.
- All women with a single cephalic pregnancy <37 weeks gestation including women with previous uterine scars.

If help in identifying which groups are responsible for high cesarean section rate and accordingly measures can be taken to decrease the high cesarean section rate.

CHAPTER 16

Miscellaneous

Laboratory Investigations, Normal Semen Report, Partogram, Chiranjeevi Scheme, Janani Shishu Suraksha Karyakram, PC-PNDT Act, and FDA Drug Categories are included in this chapter.

LABORATORY INVESTIGATIONS

Two basic investigations done during pregnancy are discussed here.

Hemoglobin (Hb) Estimation

Normal value: 13 to 15 g/100 mL of blood in non-pregnant adult female.

Method of Estimation

Currently it is done by automated hematology analyser, i.e., cell counter in standard laboratories and institutions where it is readily available. However at PHC level and subcenters the acid hematin method (Sahli) is the commonly used method.

Principle: Hemoglobin is converted to acid hematin by diluting it with weak acid and the color of it is matched with standard colored glass plates in a comparator.

Specimen: Blood sample may be oxalated venous blood (well mixed) or non-anticoagulated one obtained by capillary puncture.

Procedure

- Fill the calibrated Hb square tube up to the mark 20 with 0.1 N HCL.
- Draw the blood specimen into the Hb pipette up to mark 20 (µL). In a capillary method make sure that no air bubble has entered into the pipette.
- Empty the pipette into the acid in the square tube. Rinse the pipette by drawing acid in and out for at least 3 times.
- Mix the acid hematin solution in the tube with the glass rod or by shaking and keep it at room temperature for 10 minutes.
- Dilute the solution by adding distilled water drop by drop and stirring the mixture with glass rod. Keep the apparatus against the good daylight and add the water till the color perfectly matches with that of the standards. Read the Hb concentration in grams from the mark reached in Sahli Hb meter.

Drawback: Sahli method is not a standard one because all forms of Hb are not converted to acid hematin. Standard method recommended is **cyanmethemoglobin.**

Other Methods of Hb Estimation

- Cyanmethemoglobin method: Colorimetric and spectrophotometric.

- Alkaline hematin method.
- Specific gravity method using copper sulfate solution useful for quick screening of blood donors.
- Gasometric: By measuring O_2 carrying capacity.
- Chemical: By measuring the iron content of blood.
- Tallquist scale: By comparing color of fresh blood on filter paper with standards—highly unsatisfactory.

Urine Analysis

Commonly it is done by **urine test strip** or dipstick. The test strips consist of a ribbon made of plastic or paper of about 5 mm wide. Plastic strips have pads impregnated with chemicals that react with the compounds present in urine producing a characteristic color. For the paper strips the reactants are absorbed directly onto the paper. Paper strips are often specific to a single reaction, while the strips with pads allow several determinations simultaneously.

The strips can be **qualitative** strips that give results as positive or negative, or they can be **semi-quantitative** ones that in addition to providing a positive or negative reaction also provide an estimation of a quantitative result, in the latter the color reactions are approximately proportional to the concentration of the substance being tested for in the sample. The reading of the results is carried out by comparing the pad colors with a color scale provided by the manufacturer.

Urine Albumin

Urine protein estimation and proteinuria are more accurate terms, but albuminuria is still commonly used.

Following tests can be done if urine strips are not available.
- **Heat acetic acid test:** About three-fourth of a test tube is filled with urine. Keeping the tube obliquely, upper part is boiled for a minute in a flame. Cloudy precipitate indicates presence of protein. It is further checked by adding 3 to 5 drops glacial acetic acid. Upon acidification turbidity due to phosphates disappear while that due to proteins persists or intensifies.

Result	Reporting	Approximate amount of protein
Faint turbidity	Trace	<10 mg/100 cc urine
Turbidity without	+	10-100 mg/100 cc urine granules
Turbidity with	++	100-500 mg/100 cc urine granules
Granules +	+++	500-1000 mg/100 cc urine Floccules
One large clump	++++	≥1 g/100 cc urine

- **Sulfosalicylic acid test:** Mix equal amount (2 to 3 cc) of urine and 3 to 5% sulfosalicylic acid. Presence of albumin is detected by turbidity of the urine. This test does not require heating.
- **Heller's nitric acid test:** Take 3 cc of concentrated acid in a test tube. Slowly add the urine from the side of the test tube. A white precipitate at the junction of 2 layers indicates presence of protein. The test is useful when only small quantity of urine is available.
- **Esbach's test:** Protein gets precipitated with Esbach's reagent which contains picric acid + citric acid. It takes 24 hours for precipitate to form. Esbach's albuminometer gives quantitative estimation also.

Urine Sugar

Benedict's test: It detects any reducing substance in the urine. As glucose is the major component amongst the all reducing substances present in urine, it is widely used method for detecting glycosuria.

Procedure: Urine sample is collected in a clean container at a required time (e.g., fasting, random, etc.)

To 5 cc of Benedict's reagent in a test tube 8 drops of urine is added with the help of a pipette. Boil the mixture vigorously for 2 minutes and allow it to cool. The test is positive if a color change occurs and precipitate appears as follows:

Result	Reporting	Approx. glucose level in urine
Faint green color	Trace	0 —100 mg%
Green precipitate	+	100—500 mg%
Yellow precipitate	++	500—1.0 g%
Yellowish orange precipitate	+++	1.0—2.0 g%
Red precipitate	++++	>2.0 g%

Drawback: In pregnant woman other reducing substances may be found in urine, i.e., lactose, uric acid, creatinine, ascorbic acid, etc., and give false positive result

Fehling's test: Equal parts of Fehling no. I and II solutions are taken in a test tube and heated. Equal volume of urine is added and heated. Color change of the solution and precipitate gives positive result. Like Benedict this also gets reduced by other substances than glucose.

Glucose oxidase test: This is specific for glucose. The enzyme glucose oxidase in presence of oxygen catalyzes the oxidation of glucose to gluconic acid. The presence of hydrogen peroxide gives color change. Strip containing this enzyme is dipped in urine and removed immediately. Color change after 1 minute gives positive result. It is simple and quick method. However, these strips may be rendered less sensitive during pregnancy due to increased quantity of ascorbic acid in urine.

Commonly used **urocolor** 2 test strips detect both protein as well as glucose in the urine.

Osazone test: It detects glucose or lactose.

NORMAL SEMEN REPORT

Husband semen examination is the commonly advised investigation in infertile couple.

Normal Semen Report (WHO 2010)

Volume	2–5 mL
Color	Whitish gray
pH	Alkaline 7.2–7.8
Liquification	Within 30 minutes
Sperm concentration	15 million/mL
Total sperm count	40 million/ejaculate
Motility	>50% progressively motile
Viability	>60% live spermatozoa
Morphology	>4% Normal
WBC	<1 million/mL
Fructose	>120 mg%
No Significant sperm agglutination	

Abnormalities (Terminology)

Aspermia	Absence of semen
Azoospermia	Absence of sperm
Hypospermia	Low semen volume
Hyperspermia	High semen volume
Oligozoospermia	Very low sperm count
Asthenozoospermia	Poor sperm motility
Teratozoospermia	Sperm carry more morphological defects than usual
Necrozoospermia	All sperm in the ejaculate are dead
Leukospermia	A high level of white blood cells in semen

PARTOGRAM

It was first devised by EA Friedman in 1955. It is the graphical record of cervical dilatation in centimeter (cm) against duration of labor in hours. It is a useful tool in the management of labor.

Hugh Philpott in 1972 further developed the partogram and added the Alert and Action lines.

Modern partgoram as developed by WHO is a composite record of all the important features of labor plotted along the 'y' axis against time in hours along the 'x' axis.

Components of Modern Partograph

Broadly, it has three components. The topmost is the fetal record, which includes the fetal heart rate, the presence or absence of fetal membranes, the nature of the liquor and presence of molding, if any.

The middle component depicts the progress of labor where cervical effacement, dilatation, descent of the fetal head (represented as fifths palpable per abdomen) and the frequency, strength (intensity) and duration of uterine contractions are recorded.

The lowermost allows for recording of any medication or fluids administered including oxytocin augmentation, maternal pulse, blood pressure and temperature, the volume of urine passed and the presence of albumin and acetone, if any, in the urine.

- The **'Alert line'** drawn from 3 to 10 cm represented the rate of dilatation of cervix at approximately 1 cm/h.
- **'Action line'** is drawn 4 hours to the right of the Alert line.

Modified WHO Partograph (Introduced in 2000)

Since a prolonged latent phase is relatively infrequent and differentiating the latent phase from false labor is often difficult, a modified WHO 'partograph' was introduced and incorporated **removal of the latent phase** and defined the **beginning of the active phase at 4 cm cervical dilatation** instead of 3 cm.

Recording

Progress of Labor

In the center of the partograph is a graph along the left side are the figure 0-10 against squares. Each square represents 1 cm dilatation. Along the bottom of the graph are number 0-24. Each square represents one hour. Dilatation of the cervix is measured in cm. The first vaginal examination is done on admission, includes a pelvic assessment and findings are recorded. Then after vaginal examinations are made every four hours or frequently, if needed.

Descent of the fetal head: It is measured as fifths palpable per abdomen. This is done immediately before vaginal examination and plotted on the graph. On left side of graph word descent with Nos. 5 to 0 are there.

The rule of fifth means the palpable fifth of the fetal head felt by abdominal examination above the level of symphysis pubis. When 2/5 or less of fetal head is felt from above it means that the head is engaged and by vaginal examination, the lowest part of vertex has passed or is at the level of ischial spines.

Fifth Palpable

5/5	—	Sinciput and occiput above the brim
4/5	—	Sinciput high, occiput easily felt
3/5	—	Sinciput easily felt, occiput felt
2/5	—	Sinciput felt, occiput just felt
1/5	—	Sinciput just felt, occiput not felt
0/5	—	No pole felt

Uterine contractions: On partograph below time line there is vertical column of 5 squares. The squares are shaded according to the number of contractions per 10 minutes. The density of shading correlates with intensity of uterine contractions.

Fetal Condition

Fetal heart rate: it is recorded every half hourly. Normal heart rate is between 120 and 160 per minute, 1 square on the graph represents 1/2 hour.

Liquor amnii: Membranes intact is recorded as **I**, membranes ruptured as **R**, clear liquor **C**, meconium stainted as **M**.

Molding: Degree of molding is recorded as +, ++ or +++.

Maternal Record

Pulse	1/2 hourly.
BP and temperature	4 hourly or more frequently, if indicated.
Urine	Note for presence of protein or acetone.
	Volume: Encourage woman to pass urine 2-4 hourly.
Drugs and I/V fluids	Charted in appropriate column.
Oxytocin	Charted in the column for oxytocin titration.

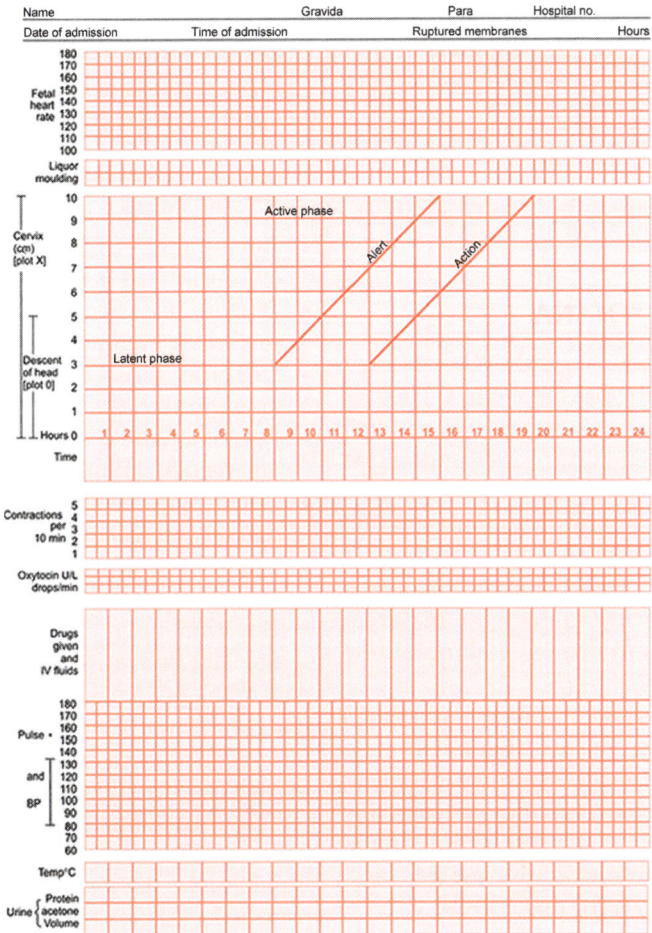

Abnormal Progress of Labor

- **Prolonged active phase:** If cervical dilatation is <1.2 cm/h in nullipara and <1.5/h in multipara. Here if plotting moves on the right side of **alert line** and if adequate facilities are not available to deal with obstetric emergencies, she must be transferred to hospital.

  If women's labor reaches **action line** decision must be made about the cause of slow progress and appropriate action taken. This is only possible in a hospital with facilities to deal with obstetric emergencies. So timely reference in prolonged latent phase or when alert line is crossed is important.

- It is important to note that partograph is a tool for managing labor only. It does not help to identify other risk factors which may have been present before labor started. Start partograph only when you have checked that there are no complications of pregnancy that require immediate attention, e.g., contracted pelvis, malpresentation, multiple pregnancy, severe anemia, PIH, etc.

Advantages of Partogram

- It is a composite record. A single sheet of paper can provide all necessary information.
- Repeated recordings of labor events are avoided.

- Early detection of abnormality, so timely correction and intervention can be done.
- Grace period of 4 hours between alert line and action line avoids unnecessary intervention.
- Helps in handover procedures of the patients.
- It helps for records purpose and medicolegal purpose.

CHIRANJEEVI YOJANA

It is the scheme implemented by Government of Gujarat involving private sector Obstetrics and Gynecology specialists to reduce maternal mortality. It started in April 2005 and in first phase it was implemented in 5 pilot districts which were having maximum number of BPL families.

The objective of the scheme is to encourage institutional delivery to decrease maternal and perinatal mortality by making public private partnership.

Experiencing good response and results from first 5 districts the scheme is now extended to cover all the 26 districts of state of Gujarat. Chiranjeevi Yojna has substantially decreased maternal mortality and perinatal mortality and has won the awards and appreciation form WHO and UNFPA.

Benefits of the Scheme

This scheme empowers the poor in several ways:

It provides them entitlement for free delivery care in private sector.

It provides immediate access to Emergency Obstetric Care (EmOC) when needed.

Reduction in out of pocket expenditure.

It also provides them choice of several providers nearby from which they can choose from.

It also shows that it is possible to develop large scale partnership with private sector to provide skilled birth attendance and EmOC to poor women at a relatively small expenditure.

The Chiranjeevi scheme is now linked with Emergency Management and Research Institute (EMRI) services for elimination of transportation time delay. EMRI is providing free ambulance services to all sections of the society in entire Gujarat state.

Private doctor fulfilling following criteria are enrolled for the scheme.

- Doctor must be having PG qualification in Obstetrics and Gynecology.
- Doctor must have his or her own hospital, preferably minimum 15 beds.
- Hospital must have labor room and operation theater.
- Doctor must be able to access blood in emergency situation.
- Doctor must be able to arrange anesthetic and do emergency surgery.
- Facility should be preferably accredited for sterilization procedures by the Government.

For 100 deliveries total 3,80,000 ₹/- are paid to the private doctor (i.e., 3800 per case) irrespective of type of delivery—normal, instrumental or cesarean. Out of this money in each case Rs. 200 is given for the transport.

The main difference from Janani Suraksha Scheme of Central Government is that money is paid to the doctor and not the patient and private doctors are enrolled and not only the Government Institutions.

Bal Sakha Yojana is now linked with Chiranjeevi Yojana. It is a scheme to provide treatment by private pediatrician to children aged upto 1 month.

JANANI SHISHU SURAKSHA KARYAKRAM (JSSK)

JSSK was launched on 1st June 2011 started under National Rural Health Mission (Now NHM). This scheme supplements to cash assistance given to a pregnant woman under Janani Suraksha Yojana (JSY) and is aimed at mitigating the burden of out of pocket expenses incurred by pregnant women and sick newborns.

The initiative entitles all pregnant women delivering in public health institutions the following:
- Absolutely free and no expense delivery including cesarean section
- Free drugs and consumables
- Free diet up to 3 days in normal deliveries and 7 days in cesarean section
- Free essential diagnostics
- Free blood wherever required
- Free transport from home to institution
- Free transport between facilities in case of referral
- Free drop back from institution to home
- Exemption from all kind of user charges

Similar entitlements have been put in place for all sick newborns treatment accessing public health institutions for treatment till 30 days after birth. This has now been expanded to cover sick infants:
- Free treatment
- Free drugs and consumables
- Free diagnostics
- Free provision of blood
- Exemption from user charges
- Free transport from home to health institutions
- Free transport between facilities in case of referral
- Free drop back from institutions to home.

PC-PNDT ACT

The Pre-Natal Diagnostic Techniques (Regulation and Prevention of Misuse) Act, 1994 came into effect from January 1996. The act was amended in 2002 and amendment rules were in force from 2003. With the amendment the name "The Pre-Natal Diagnostic Techniques (Regulation and Prevention of Misuse)" is substituted by "Pre-Conception and Pre-Natal Diagnostic Techniques (Prohibition of Sex Selection) Act".

It is an Act to provide for the regulation of the use of pre-natal diagnostic techniques for the purpose of detecting genetic or metabolic disorders or chromosomal abnormalities or certain congenital malformations or sex-linked disorders and for the prevention of the misuse of such techniques for the purpose of pre-natal sex determination leading to female feticide; and for matters connected there with or incidental thereto.

This became necessary as with availability of detection of sex antenatal by USG, chorionic villus biopsy and amniocentesis female feticides increased rampantly in our country during 19th century, changing the female/male sex ratio to a dangerous low level.

Certain definitions under this act are important as follows:
- Appropriate authority: An authority appointed by government for the purposes of this act.
- Genetic counseling center: It means an institute, hospital, nursing home or any place, by whatever name called, which provides for genetic counseling to patients.
- Genetic clinic: It means a clinic, institute, hospital nursing home or any place by whatever name called which is used for conducting prenatal diagnostic procedures.
- Genetic laboratory: It means a laboratory and includes a place where facilities are provided for conducting analysis or tests of samples received from genetic clinic for pre-natal diagnostic test.
- Pre-natal diagnostic procedures: It means all gynecological or obstetrical or medical procedures such as ultrasonography, fetoscopy, taking or removing samples of amniotic fluid, chorionic villi, blood or any tissue of a pregnant woman for being sent to—genetic, prenatal diagnostic techniques includes all pre-natal diagnostic procedures and pre-natal diagnostic tests.
- Under this act, all genetic counseling centers, genetic laboratories and genetic clinics require to be registered. Registration should be renewed every 5 years. Copy of certificate of registration (Form-B) should be displayed at a conspicuous place at the center.

- No prenatal diagnostic techniques shall be used or conducted unless the person qualified to do so is satisfied that any of the following conditions are fulfilled, namely:
    - Age of the pregnant woman is above 35 years
    - The pregnant woman has undergone of two or more spontaneous abortions or fetal loss
    - The pregnant woman had been exposed to potentially teratogenic agents such as drugs, radiation infection or chemicals
    - The pregnant woman has a family history of mental retardation or physical deformities such as spasticity or any other genetic disease
    - Any other condition as may be specified by the Central Supervisory Board.
- Written consent of pregnant women for USG or invasive procedures and not wanting to know the sex of the fetus is must
- Form-F for maintenance of record by genetic clinic/USG clinic/imaging center should be filled in triplicate out of which one is sent to appropriate authority every month before 5th of next month.
- Maintenance of records: All records charts, forms reports, consent letters and all other documents required to be maintained under this act and the rules shall be preserved for a period of two years and kept ready for inspection whenever demanded by appropriate authority.
- Offences and penalties: The person who contravenes any of the provisions of the act or rules made thereunder shall be punishable with imprisonment for a term which may extend to three years with fine which may extend to 10,000 rupees and on any subsequent conviction, with imprisonment which may extent to 5 years and with fine which may extend to 50,000 rupees.

On reporting by the appropriate authority to the respective state medical council the name of the registered medical practitioner will be removed from the register of the council for a period of 5 years for the first offence and permanently for the subsequent offence.

Pregnant woman herself or person compelling her to undergo prenatal diagnostic techniques is also punishable in the same manner as medical practitioner.

FOOD AND DRUG ADMINISTRATION'S USE IN PREGNANCY RATINGS

FDA Categories

Category	Interpretation
A	Controlled studies show no risk. Adequate, well-controlled studies in pregnant women have failed to demonstrate risk to the fetus.
B	No evidence of risk in humans. Either animal findings show risk but human findings do not or if no adequate human studies have been done, animal findings are negative.
C	Risk cannot be ruled out. Human studies are lacking and animal studies are either positive for fetal risk or also lacking. However, potential benefits may justify the potential risk.
D	Positive evidence of risk. Investigational or post-marketing data show risk to the fetus. Nevertheless, potential benefits may outweigh the potential risk.
X	Contraindicated in pregnancy. Studies in animals or humans have shown fetal risk that clearly outweighs any possible benefit to the patient.

*Most of the drugs used in practice fall in C category.

Course of Practical Exam

A. GYNECOLOGY TABLE

- Gynecology instruments including catheters, suture materials, needles, knives, pessaries, instruments of laparoscopy with Falope ring and clips
- Gynecology specimens
- Contraceptive pills, IUCDs, condoms, injections, etc.
- Drugs for MTP and MVA syringe
- Gynecology drugs
- Gynecology X-rays—HSGs
- Sonography plates or prints

B. OBSTETRIC TABLE

- Obstetric instruments including catheters, obstetric forceps, vacuum extractor
- Obstetric specimens
- Bony female pelvis, dummy pelvis and baby (plastic), fetal skull
- Obstetric drugs—injections, tablets, gel, etc.
- Obstetric X-rays
- Sonography plates or prints
- Miscellaneous: IV set, BT set, scalp vein set, intracath (plastic IV cannula), IV pints (e.g., 5% glucose, glucose saline, Ringer's lactate), spinal needle.

C. OBSTETRIC CASES

- Antenatal case (usually second half of pregnancy)
- Postpartum (vaginal delivery or cesarean section) case.

D. GYNECOLOGY CASES (PG EXAM)

- Case of gynecology diseases, e.g., fibroid, dysfunctional uterine bleeding (DUB), prolapse, carcinoma, etc.
- Postoperative gynecology cases.

Index

Page numbers followed by *f* refer to figure.

A

Abdominal circumference 188
Abdominal hysterectomy 148
Abortion specimen qs 203
　USG 186
Abruptio placentae specimen 208
Adenomyosis specimen 209
Allis' forceps 13
Alpha methyldopa 113
Anencephaly 198
Anterior vaginal wall retractor 3
Antihypertensive drugs 113
Antimalarial drugs 102
Anxol 96
Apgar's score 214
Artery forceps 11
Aspirin 115
Aspirotomy 86
Atenolol 114
Atropine 104
Ayre's spatula 28

B

Babcock's forceps 14
Berkley-Bonney's round ligament forceps 28
Beta-blockers 114
Betnesol 103
Biophysical profile score 190
Biparietal diameter 188
Bishop's score 214
Bishop score - modified 214
Bladder sound 22
Bonney's myomectomy clamp 14
Breech X-ray 196
Bromocriptine 111
Bupivacaine 104
Buscopan 95

C

Cabergoline 111
Camylofin 95
Caput succedaneum 163
Carcinoma body uterus staging 212
Carcinoma cervix staging 212
Catgut 38
　plain 39
　chromic 39
Catheters 32
　simple 32
　Foley's 34
　malecot 37
　metal 37
　Plastic (K-90) 34
Centchroman 72
Cervarix 118
Cervical cauterization 133
Cervical incompetence 123
Cervical punch biopsy forceps 24
Cerazette 67
Cervical score 216
Cerviprime 94
Cesarean hysterectomy 129
Cesarean section 124
Chiranjeevi yojana 230
Clomiphene citrate 110
　enclomiphene 110
Clotrimazole 116
Colposcopy 136
Condom 57
　male 57
　female 59
Contraceptive pills 66
Contraction stress test 218
Copper T 61
　TCu 380A 61*f*
Cotton thread 42
Craniotomy 131
Crown rump length 188, 189, 189*f*
Cryosurgery 134
Curettes flushing 8
Cu-7 61

D

Danazol 112
Dartigue's forceps 16, 16*f*
Destructive operations 130

Dexon 40
Dexona 103
Diabetes classification 222
Diazepam 96
Diaphragm vaginal 60
Diagonal conjugate 158
Dienogest 113
Dilatation and curettage (D&C) 137
Dilatation and evacuation (D&E) 120
Dilators
    Fenton's 5, 6*f*
    Hegar's 6, 6*f*
    Hawkin-Ambler's 6, 6*f*
Dilex-C 7
Dinoprostone gel 94
Dissecting forceps 27
DMPA 73
Drotin 95
Drugs for leukorrhea 116

E

Ectopic pregnancy 186, 186*f*, 205
    specimen 205
Emergency contraception 75
Emdopa 114
Endometriosis classification 222
Enoxaparin 102
Epidosin 95
Episiotomy 119
Episiotomy scissors 17
Ergometrine 88
Estrogens 105
Ethacridine lactate-emcredil 82

F

Falope ring 142, 143*f*
FDA–Drug category 225
Fontanelle
    anterior 175
    posterior 175
Femilon 68
Femur length 188
Fenticonazole 116
Fetal skull 161
Fibroid specimen 203, 208
Filshie clip 142, 143*f*
Flexiguard 66
Flexion point 54*f*, 55
Foley's catheter 34
Forceps obstetric 45

Fortwin 100
Fractional curettage 138
Furosemide 97

G

Gardasil 118
Gestrinone 112
GnRH analogues 109
Gonadotropins 107
Green-Armytage hemostatic forceps 20
Glycopyrrolate 105

H

Hb estimation 225
HCG 108
Head circumference 188
Heaney's clamp 13
Heart disease
    NYHA grades 222
History taking
    antenatal 164, 170
    postnatal 170
HMG 108
Hodge pessary 30
Hulka–Clemens clip 142
Hulka's manipulator 23
Hydralazine 114
Hydrocephalus 200
Hydrocortisone 103
Hydrosalpinx specimen 212
Hypertonic saline 83
Hysterectomy 148
    abdominal 148
    vaginal 151
Hysterosalpingography 195
Hysteroscopy 146
Hysterotomy 86

I

Imferon 90
Intra-amniotic saline 83
Intrauterine death X-ray 196
Iron sucrose 89
Isoxsuprine 92
IUCD 61
IUCD removing hook 28
IUGR 189
    USG 189

Index

J

JSSK 230
Jectocos 90
Johnson's formula 167

K

Karman's suction cannula 18
Kielland's forceps 51
Kleihauer–Betke test 96
Kobayashi silastic cup 52, 53f
Kocher's clamp 12
Kuppuswamy classification 169

L

Labetalol 114
Lamicel 8
Laminaria tent 7
Laparoscopy 141
Laparoscopic TL 142
LASER 147
Lasix 97
Leech Wilkinson's cannula 17, 17f
Letrozole 111
Lippes loop 61, 61f
LSCS 88
Lytic cocktail 99

M

McDonald's operation 121
Magnesium sulfate 91
Maingot's clamp 13
Manchester operation 154
Manual vacuum aspiration 81
McDonald's rule 167
Menstrual regulation 82
Methergine 89
Metronidazole 116
Midazolam 97
Mifepristone 78
Minipill 66
Mirena 65f
Misgav Ladach technique 128
Misoprostol 182
Monocryl 41
Mosquito forceps 12
Molding 163
MTP Act 77
Multiload copper 65

Myoma screw 14f, 15
Myomectomy clamp 14

N

NACO guidelines 117
Naegele's formula 164
Needle holder 24
Needles suture 43
NET-EN 73
Nevirapine 117
Nifedipine 113
Nonstress test 216
Norplant 74
Novafil 74
Novelon 67
Nova-T 66
Nylon 41
Nuchal translucency USG 185

O

Obstetric examination 166
Obstetric forceps 45
Obstetric grips (Leopold) 167
Ochsner's clamp 13
Odon device 53
Ondansetron 101
Ovaries at hysterectomy 153
Ovarian cancer staging 220
Ovulation detection methods 9
Ovum forceps 17
Oxytocin 87
Oxytocin challenge test 218

P

Pap smear 29
Partogram 227
PC-PNDT Act 231
Pelvis female bony 157
Pentazocin 100
Perinorm 101
Pessary
   Hodge 30
   ring 29
Pethidine 99
Phenergan 100
Pills
   minipill 66
   oral-combined 66
   post-coital 68

Pinard's fetal stethoscope 21
Placenta specimen 204
    USG 204
Polyp forceps 23
Pomeroy modified 139
Post-exposure prophylaxis 117
Postpartum case porforma 164
Prasad classification (modified) 169
Pritchard regimen 91
Progestasert 66
Prolapse operation 155
Prolene 42
Prostaglandins–MTP 94
Prostodin 85
Purandare's cervicopexy 154

R

Rasmin 68
Retractors 25
    Doyen's 26
    Landon's 26
    Morris 16
Rh-anti-D immunoglobulin 96
Ritodrine 93
Robson classification 223
Roll over test 219
Rubin's cannula 16
Rubin's test 135
RU 486-Mifepristone 76

S

Seasonale 68
Semen report 227
Shake test 219
Shirodkar's cannula 17
Shirodkar's sling 154
Shirodkar's uterus holding forceps 16
Silk 41
Simple endometrial biopsy 9
Simpson's perforator 130f, 131
Sims' anterior vaginal wall retractor 3
Sodium bicarbonate 99
Sonosalpingography 192
Sound
    bladder 22
    uterine 3
Spalding's sign 197
Spencer-Well's hemostat 11

Speculum
    Cusco's 2
    Sims' 1
Sponge holding forceps (Swab holder) 5
Sterilization operations female 138
Suction cannula 18
Suction MTP 18
Suture materials 38
Suture needles 43

T

Tamoxifen 110
Tcu 380 A 61
Tetanus 98
    antitoxin 98
    Tdap 99
    toxoid 98
Tenaculum 11
TL Operations 139
TOLAC 129, 206
Toothed forceps 27, 27f
Toothless forceps 27
Towel clip 27
Tramadol 100
Tranexamic acid 115
Triquilar 67
Tubal patency tests 135
Twins USG 190

U

Urine albumin, sugar collecting bag 226
Ultrasonography 184
    Gynec 191
    Obstetric 186, 187, 189
Umbilical
    cord scissors 21
    cord clamps 21
Uterine dressing forceps 18
Uterine manipulator 23
Uterine packing forceps 18
Uterine sound 3
Uterus perforation of 19
    rupture, specimen 206

V

Vaginal hysterectomy 151
Vaginal TL 141

Valethamate 95
Vacuum extractor (ventouse) 52
    Bird's modifications 52
Vault prolapse operations 155
VBAC 129
Veress needle 141
Vertex 161
Vesicular mole specimen 205
Vicryl 39
    plus 40
    rapide 40
Vulsellum 10
Vulva cancer staging 221

W

White classification 222

WHO MEC Wheel 69, 70
Wrigley's forceps 46

X

X-rays 193
    Gynecology 193
    Obstetric 195
Xylocaine 104

Y

Yuzpe method 76

Z

Zicoid 65f, 66